NUTRITION AND DIET RESEARCH PROGRESS

CHEESE: TYPES, NUTRITION AND CONSUMPTION

NUTRITION AND DIET RESEARCH PROGRESS

Additional books in this series can be found on Nova's website under the Series tab.

Additional E-books in this series can be found on Nova's website under the E-books tab.

FOOD AND BEVERAGE CONSUMPTION AND HEALTH

Additional books in this series can be found on Nova's website under the Series tab.

Additional E-books in this series can be found on Nova's website under the E-books tab.

NUTRITION AND DIET RESEARCH PROGRESS

CHEESE: TYPES, NUTRITION AND CONSUMPTION

RICHARD D. FOSTER
EDITOR

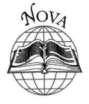

Nova Science Publishers, Inc.
New York

Copyright © 2011 by Nova Science Publishers, Inc.

All rights reserved. No part of this book may be reproduced, stored in a retrieval system or transmitted in any form or by any means: electronic, electrostatic, magnetic, tape, mechanical photocopying, recording or otherwise without the written permission of the Publisher.

For permission to use material from this book please contact us:
Telephone 631-231-7269; Fax 631-231-8175
Web Site: http://www.novapublishers.com

NOTICE TO THE READER

The Publisher has taken reasonable care in the preparation of this book, but makes no expressed or implied warranty of any kind and assumes no responsibility for any errors or omissions. No liability is assumed for incidental or consequential damages in connection with or arising out of information contained in this book. The Publisher shall not be liable for any special, consequential, or exemplary damages resulting, in whole or in part, from the readers' use of, or reliance upon, this material. Any parts of this book based on government reports are so indicated and copyright is claimed for those parts to the extent applicable to compilations of such works.

Independent verification should be sought for any data, advice or recommendations contained in this book. In addition, no responsibility is assumed by the publisher for any injury and/or damage to persons or property arising from any methods, products, instructions, ideas or otherwise contained in this publication.

This publication is designed to provide accurate and authoritative information with regard to the subject matter covered herein. It is sold with the clear understanding that the Publisher is not engaged in rendering legal or any other professional services. If legal or any other expert assistance is required, the services of a competent person should be sought. FROM A DECLARATION OF PARTICIPANTS JOINTLY ADOPTED BY A COMMITTEE OF THE AMERICAN BAR ASSOCIATION AND A COMMITTEE OF PUBLISHERS.

Additional color graphics may be available in the e-book version of this book.

Library of Congress Cataloging-in-Publication Data

Cheese : types, nutrition, and consumption / [edited by] Richard D. Foster.
   p. cm.
Includes bibliographical references and index.
ISBN 978-1-61209-828-9 (hardcover : alk. paper)
 1. Cheese products. 2. Cheese--Varieties. I. Foster, Richard D. (Richard David), 1966-
   SF271.C436 2011
   641.3'73--dc22
                                                                2011004578

Published by Nova Science Publishers, Inc. ✝ New York

CONTENTS

Preface		ix
Chapter 1	Technological and Health Aspects of Probiotic Cheese *Barbaros Özer and Hüseyin Avni Kırmacı*	1
Chapter 2	The Relationship between Genetic and Technological Aspects and Cheese Quality *M. Fresno and S. Álvarez*	43
Chapter 3	Authentication of Local Cheeses: A Global Perspective *Ahmet Koluman, Rind Kürşat Aktaş and Abdullah Dikici*	71
Chapter 4	Spanish Blue Cheeses: Functional Metabolites *Sivia M. Albillos, Carlos García-Estrada and Juan-Francisco Martín*	89
Chapter 5	Sodium in Different Cheese Types: Role and Strategies of Reduction *Mamdouh El-Bakry*	105
Chapter 6	Investigation on a Typical Dairy Product of the Apulia Region (Italy), The Garganico Cacioricotta Cheese, by Means of Traditional and Innovative Physico-Chemical Analyses *A. Sacco, D. Sacco, G. Casiello, A. Ventrella, and F. Longobardi*	119
Chapter 7	Slovak Bryndza Cheese *Roman Dušinský, Libor Ebringer, Mária Mikulášová, Anna Belicová, and Juraj Krajčovič*	143
Chapter 8	Processed Cheese: Relevance for Low Sodium Cheese Development *Adriano G. Cruz, Adriane E. C. Antunes, Renata M.S. Celeguini, Jose A. F. Faria and Marise Aparecida Rodrigues Pollonio*	157
Chapter 9	Italian Cheese Types and Innovations of Traditional Cheeses *Palmiro Poltronieri, Maria Stella Cappello, Federico Baruzzi and Maria Morea*	171

Chapter 10	NMR Spectroscopy in Dairy Products Characterization *Elvino Brosio and Raffaella Gianferri*	183
Chapter 11	Cheese Flavors: Chemical Origins and Detection *Michael H. Tunick*	207
Chapter 12	Antihypertensive Peptides Found in Cheese *F. Javier Espejo, M. Carmen Almécija, Antonio Guadix and Emilia M. Guadix*	221
Chapter 13	New Approachment on Cholesterol Removal in Cheese *Hae-Soo Kwak*	247
Chapter 14	Nutritional Benefits in Cheese *Hae-Soo Kwak, Palanivel Ganesan and Youn-Ho Hong*	267
Chapter 15	Cheese Types *Jee-Young Imm and In-Hyu Bae*	289
Chapter 16	World Production and Consumption of Cheese *Suk-Ho Choi and Se-Jong Oh*	301
Index		309

PREFACE

Cheese is a versatile, nutrient-dense dairy food which is an important component in highly consumed convenience foods. In this new book, the authors present current research in the types, nutrition value and consumption of cheese. Topics discussed include the technological and health aspects of probiotic cheese; authentication of local cheeses; the functional metabolites of Spanish blue cheese; the role of sodium in cheese manufacture; sheep farming and Bryndza Slovak cheese; low sodium processed cheese developments; Italian cheese types and innovations and cheese flavors.

Chapter 1 - There have been numerous scientific studies on the incorporation of probiotic bacteria into foods in the literature since their health promoting effects have been well established about two decades ago. Among the foods, dairy products have a distinct place in delivering probiotics into human gut, as these products provide probiotic bacteria with a suitable environment in which their growth are stimulated. During the last two decades, significant attention has been paid to fermented dairy products containing probiotic bacteria originating from the human intestine. Up until now, physical, chemical and sensory properties of such products have been well documented and some products have already been commercialized. However, probiotics may show rather low viability in yogurt and other fermented dairy products due to their acidic nature. Because of its higher pH, fat content and more solid consistency, cheese offers certain advantages over fermented milk products in terms of delivering viable probiotics to the human gut and, therefore, has been considered to be an ideal vehicle for probiotic uptake. Although, cheese provides many advantages regarding probiotic uptake, the growth and viability of probiotics in cheese depend largely on manufacturing practices. Cheddar type scalded cheeses, for example, have been proved to be more suitable for inclusion of probiotics than brined or high cooked cheeses. Stimulative or inhibitive effect(s) of metabolites generated by classical cheese starters and/or natural cheese flora on the probiotics is another issue that needs to be investigated in detail. The relationship between probiotic adjuncts and the quality of the cheeses after ripening or maturation is yet to be established for many varieties. Finally, in the most recent works, some probiotic strains have been shown to be able to produce bioactive peptides and angiotensin converting enzyme-inhibitor peptides (ACE-I) which further contributes to their already established health promoting effects. This review details technological advances shown to be effective in the incorporation of probiotic bacteria into cheeses and techniques for the accurate enumeration of these bacteria in the presence of complex cheese flora. The systematic approach for the screening probiotic effect in fresh and mature cheeses, impact of the processing parameters on viability of probiotics, methods of protecting probiotics against harsh environmental conditions in cheese (i.e. microencapsulation, addition of probiotics, effective packaging etc.) and health aspects of probiotics with specific reference to cheese applications are also included in this review.

Chapter 2 – Cheese quality is dependent on its physiochemical composition and sensory properties. These factors are influenced by milk composition, which, in turn, depends on the structure of the feed ingested by the dairy animals. However, technological and genetic aspects can also interact and can often mask the effect of diet in addition to being an important source of quality variation. Studies investigating the role of genetic factors (species and breed) in cheese quality frequently take place looking at differences between cheeses made with a local breed's milk and those elaborated with milk from international breeds. In addition, the autochthonous genotypes are usually linked to labelled products and normally have higher concentration of certain milk components, such as protein and casein. The relationship between genotype and quality is mainly linked to changes in milk quality that modify the physicochemical composition of cheeses that affect the nutritional value of the product. Furthermore, technological parameters also influence changes of cheese quality. The two traditional cheese-making practices, type of rennet and smoking process, can play an important role in cheese quality in two different ways: to recover traditional characteristics of Protected Denomination of Origin cheeses or other labelled products, and to impart different organoleptic properties to new products. These cheese-making practices can be useful commercial tools for cheese producers to identify and differentiate their products in current global market. The type of rennet used has an important influence in milk clotting and cheese quality. Artisan rennet (kids or lambs) pastes and traditional vegetable coagulants, especially different species of the *Cynara* genus, affect fat, protein fraction and sensory profile. Smoking, together with drying and salting, is one of the oldest food preservation techniques. Smoke has an antioxidant and bacteriostatic action; it also dries the rind of the cheeses and contributes to their conservation. In modern food technology, smoking is no longer considered as food preservation practice and the primary purpose of this technique is to give the product a characteristic taste, texture and appearance. Where smoked products are concerned, the most important feature of consumer choice is distinctiveness in the sensory properties. The purpose of the present chapter is to analyze how genetic aspects and some technological practices (type of rennet and smoking process) affect cheese quality.

Chapter 3 - Globalization of food sources triggered a demand and public tendency for organic foods and local products. This demand caused a massive application for patenting the local products. With this perspective, authentication studies for all food products have been started globally. Like all food other types cheese has become one of the major subject for authentication process. Authentication includes patenting and under the defined names are: Protected Designation of Origin (PDO) and Protected Geographical Origin (PGO). "Geographical indications (GI)" is also a term for proving the authentication with geographical parameters. European Union (EU) has started to use the patenting approach at their local products on 12 June 1996 with "Commission Regulation (EC) No 1107/96" of the registration of geographical indications and designations of origin under the procedure laid down in "Article 17 of Council Regulation (EEC) No 2081/92". This regulation leads to PDO and PGO patenting of different food products including cheese. Some samples for patenting of authentic cheeses can be listed as; Beacon Fell traditional Lancashire cheese (PDO), Bonchester cheese (PDO), Buxton blue (PDO), Dorset Blue cheese (GI), Dovedale cheese (PDO), Exmoor Blue cheese (PGO), Single Gloucester (PDO), Staffordshire Cheese (PDO),

Swaledale cheese (PDO), Swaledale ewes' cheese (PDO), Teviotdale cheese (GI), Stilton - White cheese (PDO), Stilton - Blue cheese (PDO), West Country farmhouse Cheddar cheese (see Cheddar cheese) (PDO).

This chapter aims to summarize definitions of authentic and local products, PDO, PGO, and GI. On the other hand, it underlines the regulations for authentication, makes a comprehensive review for PDO, PGO and GI procedures and sustainability for authentic cheese production. Global supply and demand for authentic cheeses and labeling of these cheeses is also given under this chapter.

Chapter 4 - Blue cheeses are produced from cow's milk, sheep's milk, or goat's milk depending on the variety. They always have *Penicillium* cultures added, along with the lactic acid bacteria starter cultures (*Lactococcus lactis* and *Leuconostoc cremoris*), so that the final product is spotted or veined throughout with blue, blue-gray or blue-green mold. The aftertaste is a little salty and sharp and its characteristic smell is often produced by metabolites released by the bacteria *Brevibacterium linens*. *Penicillium roqueforti* utilizes □-ketoacyl-CoA deacylase (thiohydrolase) and β-ketoacid decarboxylase to provide the compounds typical for the aroma of the blue semi-soft cheeses. The production of blue cheeses is basically concentrated on a few countries around the world, such as France, Spain, Italy, England and Denmark. Throughout history, there are vestiges that the Roquefort region produced cheese as long as 3,500 years ago, being often considered a delicatessen and prohibitive because of its costly price and political reasons. Roquefort has been named as the "king of cheeses" or the "cheese of the king" due to the veneration that the emperor Charlemagne and several French kings had for this type of product.

In Spain, several blue-veined cheeses of excellent quality are produced, being the region on the north area of Picos de Europa the one with more varieties (Cabrales, Valdeón, Bejes-Tresviso, Picón, among others that carry a legally Protected Designation of Origin). Our research group has recently studied some of these varieties and characterized the *Penicillium* species present in the blue cheese. Interestingly, we have found that *P. roqueforti*, the main of these species, produces important secondary metabolites with functional properties, such as the antitumor andrastins and mycophenolic acid, together with mycotoxins (roquefortine C and PR toxin). Efforts have been made by our group in order to shed light on the biosynthetic pathways for those secondary metabolites with the aim of engineering *P. roqueforti* strains with an added value for the cheese industry.

Chapter 5 - Cheese is a versatile, nutrient-dense dairy food, i.e. a good source of protein, vitamins and minerals particularly calcium and phosphorus, which is an important component in highly consumed convenience foods (O'Brien and O'Connor, 2004). However, cheese is perceived as being high in saturated fat, which might contribute to risks of atherosclerosis, and sodium (Johnson et al., 2009). There is considerable evidence that high sodium intake, which is the case in Western countries, is associated with hypertension and strokes, hence, dietary guidelines recommend that sodium intake be reduced.

This chapter covers the scientific and technological aspects of the role of sodium in cheese manufacture and functional properties and highlights various strategies for reducing the sodium. The focus is on natural cheese, made from milk by acid and/or rennet-coagulation, and process cheese. This cheese differs from natural cheese in that it is made from natural cheese or casein, which is blended with the necessary emulsifying salts and in the presence of heat, leading to the formation of a homogeneous product with extended shelf-life (Zehren and Nusbaum, 2000). Process cheese has numerous end-use applications in processed foods, which counts for ~75% of the dietary sodium in industrialized diets (Doyle and Glass, 2010).

The source of sodium in cheese is mainly the added salt (sodium chloride). Salt acts primarily as food preservative and flavor enhancer and also interacts with major components in the cheese and thereby affecting the functionality, e.g. salt increases the protein hydration during manufacture which affects the stability and textural properties (Johnson et al., 2009). Process cheese contains much higher sodium content, compared to natural cheese, due to the necessity of using emulsifying salts, such as sodium citrate and phosphate. These salts are crucial for the hydration of the protein, emulsification of fat and the stability of the final product.

Strategies for reducing sodium in cheese are mainly outlined in the reduction of the salt and/or emulsifying salts used and their substitution by the potassium equivalents salts. However, these strategies present many challenges, such as adverse effects on flavor and microbiological stability. In process cheese, a high reduction of emulsifying salts does not allow for the formation of a homogeneous end product. Recent approaches of reducing emulsifying salts used are also discussed, such as utilizing of emulsifiers or protein hydrolyzates in the manufacture of cheese (Zehren and Nusbaum, 2000).

A final section in this chapter is about the future of low sodium cheese manufacture, including suggestions for reducing sodium which has not been systematically investigated in research on various cheese types.

Chapter 6 - This work deals with the characterization of a typical goat cheese, cacioricotta, produced in a restricted area (Promontory of Gargano) of the Apulia Region in Southern Italy. For this purpose, conventional (fat, protein, casein, urea, cryoscopy, metals content, fatty acid composition, solid content, moisture, ashes, pH) and innovative physico-chemical analyses, such as Nuclear Magnetic Resonance (NMR) Spectroscopy and Isotope Ratio Mass Spectroscopy (IRMS), have been carried out. The determinations have been done both on the starting goat milk and on the obtained cheese after 20 and 60 days of ripening. The conventional analysis has allowed to follow compositional changes of some elements occurred during the ripening of cacioricotta cheese. The NMR spectra were recorded using two different procedures. In the former, the sample was prepared by means of an aqueous extraction of the cacioricotta, while in the latter, the analysis was performed directly on the cacioricotta sample by using the ^{1}H HR-MAS NMR technique. All spectroscopic results have allowed the identification of the metabolic profile of cacioricotta cheese. Finally, for the first time, the IRMS has been applied on goat milk and cheese. The obtained isotopic results were not easy to understand and required further investigations on a higher number of samples. Moreover, a comparison of results of cacioricotta samples coming from different areas of production could be very interesting.

Chapter 7 - Slovak Bryndza cheese is a traditional type of cheese closely associated with the history and culture of Slovakia. "Slovenská bryndza" (Slovak Bryndza cheese) has been granted European Protected Geographical Indication (PGI) status. The matured sheep lump cheese alone or mixed with cow cheese is crushed and ground to give rise to soft, spreadable, salty Bryndza cheese. At present, commercially available Bryndza cheese can legally contain up to 49% cow cheese and the traditional technology is influenced by sophisticated milking machines and by thermal processing of the ewes' milk. Characteristic aroma and taste of the traditional Bryndza cheese are the result of the presence of a high amount of natural microorganisms, especially lactic acid bacteria (*Lactobacillus, Enterococcus, Lactococcus*) and partly micromycetes (*Kluyveromyces, Galactomyces, Mucor*) as well. Food safety of the unpasteurized product is ensured by a technological process of fermentation. Keeping sheep on the mountainous meadows makes Bryndza cheese really healthy because of the rich content of unsaturated fatty acids (ALA – alpha linolenic acid, CLA – conjugated linoleic acid), an appropriate amount of minerals and a relatively high content of vitamins and natural positive microflora. Beneficial attributes of the traditional Bryndza cheese in human health and nutrition are being researched. Bryndza cheese is mostly eaten as a topping on small boiled potato dumplings (with pieces of fried bacon) as a Slovak national meal called "Bryndzové halušky" (Bryndza cheese dumplings). It is also often used as a spread on a piece of bread or as a compound of more complex spreads, filling for pasta and pies, or used in a soup. Sheep farming and Bryndza cheese is a part of the unique and specific Slovak folk culture tradition which influenced and boosted tourism, including various annual festivals, e.g. the World Championship of Cooking and Eating Bryndza Cheese Dumplings or "Ovenalie" – Shepherd's Sunday.

Chapter 8 - Sodium is a mineral widely consumed in human diets, bestowing pleasant sensory characteristics when added to foods at certain concentrations.

Besides, salt was a precious commodity and was also an emblem of immortality and a symbol of immutable loyalty. This is reflected for instance by the act of sharing bread and salt with a guest—still practised in Slavic countries (Ritz, 2006). Sodium consumption is even quoted in the Holy Bible in three of the four Gospels (Matthew 5: 13-14, Mark 9, 50 and Luke 14, 34): "You are the salt of the earth. But if the salt loses its saltiness, how it be made salty again?". Certainly, the motivation of biblical quotations were using elements of daily life to explain the religious values and not properly discuss salt consumption in the population.

Chapter 9 - Dairy productions in the Italian area are rich in fresh soft cheeses, spreadable cheese, like Crescenza and Gorgonzola, fresh type cheeses, like Primo sale and Cacioricotta, and ripened cream types, such as Ricotta forte.

Manufacturing trends and consumer novel products influenced the development of different innovative dairy products such as cheeses containing probiotic microorganisms. These cheese productions help the sustainable development and growth of local producers increasing the economy of dairy factories through the development of products dedicated to individuals with special dietary requirements.

Chapter 10 - A low- and high-resolution nuclear magnetic resonance spectroscopy based protocol to characterise traditional Italian cheese as *Mozzarella di Bufala Campana* and *Grana Padano* is reported. Low-resolution relaxometry was used for studying the state and distribution of water in different structural elements of cheese resulting from the production process. High-resolution NMR allowed definition of the "chemical fingerprint", the cheese complex matrix profile of low molecular weight metabolites extracted from *Mozzarella* and *Grana Padano*. Both low-resolution and high-resolution NMR seem to provide useful parameters that could be used for monitoring structure and evolution of PDO Italian cheese.

Chapter 11 - The hundreds of flavor compounds found in cheese arise from the proteins, lipids, and carbohydrates it contains. Flavor compounds are products of diverse reactions that occur in milk during processing, in curd during manufacture, and in cheese during storage, and are detected by a number of methods. Acids, alcohols, aldehydes, esters, ketones, and lactones may all form in cheese depending on the variety. The different pathways of flavor compound formation result from the feed or grass consumed by the animals, enzymes present in the starter culture microorganisms, any adjunct cultures or molds that have been added, the action of the coagulant, and the time and temperature of aging. An assortment of techniques for extracting and identifying flavors has been developed over the years. Gas chromatography and sensory analysis are used to examine these compounds. This chapter will cover the origins of cheese flavors and the ways that scientists can examine them.

Chapter 12 - The production and ripening of cheese involves some biochemical transformations such as the proteolysis of caseins by enzymes associated to lactic acid bacteria. It has been found that these hydrolytic processes may promote the release of a significant amount of peptides with biological activity.

Among the bioactivities described in the scientific literature, peptides which inhibit the angiotensin converting enzyme (ACE) are highlighted because their potential health benefit for hypertension. ACE is a zinc metallopeptidase which converts a biologically inactive polypeptide, angiotensin I, to a potent vasoconstrictor, angiotensin II. Furthermore, ACE catalyses the degradation of bradykinin, a blood pressure lowering nonapeptide. By these actions, ACE raises blood pressure, and therefore, inhibition of this enzyme results in an antihypertensive effect.

In this chapter, it will be reviewed the presence and bioavailability of ACE-inhibitory peptides in a wide array of cheeses from different world regions, including some well-known types such as Cheddar, Mozzarella, Camembert or Manchego. The analytical techniques for quantification and purification of these peptides will be presented. Moreover, procedures for the determination of the antihypertensive effect will be explained for both in vitro and in vivo methods.

Chapter 13 - Cheese is a nutritious food with various balanced nutrients, such as proteins, peptides, amino acids, fats, fatty acids, vitamins and minerals. However, the amounts of cholesterol is very high, e.g. 102mg/100g Cheddar cheese. Most of consumers are not prefer the cholesterol. Dairy scientists have been tried for lowering the cholesterol in cheeses for a long time. The method found initially is reducing fat in cheese that is poor in taste. Recently, we have been studied about removing specifically cholesterol during cheese making without changing anything from cheese including nutrients, flavor, taste and texture. The method developed is entrapping cholesterol by crosslinked β-cyclodextrin (β-CD). Cholesterol can be removed from milk for soft cheeses and from cream for semi hard and hard cheeses. In cholesterol-removed Cheddar cheese ripening, ripening time could be shortened about 50%. Crosslinked β-CD is lower solubility than β-CD, and particle size is bigger. So entrapment and separation from cream are possible and the β-CD is recyclable about 10times. We developed various cholesterol-removed cheeses, such as Cheddar cheese, Mozzarella cheese, Camembert cheese, blue cheese, Gouda cheese, Feta cheese and process cheese. Cholesterol-removed cheeses will be commercialized in near future. I will describe the developed technique in detail in this chapter.

Chapter 14 - Cheese serves as a one of the good sources for essential nutrients, such as proteins, lipids, minerals and vitamins. It can enhance health benefits by the production of certain peptides and free amino acids which has various bioactive properties, such as anti-microbial, anti-carcinogenic, anti-thrombotic and so on. Certain biologically active lipids, such as conjugated fatty acid (CLA) and milk fat globule membrane (MFGM), present in cheeses are also found to be health beneficial. Thus, it plays a very important role in the diet of human; however, it suffers from adverse nutritional image due to the presence of saturated fatty acid, cholesterol and salt content. It can be overcome by the production of cheese with low fat or cholesterol removal and by the addition of certain functional living materials, such as probiotic bacteria. The non-starter lactic acid bacteria (NSLAB) used in the cheeses found to be bioactive, such as inactivation of antigenotoxins and production of gamma-aminobutyric acid generation of bioactive peptides. This chapter describes the nutritional significant of cheese components, and their role in enhancing the health benefits.

Chapter 15 - Classification of more than 500 cheeses is very difficult task. Although classification of cheeses based on single criterion is not perfect or satisfactory grouping of cheese would be necessary to understand similarities and differences of a variety of cheeses. Cheese can be commonly classified by texture (water content) or rind and further classified by ripening microorganism such as bacteria, mold or combination. The most common classifications for cheese are fresh, soft, semi-soft, firm and hard. Within the same classification they have similarities in taste and textures. Fresh cheese includes world famous mozzarella, cottage, those are particularly used for Pizza and Italian dishes. Brie and Camembert belongs to pungent soft cheese. Semi-hard cheeses are recognized by texture of "not too hard" and" not too firm." Blue cheese such as Roquefort, Gorgonzola is characterized by distinctive blue greens color and strong flavor. Emmental and Gruyeres cheeses are representative firm Swiss cheese and contain medium size holes formed by propionic fermentation. World reknown Cheddar cheese also belongs to this class. Hard cheese such as Grana Padano and Pecorino Romano cheeses have the lowest water content and typical grainy texture. They have long aging time and produced for grating purpose.

Chapter 16 - World production of industrial cheeses has reached 17.0 million tons in 2009. The countries in Europe and northern America produced and consumed about 80% of cheeses in the world. Cheese production and consumption worldwide steadily increased during the period from 2000 to 2007 due both to demand for commodity cheeses, such as Mozzarella, Cheddar, and other cheeses of prospering fast food outlets and restaurants and to rising incomes in both non-EU European countries, such as Russia, Belarus and Ukraine, and developing countries, such as Brazil, Republic Korea. Cheese production and consumption of New Zealand and Australia stagnated and decreased, which can be attributed to both to stagnating milk supplies and to decreasing cheese export. The cheese production and consumption were negatively affected by the financial crisis and following economic depression in 2008. The cheese trade outpaced cheese production during the period from 2000 to 2009. EU, New Zealand and Australia are leading cheese exporters, while Russia and Japan are noticeable cheese importers. Cheese importing countries are located rather widely throughout the world.

In: Cheese: Types, Nutrition and Consumption
Editor: Richard D. Foster, pp. 1-42
ISBN 978-1-61209-828-9
© 2011 Nova Science Publishers, Inc.

Chapter 1

TECHNOLOGICAL AND HEALTH ASPECTS OF PROBIOTIC CHEESE

Barbaros Özer[1] and Hüseyin Avni Kırmacı[2]*

[1] Abant Izzet Baysal University Faculty of Engineering and Architecture, Department of Food Engineering, 14280 Golkoy, Bolu, Turkey
[2] Harran University Faculty of Agriculture Department of Food Engineering, 63040, Sanliurfa, Turkey

ABSTRACT

There have been numerous scientific studies on the incorporation of probiotic bacteria into foods in the literature since their health promoting effects have been well established about two decades ago. Among the foods, dairy products have a distinct place in delivering probiotics into human gut, as these products provide probiotic bacteria with a suitable environment in which their growth are stimulated. During the last two decades, significant attention has been paid to fermented dairy products containing probiotic bacteria originating from the human intestine. Up until now, physical, chemical and sensory properties of such products have been well documented and some products have already been commercialized. However, probiotics may show rather low viability in yogurt and other fermented dairy products due to their acidic nature. Because of its higher pH, fat content and more solid consistency, cheese offers certain advantages over fermented milk products in terms of delivering viable probiotics to the human gut and, therefore, has been considered to be an ideal vehicle for probiotic uptake. Although, cheese provides many advantages regarding probiotic uptake, the growth and viability of probiotics in cheese depend largely on manufacturing practices. Cheddar type scalded cheeses, for example, have been proved to be more suitable for inclusion of probiotics than brined or high cooked cheeses. Stimulative or inhibitive effect(s) of metabolites generated by classical cheese starters and/or natural cheese flora on the probiotics is another issue that needs to be investigated in detail. The relationship between probiotic adjuncts and the quality of the cheeses after ripening or maturation is yet to be established for many varieties. Finally, in the most recent works, some probiotic strains have been shown to be able to produce bioactive peptides and angiotensin converting

---

* Corresponding author: adabarbaros@gmail.com.

enzyme-inhibitor peptides (ACE-I) which further contributes to their already established health promoting effects. This review details technological advances shown to be effective in the incorporation of probiotic bacteria into cheeses and techniques for the accurate enumeration of these bacteria in the presence of complex cheese flora. The systematic approach for the screening probiotic effect in fresh and mature cheeses, impact of the processing parameters on viability of probiotics, methods of protecting probiotics against harsh environmental conditions in cheese (i.e. microencapsulation, addition of probiotics, effective packaging etc.) and health aspects of probiotics with specific reference to cheese applications are also included in this review.

1. INTRODUCTION

Functional foods are those foods or food components that are scientifically recognized as having physiological benefits beyond those of basic nutrition (Gibson and Williams, 2000). Functional foods are also called nutraceuticals and can include foods that are genetically modified. The global functional foods market continues to be a dynamic and growing segment of the food industry. The major driving force behind this growth is the growing consumers' interest in the role of nutrition for health and well-being. Additionally, today consumers desire to take a more proactive role in optimizing personal health and well-being, without relying on pharmaceuticals. According to Champagne and Molgaard (2008), in North America, up to 93% of consumers believe certain foods have health benefit that may reduce the risk of disease. Today, consumers care more about their health spans than their life spans (Özer and Kırmacı, 2010). Especially, in recent years, increasing medical costs have forced people to find cheaper and effective means of protecting their health and, therefore, interest in functional foods, with specific emphasize on functional dairy foods, has increased. The growing consumers' demand over functional foods has triggered the innovative nature of food industry. In the past two decades, many examples testify to innovation in the food and drink industry, and arguably, manufacturers and retailers are more innovative than before. As a result of the fast development of the food and drink industry, and technology, the variety of products presented to the markets has increased marginally.

Among the functional foods, functional dairy products have a distinct place. The functional dairy products market has increased by 43% during 2004-2009 to reach $ 4.840 million in 2009 (Mintel, 2009). Although, in recent years, the number of commercial dairy products (both dairy based beverages and set type products) containing bioactive components (*e.g.* phytosterols, bioactive peptides, minerals, vitamins, vegetable and fish oils etc.) has increased dramatically, the probiotic dairy products are still in the forefront of innovation in the functional food sector (Champagne, 2009). The global probiotic products market reached $ 15.9 million in 2009 (Anonymous, 2010a). According to Heller (2008), more than 500 probiotic food and beverage products have been introduced into the market in the past two decades. These products have received varying levels of success, mostly in congruence with their overall health benefits. Probiotic yogurts lead to the probiotic dairy products segment. Today, probiotic yogurt and beverages market is growing at a pace of 5 to 30% depending on the country and product type. The probiotic yogurt market in Latin America, for example, expanded 32% per annum between 2005 and 2007 (Crowley, 2008). The sales growth rate of fresh probiotic dairy products in the USA in 2004 was much higher than cheese (9-10% *vs.* 2%) (Fletcher, 2006). Europe is currently the largest probiotics market, owing to its high awareness of the benefits of probiotic yogurts and fermented milks. The European probiotic food and beverage market is estimated to reach $163 million by 2013. The US market is also growing rapidly due to the general affinity of the US population towards the probiotic dietary supplements.

Taking advantage of the growing market for functional dairy products and the opportunity to develop a commercially viable probiotic cheese, several cheese brand and dairy entrepreneurs have tried to penetrate into the functional dairy products market with probiotic cheese (Anonymous, 2010b). In March 2007, Kraft Food Inc. became the first major North American food company to introduce a Cheddar cheese product with probiotics in the Canadian market, launching Kraft LiveActive. The company later introduced medium Cheddar (in 300 g block format), marble Cheddar and cheese snacks (Kraft LiveActive Marble). Later, another cheese company, DCI Cheese Co., offered probiotic cheeses under County Line brand in 2007 (Anonymous, 2008). In 2009, Next Generation Organic Dairy introduced raw milk Cheddar as probiotics under its gourmet line. In more or less similar period, a Californian company, Cheese Well, started production of probiotic Cheddar and Monterey Jack cheeses. According to Euromonitor, fortified cheeses account for only about one percent of the $100 billion global cheese market, with probiotic versions faring very poorly (Starling, 2009; Anonymous, 2010b).

2. CHARACTERISTICS OF CHEESE BENEFICIAL TO THE GROWTH OF PROBIOTIC

Bacteria

According to FAO/WHO (2001), probiotics are defined as live organisms which when administrated in adequate amounts confer a health benefit on the host. It has been established that maintaining the viability and metabolic activities of probiotics during food processing, at the point of sale (Kailasapathy, 2002; Stanton et al., 2003; Sarkar, 2010) and in host gastro-intestinal tract (Hamilton-Miller et al., 1996) are essential for extending health benefits. It is the major challenge for the probiotic food industry that the identity and the number of incorporated species do not always correspond to those declared on the product labels (Shah, 2000; Hamilton-Miller and Shah, 2002; Temmerman et al., 2002; Coeuret et al., 2004). The food industry considers 10^6 cfu/g at the time of consumption as the minimum level of probiotic bacteria necessary to perform their nutritional benefits (Bolyston et al., 2004). On the other hand, several scientific studies propose a minimum daily dose of 10^8-10^9 cfu which corresponds to 100 g of food containing 10^6-10^7 cfu/g per day (Blanchette et al., 1996; Hoier et al., 1999; Talwalkar et al., 2004; Moreno et al., 2006). The probiotics incorporated into foods should be considered as GRAS (generally recognized as safe) (da Cruz et al., 2009) and the probiotic-containing products should retain their sensorial and related properties during storage (Souza et al., 2008). Overall, probiotic bacteria must simultaneously survive in the food in high numbers, withstand gastric pH and survive intestinal bile acids, adhere to or interact with intestinal surface, colonize the intestinal environment, displace pathogenic bacterial competitors, and prevent immune sensitization by the host (Table 1) (Gürakan et al., 2010). According to globally accepted definition of probiotics, the viability and metabolic activity of probiotics must be maintained during food processing and these organisms must be able to survive in the GIT (da Cruz et al., 2009; Sanz, 2007). There are a number of methods that are employed in improving the viability of probiotics during passage through GIT. One recent approach is to add growth promoters (inulin, fructooligosaccharides etc.) into cheese base. Araujo et al. (2009) demonstrated that *Lb. delbrueckii* UFVH2b20 showed a good resistance against high bile salt level in GIT when it was used with inulin (raftilin) in the manufacture of Cottage-like symbiotic cheese. Viability of probiotics is the prime criteria for efficacy of probiotic products (Grattepanche et al., 2008). Therefore, the food manufacturing process may need to be modified and adapted to the requirements of the strains used (da Cruz et al., 2009). The oxygen concentration and pH of the foods are the major factors limiting the growth of probiotic bacteria. In general, both bifidobacteria and lactobacilli are strictly anaerobic or microaerophilic but their resistance to oxygen is strain or species-dependent (Talwalkar and Kailasapathy, 2004). For example; *Lactobacillus* strains, *B. infantis*, *B. brevis* and *B. longum* are able to grow under partial aeration, while *B.adolescentis* is suppressed by low oxygen concentration (Bolyston et al., 2004). *Bifidobacterium* spp. is more sensitive to oxygen than *Lb. acidophilus* (da Cruz et al., 2009). Similarly, survival of probiotics is restricted in the foods with pH values lower than 5.0 and acid resistance of the probiotics is strain-dependent.

Table 1. Selection criteria of probiotic microorganisms

Properties	*Related to*
Origin (human origin preferred)	Strain property
Well characterized	Strain property
Strain and genus safety	Safety
Able to active and able to survive in products	Stability
Low pH resistance	Stability
Stomach acid resistance	Stability
Bile resistant	Stability
Able to adhere to human intestinal surface	Stability
Able to colonize and grow in the human gastrointestinal system	Stability
Able to inhibit the growth of pathogenic bacteria	Antagonism

Source: Gürakan et al. (2010).

It is clear that the probiotics are dominated by yogurts and fermented milks, but scientific studies suggest that cheese can be a good but underused alternative food vehicle for the delivery of viable probiotic bacteria conferring health benefits in the host, with specific advantages compared with fermented milks and yogurts such as high cell viability (Ong and Shah, 2009; Özer et al., 2009; Grattepanche et al., 2008). The reduced acidity of cheese compared with yogurt, the high fat content and texture of cheese may offer further protection to microorganisms during passage through the gastrointestinal tract (GIT) (Stanton et al., 1998; Gardiner et al., 1998; Vinderola et al., 2002b; Corbo et al., 2001; Bergamini et al., 2005; Ross et al., 2002). However, in contrast to the short shelf life of probiotic fermented milks and yogurts, hard cheeses such as Cheddar have long ripening period of up to 1-2 years, hence the development of probiotic cheese requires stringent selection of probiotic strains to maintain viability in the cheese throughout processing, maturation and storage period till consumption (Phillips et al., 2006). The initial acidity of most cheese varieties is around pH 5.0 and the pH of cheese increases rapidly during ripening, being less pronounced in the hard and semi-hard varieties (Choisy et al., 1997). The increase in pH (reduction in acidity) is favored by probiotic bacteria for their growth. Depending on the size of the cheese blocks, the acidity of the core and outer layer of the cheeses can be different. Abraham et al. (2007) for example, demonstrated that the pH values of outer and inner parts of Camembert cheese were 6.8 and 7.5, respectively. Sharp et al. (2008) further confirmed this claim by comparing the growth patterns of *Lactobacillus paracasei* 334e, an erythromycin-resistant derivative of the strain ATCC334, both in yogurt and low-fat Cheddar cheese. It was demonstrated that the bacteria showed a good stability in Cheddar cheese after 3 months and in yogurt after 3 weeks of storage. Cheddar cheese was able to protect the viable cells against acidic conditions (pH 2) of gastric environment, as the viable cell count decreased from 10^7 cfu/g to 10^4 cfu/g after 120 min. On contrary, the counts of the probiotic bacteria in yogurt decreased to less than 10 cfu/g within 30 min of exposure. Storage conditions of many cheese varieties provide a suitable environment for long-term survival of probiotics (Bolyston et al., 2004). The oxidation-reduction potential of cheese is about -250 mV and, therefore, cheese is essentially an anaerobic system, in which only facultatively or obligatory anaerobic microorganisms can grow (Fox et al., 2000). Abraham et al. (2007) showed that the redox potential (E_h) of inner and outer parts of Camembert cheese varied during ripening period. While the E_h values of the outer part increased from +330 to +360 mV, the E_h value of the inner part reduced from -300 mV to -360 mV. This variation is related with the metabolic activity of cheese microflora. Cheese microflora consumes oxygen in cheese matrix within a few weeks providing almost anaerobic environment which is favorable for especially bifidobacteria (van den Tempel et al., 2002). On the other hand, manufacturing and/or ripening practices of many cheese varieties including high cooked cheeses and/or salted in dense brine solution are less suitable for the growth of probiotic bacteria, due to the detrimental effects of heating and salting on the survivability of probiotic cells. Probiotic cheeses should meet the expectations that the product has cell count high enough for therapeutic effect and the overall quality of the end product is maintained or improved (Ross et al., 2002). To achieve these goals some modifications in the production lines may be required. These modifications may include lowering salt level in brine, vacuum packaging, pre-incubation of milk with probiotic bacteria, addition of growth stimulators (*i.e.* inulin, oligofructose) and protection of cells against undesired environmental conditions (*i.e.* microencapsulation, cell incubation under sub-lethal conditions or cell propogation in an immobilized biofilm). Availability of these techniques for the production of probiotic cheese will be discussed later.

3. CHEESE MATRIX AND POPULATION DYNAMICS OF PROBIOTICS

Bifidobacterium spp. (*B. adolescentis, bifidum, animalis, longum*) and *Lactobacillus* spp. (*Lb. acidophilus, fermentum, casei, rhamnosus, reuteri, lactis, paracasei*) are the most widely used strains in the production of probiotic cheeses (Table 2) and as stated earlier, the growth of probiotic bacteria in cheese is largely affected by the manufacturing conditions and type of cheese (*e.g.* cheese matrix). Fresh cheeses, for example, are considered to be more suitable vehicles for the delivery of probiotic bacteria as they have no ripening stage and shorter shelf life (Heller et al., 2003; Fritzen-Freire et al., 2010). However, higher pH and more compact texture of hard and semi-hard varieties offer extra advantages for probiotics. On the other hand, one should bear in mind that metabolic products that are produced during long term ripening may affect the survivability of probiotics as well. In a long-term study carried out by Jatila and Matilainen (2008) from Valio Ltd. (Finland), *Lactobacillus* GG (LGG) counts in hard cheese at the beginning of sales period were followed for 5 years. The LGG counts remained at the level of 2×10^7 cfu/g throughout the years with no adverse effect on the overall quality of the product. Probiotic bacteria can be incorporated into cheese production in different ways including addition into cheese milk directly with the cheese starters or into cheese curd after removal of whey. In some cases, cheese milk is pre-incubated with probiotics to allow them to multiply fastly then cheese starters are added. However, Bergamini et al. (2010) showed that the direct addition of the probiotic cultures into Pategras cheese milk was more efficient than pre-incubation step in terms of chemical composition of cheese. In an earlier study, the same authors found that inoculation of cheese milk with a substrate pre-incubated with probiotic bacteria resulted in an end product with crumbly texture and lower pH (Bergamini et al., 2005). Regarding chemical and sensorial quality of the semi-hard cheese, direct addition of the probiotic culture was suggested as the methodology with the best performance; however, pre-incubation presented some advantages such as an increased population of lactobacilli in the initial inoculum (Bergamini et al., 2005, 2010). In an earlier attempt, Daigle et al. (1999) produced a Cheddar-like probiotic cheese from microfiltered milk standardized with cream enriched with native phosphocaseinate retentate and fermented by *B. infantis*. This method stimulated the growth of probiotic bacteria with no adverse effect on the cheese quality during 12 weeks of ripening.

Cheddar cheese was shown to be a good medium for the growth of *Lb. paracasei* inoculated into cheese milk at rather lower concentrations (*i.e.* 0.5%) (Ross et al., 2005). Similarly, Daigle et al. (1999) found that *B. infantis* survived very well in Cheddar cheese packed in vacuum-sealed bags kept at 4 °C for 84 days and remained above 3×10^6 cfu/g cheese. Gomes et al. (1998a) found that the number of *Bifidobacterium lactis* and *Lactobacillus acidophilus* declined gradually in Gouda cheese during the first three weeks of storage. The growth capacity of *Lb. paracasei* A13 in Argentinian probiotic cheese stored at 5 °C or 12 °C for 60 days was study by Vinderola et al. (2009). The authors demonstrated that *Lb. paracasei* A13 grew a half log order at 43 °C during manufacturing process of probiotic cheese and another half log order during the first 15 days of storage at 5 °C. It is difficult to generalize the growth trend of probiotic bacteria in cheese as it is affected by a number of parameters including cheese type, production practices of cheese, strain or species of probiotics and symbiosis of probiotics with other cheese microflora. Zehntner (2008), for example, tested two strains of *Lb. gasseri* for their suitability as probiotic additive to semi-hard cheese (Tilsit-type cheese and Swiss-type cheese) together with the starter cultures. It was shown that one strain (strain K7, a bacteriocin-gassericin K7- producing strain) had the ability to remain in concentrations above 10^6 cfu/g during entire 90-day storage, but the other strain lost its viability within a shorter period. Matijasic (2008) reported that the use of *Lb. gasseri* K7 in combination with *Str. thermophilus* gave much better results regarding the probiotic counts and overall quality of probiotic cheese at the end of ripening.

Table 2. Some examples of non-commercial probiotic cheeses

Cheese type	Bacteria	Ripening conditions			References
Cheddar	B. longum 1941, B. animalis ssp. lactis LAFTI®B94 L. casei 279, L. casei LAFTI® L26, Lb.acidophilus 4962, Lb.acidophilus LAFTI®L10	24 wk at 4 °C or 8 °C	9.10-9.74 $\log_{10}$	6.81-7.53$\log_{10}$	Ong and Shah (2009)
	B. bifidum	6 mo at 7 °C	1.0x10^6	1.4-2.6 x 10^7	Dinakar and Mistry (1994) Daigle et al. (1999)
	B. infantis ATCC 27920G Bifidobacterium sp. DR10	32 wk at 10 °C	>10^8	4.0x10^7-5x10^8	Phillips et al. (2006)
	Lb. acidophilus L10		>10^8	9.0x10^3	
	Lb. acidophilus La5		>10^8	3.6x10^3	
	Lb. paracasei L26		>10^8	1.6x10^7	
	Lb. casei Lc1		>10^8	2.0x10^7	
	Lb.rhamnosus DR20		~10^8	9.0x10^8	
	Enterococcus faecium	15 mo at 8 °C	2.0 x 10^{10}	4.0 x10^8	Gardiner et al. (1999)
	Lb. paracasei	8 mo at 8 °C	2.7 x 10^7-1.1x10^7	2.9x10^8-1.5x10^8	Gardiner et al. (1998)
Low fat Cheddar	Lb. casei 334e	3 mo at 8 °C	~10^7	>10^7	Sharp et al. (2008)
Probiotic rennet cheese	B. animalis BB12, Lb. acidophilus LA5	8 wk at 6 °C		>10^7	Ziarno et al. (2010)
Pategras cheese	Lb. casei, Lb. paracasei, Lb. rhamnosus	60 days	5x10^7	>10^7	Bergamini et al. (2010)

Table 2. (Continued)

Cheese	Strains	Storage	Initial count	Final count	Reference
Turkish white cheese	Lb. acidophilus LA5, B. animalis BB12	90 days at 4 °C	$\log_{10} 9.00$	$\log_{10} 8.04\text{-}\log_{10} 8.55$	Özer et al. (2009) Yilmaztekin et al. (2004)
	Lb. fermentum AB5-18, Lb. fermentum AK4-120, Lb. plantarum AB16-65, Lb. plantarum AC18-42	120 days at 4 °C	2.7×10^9	7.4×10^7	Kılıç et al. (2009)
	Lb. acidophilus	90 days at 4 °C	$4.0 \log_{10}$	$>10^7$	Kasımoğlu et al. (2004)
	Ent. faecium, Lb. paracasei ssp. paracasei, B. bifidum				Gürsoy and Kınık (2010)
Lamb rennet paste Pecorino cheese	Lb. acidophilus, B. longum, B. lactis	40 days	$7\log_{10}$	-	Santillo et al. (2009)
Semi hard cheese	6 strains of probiotic bacteria (3 of Lactobacillus acidophilus and 3 of Lactobacillus casei group)	2 mo at 12 °C	5×10^7	$7.98\text{-}9.23\log_{10}$	Bergamini et al. (2009a)
	Lb. acidophilus, Lb. paracasei, B. lactis	2 mo at 12 °C	1×10^6	$1 \times 10^7\text{-}1 \times 10^9$	Bergamini et al. (2009b)
	Lb. acidophilus, Lb. paracasei	60 days at 4 °C	10^6	1.6×10^9	Bergamini et al. (2005) Bergamini et al. (2006)
Cottage-like Gouda, Camembert	Lb. acidophilus UFVH2b20 Lb. acidophilus, Lb. paracasei, Lb. rhamnosus, Bifidobacterium spp.	3 mo at 5 °C		$>10^8$	Araujo et al. (2009) van de Casteele et al. (2003)
Semi soft cheese	Lb. acidophilus NCFM, Lb. rhamnosus HN001	60 days at 5 °C	$6.5 \log_{10}$ for A3 $7.2 \log_{10}$ for A1	$71.7 \times 10^9\text{-}1.85 \times 10^7$ $2.03 \times 10^8\text{-}3.43 \times 10^6$	Makelainen et al. (2009)
Argentinian Fresco cheese	Lb. paracasei A13, B. bifidum A1, Lb. acidophilus A3			$7.3 \log_{10}$ for A3 $6.7 \log_{10}$ for A1	Vinderola et al. (2009) Vinderola et al.

Cheese	Strain	Storage	Initial count	Final count	Reference
Crescenza	*Lactobacillus* sp.	12 days at 4 °C	8.0 log10 A13 7.2 log10 H5	7.9 log10 A13 7.0 log10 H5	Burns et al (2008)
Petit-suisse cheese	*B. animalis* ssp. *lactis*, *Lb. acidophilus*	28 days at 4 °C	6.49-6.99 log₁₀ for *Lb. acidophilus* 7.40-7.69log₁₀ for *B. animalis*	6.08-6.62log10 *Lb. acidophilus* 7.34-7.21log₁₀ *B. animalis*	Cardarelli et al (2008)
Minas fresh cheese	*Lb. acidophilus* *Lb. acidophilus* La5 *Bifidobacterium* BB12	14 days at 5 °C 21 days at 5 °C 28 days at 5 °C	6 log₁₀ 6.6 log₁₀ 7.74 log₁₀	7.04 log₁₀ 8.4 log₁₀ 7.93 log₁₀	Souza et al (2008) Buriti et al. (2005) Fritzen-Freire et al. (2010)
Sweet whey cheese	*Lb. paracasei* LAFTI® L26	21 days at 7 °C	10⁹-10¹⁰	increased by 1.5 log cycle	Madureira et al. (2008)
Cheese spreads	*Lb. fermentum* ME-3	28 days at 5 °C	3.4-8.0x10⁷	2.0-4.8x10⁷	Jarvenpaa et al. (2007)
Ras cheese	*Lb. reuteri, Lb. casei, Lb. gasseri*				Dabiza and Fathi (2006)
Hard cheese	*Lb. rhamnosus* LC705, *Lb. paracasei* ssp. *paracasei* DC412	3 mo at 4 °C	8.63-8.99 log₁₀	7.91-8.04 log₁₀	Kalavrouzioti et al. (2005)
Cream cheese Kasar cheese	*Lb. casei, Lb. reuteri, B. bifidum* *Lb. acidophilus* LA5, *B. animalis* BB12	3 mo at 4 °C	4x10⁹ for each bacteria	7.17-7.32 log₁₀ for BB12 6.04 log₁₀ for LA5	Ortega et al. (2005) Özer et al. (2008)
Queijo de Cabra	*B. bifidum* BB02, *B. longum* BB46 *Lb. acidophilus*	70 days	3x10⁷ for *Bifidobacterium* 7.5x10⁶-1.0 x10⁷ for *Lactobacillus*	3x10⁸ for *Bifidobacterium* 6x10⁷ for *Lactobacillus*	Gomes and Malcata (1998)

Table 2. (Continued)

Vidiago cheese washed curd cheese	Lb.delbrueckii ssp. lactis UO 004	28 days at 4 °C	10^8-10^9	Fernandez et al. (2005)
Pont-L'Eveque cheese	Lb.plantarum UCMA 3037	75 days	>10^7	Coeuret et al. (2004)
Fresh cheese	B. bifidum, Lb. casei			Suarez-Solis et al. (2002)
	Lb. acidophilus JCN11047, 1132T, Lb. gasseri JCM11657	4 weeks at 7 °C	6×10^8 <10^8	Masuda et al. (2005)
Tallaga cheese	Lb. acidophilus LA-5, B. lactis BB-12	28 days	> $6 \log_{10}$	El-Zayat and Osman (2001)
Iranian White cheese	B. bifidum or B.adolescentis	60 days	>10^7	Ghoddusi and Robinson (1996)
Cottage cheese	B.infantis, B. longum, B. catenulatum, B. bifidum, B. angulatum, B. breve, B. pseudocatenulatum,	14 days at 4 °C	10^6-10^7	O'Riordan and Fitzgerald (1998)
Crescenza cheese	B. bifidum, B. longum, B. infantis	14 days	8.05 $\log_{10}$ for B.bifidum 7.12 $\log_{10}$ for B. longum 5.23 $\log_{10}$ for B. infantis	declined 3 log cycle 1 log cycle increase in B. bifidum, B. longum 1 log cycle decrease in B. infantis	Gobbetti et al. (1998)
Canestrato Pugliese cheese	B. longum, B. bifidum	56 days	7 $\log_{10}$	1 log cycle decrease	Corbo et al. (2001)

Strains of *Str. thermophilus* with high oxygen consumption ability have been shown to enhance the viability of bifidobacteria (Okonogi et al., 1984); therefore these strains could be used in cheese-making along with bifidobacteria. Similarly, a commercial strain of *Lb. acidophilus* LA-5 grew poorly in 32 week-old Cheddar cheese (Phillips et al., 2006), while this strain showed better survivability in white brined cheese (Yilmaztekin et al., 2004). Some *Enterococcus* spp. are now considered to be classified as probiotic. Gardiner et al. (1998, 1999) showed that *Enterococcus faecium* survived remarkably in Cheddar cheese after 15 months storage at 8 °C.

The characteristics of cheese matrix affect the fate of probiotic cells in GIT. Masuda et al. (2005) demonstrated that human derived strains of *Lb. acidophilus* and *Lb. gasseri* delivered to human body through fresh cheese were well-protected against bile salts and gastric conditions (Masuda et al., 2005). Physical properties of cheese matrix was also found to determinative on the survivability of *Lb. acidophilus* LAC-1 and *Lb. acidophilus* Ki, *Lb. paracasei* ssp. *paracasei* LCS-1, *Lb. brevis* LMG 6906, *B. animalis* BLC-1, *B. animalis* BB12 and *B. animalis* Bo in Requeijao cheese (a fresh whey cheese) (Madureira et al., 2005). Makelainen et al. (2009) investigated the influence of cheese matrix on the survival and metabolic activity of *Lb. rhamnosus* HN001 and *Lb. acidophilus* NCFM™, using three different models simulating the human upper gastrointestinal tract, human colon and colonocytes in cell culture. Probiotics in cheese survived in the simulated upper gastrointestinal tract model, and numbers of *Lb. acidophilus*, *Lb. rhamnosus* and total lactobacilli were increased in the colonic fermentation simulations of the probiotic cheese when compared with the non-probiotic cheese used as a control. The cheese matrix also beneficially affected cyclooxygenase-gene expression of colonocytes in a cell culture model. The authors concluded that the cheese matrix did not seem to affect the probiotic survival. Similar results were obtained by Pisano et al. (2008) who found that 6 lactobacillus strains out of 14 strains isolated from Fiero Sardo cheese showed probiotic properties and great resistance against GIT conditions.

Gobbetti et al. (1998) postulated that the viability of strains of bifidobacteria was salt dependent, and exceeding the upper limit of 4 g salt/ 100 g (w/w) caused a dramatic fall in colony counts of probiotic strains in Crescenza cheese. It was reported that *Lb. acidophilus* was susceptible to salt concentrations above 6% and a maximum 3.5% (w/w) salt in goat cheese provided counts of *B. lactis* and *Lb. acidophilus* high enough for a probiotic effect in goat cheese (Gomes and Malcata, 1998). The brined cheese traditionally contains relatively high concentrations of salt. It is thought that, with moderate modifications in the technology of manufacturing of this cheese variety, it may be possible to produce cheese containing probiotic effect (>10^6 cfu/g) without imparing the quality of final product (Samona and Robinson, 1994; Gomes et al., 1995). Yilmaztekin et al. (2004) investigated the survival of *Lb. acidophilus* LA-5 and *B. bifidum* BB-02 in white brined cheese. Authors demonstrated that the counts of both probiotic bacteria dropped gradually during 90-day ripening in brine, being more remarkable in *Bifidobacterium* BB-02, but the counts of probiotic bacteria were above the threshold for a therapeutic minimum (10^6 cfu/g). Similar results were reported for white brined cheese (Ghoddushi and Robinson, 1996; Gürsoy and Kınık, 2010), cottage cheese (Blanchette et al., 1996) and fresh cheese (Roy et al., 1997) as well. The rate of salt penetration into cheese blocks is influenced by many factors including concentration of brine solution, temperature, pH and cheese texture. Daigle et al. (1999) found that loss of *B.*

bifidum in Cheddar cheese was more remarkable during the first week of ripening (the loss of 0.5 log cycle) and the numbers remained stable during the following 11 weeks. Salt is not the sole criteria that affects the growth of probiotic bacteria (especially *Bifidobacterium* spp.) but also the type of ions in salt may affect the growth pattern and metabolic activities of the *Bifidobacterium* spp. The calcium and sodium ions, for example, have been shown to cause morphological changes in bifidobacteria, their acid-producing ability and other growth characteristics (Misra and Kuila, 1990; Modler et al., 1990; Samona and Robinson, 1991).

Initial inoculation level of probiotic bacteria may be an alternative to reduce the adverse effect of salt on viability of probiotic cells. Gomes et al. (1995) proposed that a relatively large inocula, 3.5-7.0% (corresponding the average levels of 2.0×10^9 cfu/g and $3-4 \times 10^9$ cfu/g, respectively), of probiotic strains were required to achieve the proper acidification rates in Gouda cheese. Yilmaztekin et al. (2004) compared two inoculum levels of *Lb. acidophilus* LA5 and *B.bifidum* BB02 (2.5% and 5.0% corresponding to average levels of $1.0-1.3 \times 10^9$ cfu/g and $2.0-2.1 \times 10^9$ cfu/g, respectively) in white brined Turkish cheese. Although the trend of variation in the counts of probiotic bacteria was same in both cheeses, the sample with higher inoculum had higher cell counts for both probiotic bacteria throughout 90-day ripening.

The probiotics must not show an antagonistic effect against mesophilic or thermophilic cheese starters or *vice versa*. Ziarno et al. (2010) showed that the manufacture of probiotic cheese only with probiotics was not possible because of their weak growth in milk and the lack of proteolytic activity. The authors also observed no inhibitory effect of probiotics on the mesophilic cheese starters; however, the growth of probiotic bacteria was stimulated when the ripening temperature was increased from 6 °C to 14 °C, with more pronounced in *Lb. acidophilus* LA-5 than *B. animalis* ssp. *lactis* BB12. On contrary, Gobbetti et al. (1998) showed that the lactic acid produced by *Streptococcus thermophilus* caused a decreased in the counts of *B. infantis* within 14 days of storage in Crescenze cheese, while the numbers of *B. bifidum* and *B. longum* increased 1 to 2 log cycle under the same conditions. Souza and Saad (2009) investigated the symbiosis between thermophilic yogurt starter bacteria and *Lb. acidophilus* LA-5 with thermophilic yogurt starters in Minas fresh cheese. The authors found that thermophilic yogurt bacteria did not affect the growth of *Lb. acidophilus* LA-5 but the overall quality of cheese improved except for a slight post-acidification problem (Souza et al., 2008; Souza and Saad 2009). Probiotic ABT cultures (*Lb. acidophilus* LA-5, *B. animalis* BB12 and *Str. thermophilus*) can be used in the production of fresh probiotic cheese (e.g. Minas Frescal cheese) together with mesophilic cheese starters with no negative effect on the final product (Fritzen-Freire et al., 2010; Marcatti et al., 2009), and ABT culture can be employed as an alternative to classical O-type starter cultures (Buriti et al., 2007). Gürsoy and Kınık (2010) stated that *Lb. paracasei* ssp. *paracasei*, *Enterococcus faecium* and *B. bifidum* showed no antagonistic effect against lactococcal cheese starters in white brined Turkish cheese.

4. METHODS FOR IMPROVING VIABILITY OF PROBIOTICS IN CHEESE

There are a number of alternatives employed in protection of probiotic strains against undesirable environmental conditions. These include cell incubation under sublethal conditions, two-stage fermentation, inclusion protective agents, improved stress adaptability, cell propogation in an immobilized biofilm and microencapsulation. Each of these techniques has advantages and limitations in food applications. Among these techniques, microencapsulation has gained popularity in recent years. Compared to immobilization/ entrapment techniques, microencapsulation offers many advantages (Krasaekoopt et al., 2003). Especially, microencapsulating cells in hydrocolloid bead matrix results in an improved protection of probiotic bacteria from environmental conditions (Picot and Lacroix, 2004).

Table 3. Microencapsulation/immobilization of probiotic cells for cheese production

Bacteria	Technique	Cheese	Supporting material	Reference
Lb. paracasei	Milk fat	Cheddar	-	Stanton et al. (1998)
Lb. acidophilus+ *B. bifidum*	Extrusion	White Brined Turkish cheese Kasar cheese	Ca-alginate	Özer et al. (2009) Özer et al (2008)
Lb. acidophilus+ *B. bifidum*	Emulsion	White Brined Turkish cheese Kasar cheese	κ-carrageenan	Özer et al. (2009) Özer et al (2008)
Ent. faecium	Milk fat	Cheddar	-	Gardiner et al. (1998)
B. bifidum, *B. adolescentis*	Cream	White brined cheese		Ghoddusi and Robinson (1996)
B. bifidum *B. infantis* *B. longum*		Crescenza cheese	Ca-alginate	Gobbetti et al. (1997)
Lb. acidophilus *B. lactis*	Emulsion	Feta cheese	Ca-alginate	Kailasapathy and Masondole (2005)
Lb. acidophilus *B. infantis*	Emulsion	Cheddar	Ca-alginate	Godward and Kailasapathy (2003)
Lb. casei	Immobilization	Feta	Fruit pieces	Kourkoutas et al. (2006)
B. bifidum	Immobilization	Cheddar	κ-carrageenan	Dinakar and Mistry (1994)

The microcapsule is made up of a semipermeable, spherical, thin and strong membranous wall (Kailasapathy and Masondole, 2005). The diffuse of nutrients and metabolites in and out of the semipermeable membrane takes place easily. This technology has been successfully employed in the manufacture of whey-based products (Audet et al., 1989) and yogurt (Prevost and Divies, 1988). Microencapsulated bacterial cells are further protected against phage attacks (Steenson et al., 1987), conditions during lyophylization and freezing (Kearney et al., 1990; Sheu and Marshall, 1993; Sung, 1997) and improved stability of bacterial growth during storage (Kebary et al., 1998). There are a number of methods for the encapsulation of bacterial cells including emulsion, extrusion, interfacial polymerization and/or coacervation (Kailasapathy, 2002). Among these methods, cell entrapment in gelled biopolymers in which κ-carrageenan or calcium-alginate is used as support material, is the most commonly employed method in laboratory scale. Goderska et al., (2003) showed that while *Lb. rhamnosus* colonies microencapsulated in alginate matrix kept their viability up to 48 h at pH 2.0, free cells were inactivated completely under the same conditions. Similarly, increasing the alginate concentration led to an increase in the colony counts of *B. longum* (Lee and Heo, 2000). Table 3 shows the encapsulation conditions of the probiotic bacteria used in the manufacture of cheese.

Encapsulation by extrusion or emulsion techniques has been succesfully used for the protection of probiotic bacteria against adverse environmental conditions (Doleyres and Lacroix, 2005; Jankowski et al., 1997; Kebary et al., 1998). The viability of probiotic bacteria could be extended up to 80-95% by emulsion or extention techniques (Jankowski et al., 1997; Kebary et al., 1998; Doleyres and Lacroix, 2005). Özer et al. (2009) demonstrated that the survivability of the encapsulated probiotic bacteria in white brined cheese was higher (1 log cycle decrease after 90 days) than the cheese inoculated with probiotics in free state (3 log cycle decrease after 90 days) (Figure 1).

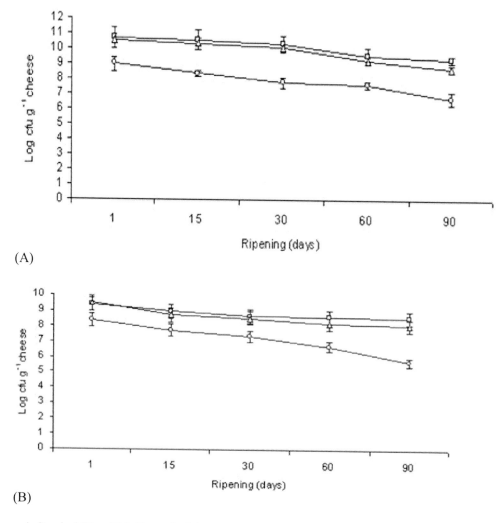

Figure 1. Survivability of (a) *Lb. acidophilus* LA-5 and (b) *B. animalis* BB-12 in white brined cheese throughout 90-day ripening period. (○) Cheese with added probiotics in unprotected state, (□) Cheese with added probiotics microencapsulated by extrusion technique, (Δ) Cheese with added probiotics microencapsulated by emulsion technique.

However, in contrast, Godward and Kailasapathy (2003) claimed that microencapsulation of probiotic cells in Feta cheese caused higher cell loss, either by preventing encapsulated bacteria from interacting with the environment for survival or inhibiting disposal of cell metabolites that may be accumulating inside the encapsulated capsules causing death. Similar conclusions were drawn by Godward (2000) for Cheddar cheese, the dense matrix of which was claimed not to be conducive for free exchange of metabolites and nutrients to and from the entrapped capsules. Later, Kailasapathy and Masondole (2005) showed that microencapsulation did not offer protection to the probiotic bacteria, due to the open texture of Feta cheese, disintegration of microcapsules in brine solution and a higher salt uptake when encapsulated cultures were incorporated. Here, the degree of disintegration of microcapsules and cheese texture are the major factors determining the success of the cell encapsulation. It may be possible that exchanging sodium ions with calcium ions binding alginate capsules together leads to disintegration of the capsules, releasing probiotic bacteria into the medium (Özer et al., 2009). During time-dependent release of probiotic bacteria, a sligth salt adaptation may develop in the probiotic cells and the death of the cells remain relatively limited. Similar results were reported by Kailasapathy and Masondole (2005) who demonstrated that microcapsules formed by calcium alginate polymers containing starch were susceptible to disintegration in Feta cheese ripened in brine. On the other hand, it should be borne in mind that apart from slow disintegration of microcapsules during ripening, the salt might penetrate into the beads and affect the viability of probiotic bacteria. The role of sodium chloride in the disintegration mechanism of κ-carrageenan or Ca-alginate capsules is not clear and need further investigation. Kasar cheese, a kind of pasta-filata cheese native to Turkey, was shown to be an ideal medium for the incorporation of microencapsulated probiotic bacteria (Özer et al., 2008). During manufacture of Kasar cheese, high heat treatment is applied to cheese curd and the viability of *Lb.acidophilus* LA-5 and *B. animalis* BB12 cells was maintained by microencapsulation (*see* Figure 2).

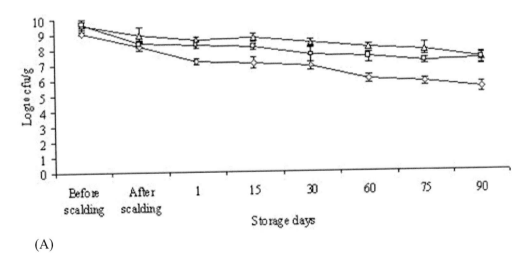

(A)

Figure 2. (Continued)

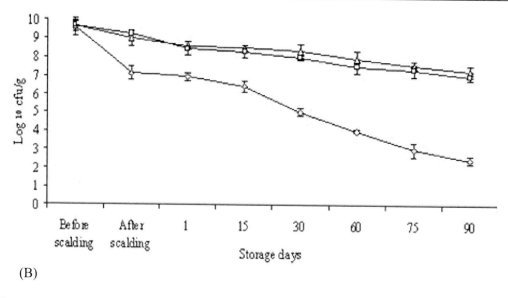

(B)

Figure 2. Survivability of (a) *Lb. acidophilus* LA-5 and (b) *B. animalis* BB-12 in Kasar cheese throughout 90-day ripening period. (○) Cheese with added probiotics in unprotected state, (Δ) Cheese with added probiotics microencapsulated by extrusion technique, (□) Cheese with added probiotics microencapsulated by emulsion technique.

In addition to the increased protection of microbial viability after microencapsulation, the chemical and physical properties of the cheeses containing probiotic bacteria in the encapsulated form may be affected as well. Özer et al., (2008) demonstrated that micro encapsulation did not affect the basic composition of Kasar cheese; however, the development of proteolysis was more pronounced in the cheeses containing probiotic bacteria in the encapsulated form. Incorporation of microencapsulated *Bifidobacterium* BB-12 and *Lb.acidophilus* LA-5 into white brined Turkish cheese resulted in much higher levels of medium- and long-chain free fatty acids than in the control cheese (Özer et al., 2009). Similarly, cheeses made with immobilized probiotics contained higher acetaldehyde and diacetyl levels than the control cheese and immobilization was reported not to affect the sensory quality of the end product. It was demonstrated that the addition of probiotic cultures, either in the free or encapsulated state, did not seem to significantly affect textural parameters such as springiness and cohesiveness of 7-week-old Feta cheese (Kailasapathy and Masondole, 2005).

The use of prebiotic agents in the manufacture of probiotic cheese is another alternative to protect the counts of probiotic cells during processing and ripening. Addition of prebiotics such as inulin, oligofructose and oligosaccharides, into yogurt has been proved to be very successful (Özer et al., 2005). On contrary, addition of prebiotic compounds into cheese milk is rather new. Cardarelli et al. (2007, 2008) investigated the effect of inulin, oligofructose and oligosaccharide from honey, combined in different proportion, on the probiotic viable count in synbiotic petit-suisse cheese. Addition of the prebiotics increased the numbers of *B. animalis* ssp. *lactis* and *Lb. acidophilus* with no adverse affect on the sensory quality of the resulting product. Similar results were obtained by Modzelewska-Kapitula et al. (2007) who investigated the effect of inulin HPX on the growth of *Lb. plantarum* 14 in soft cheese. Hayes et al. (1996), on contrary, found that fructooligosaccharides (FOS) was ineffective in stimulating the growth of bifidobacteria in Edam cheese. Both cheese starters and probiotic adjunct are not able to degrade the fructans added into cheese milk as prebiotics (Buriti et al., 2007).

Apart from prebiotics, the biopreservative compounds can also stimulate the growth of probiotic bacteria in cheese. For example, metabolites produced by *Propionibacterium thoenii* P-127 were shown to stimulate the growth of *Bifidobacterium bifidum* in Domiati cheese (El-Kholy et al., 2006). Overall, probiotic bacteria are more inhibitory towards lactic acid bacteria than *vice versa* with a few execptions (Vinderola et al., 2002a). The antimicrobial compounds produced by probiotic strains such as hydrogen peroxide, alcoholic compounds, diacetyl and bacteriocins, can create a hostile environment for pathogens (Buriti et al., 2007) and in some cases for non-pathogenic lactic acid bacteria. Tharmaraj and Shah (2009) showed antimicrobial effect of *Lb. paracasei* ssp. *paracasei*, *Lb. rhamnosus*, *Lb. acidophilus*, *B. animalis* and *Propionibacterium* sp. on *Aspergillus niger*, *Penicillium roqueforti*, *Candida albicans* and *Saccharomyces cerevisiae* in cheese-based dips. Similarly, *Lb. reuteri*, *Lb. casei* and *Lb. gasseri* were demonstrated to be effective against coliforms, *Staphylococcus* sp., and yeasts (Dabiza and El-Deib, 2007) and against moulds (Dabiza and Fathi, 2006) in Ras cheese. A strong antimicrobial effect of *Lb. fermentum* ME-3 in Pikante cheese -a traditional Estonian cheese- was shown by Songisepp et al. (2004). Similarly, *Lb. helveticus* CU631 in cream cheese had a strong antagonistic effect against *Helicobacter pylori* (Song et al., 2001) which may be useful to consume cheeses containing this bacteria by the consumer suffering from ulcer. Late blowing caused by *Clostridium* sp. is one of the major challenges of cheese industry and some probiotic strains such as *Lb. gasseri* LF221 and K7 are able to prevent late blowing during ripening (Perko et al., 2002).

Enhancement of bifidobacterial cold- and/or acid-tolerance could increase the number of viable probiotic bacteria ingested *via* refrigerated dairy products. One strategy for enhancing bacterial tolerance of stress is prior exposure to sub-lethal levels of the given stress (Maus and Ingham, 2003; Saarela et al., 2004; Roy, 2005). Collado and Sanz (2006) showed that the recovered strains of *B. breve* and *B. adolescentis* obtained after prolonged exposure of human feces to homologous lethal stress conditions were resistant to high concentrations of bile salts and sodium chloride. This indicates the potential use of these strains in the manufacture of cheese. Acid treatment at pH 3 or 4 may protect the probiotic cells against pH 2.5 or a treatment at 47 °C may protect against heat treatment at 55 °C (Sarkar, 2010; Saarela et al., 2004). Maus and Ingham (2003) demonstrated that the exposure of early stationary phase bacterial cells to combinations of reduced temperature (~6 °C), reduced pH (improved resistance against pH 3.5 when the growth medium pH decreased from 6.0 to 5.2) and starvation (30 to 60 min under reduced pH and temperature conditions) could enhance the viability of some strains of *B. longum* and *B. lactis*. These strains are considered to be suitable for the manufacture of fresh cheeses and other varieties with low pH.

Pressure pre-treatment is another alternative to improve the thermo-tolerance of probiotic bacteria. The survival of pressure treated cells of *Lb. rhamnosus* GG was higher than the untreated cells when exposed to heat treatment at 60 °C (Desmond et al., 2002; Ananta and Knorr, 2004). This strain could be employed in the manufacture of high cooked or pasta-filata type probiotic cheeses.

As stated earlier, vast majority of the probiotic strains are facultative aerobic or obligatory anaerobic and dissolved oxygen is one of the most powerful detrimental factors against probiotics. Therefore, selection of packaging materials for probiotic dairy products is of great importance. In general, high impact polystyrene containers with a wall thickness of 300-350 μm allowing oxygen diffusion at the rate of 1.0 to 5.0 cm^2/kg/d are more suitable for probiotic cultured foods (Miller et al., 2002; Sarkar, 2010; Dave and Shah, 1997). Plastic films with low oxygen permeability seem to be the ideal material for packaging of probiotic cheeses. Compared to the fermented probiotic products, much less attention has been paid on the relationship between the packaging materials and survivability or probiotics in functional cheeses. Kasımoğlu et al. (2004) monitored the viability of *Lb. acidophilus* in vacuum-packed white brined Turkish cheese stored at 4 °C for 90 days. On ripening in vacuum pack, *Lb. acidophilus* survived to numbers >10^7 cfu/g, which is necessary for positive effects on health, without imparing the overall quality of the end product. Authors concluded that *Lb. acidophilus* could be used for the manufacturing of probiotic white cheese to shorten ripening time and vacuum packaging is the preferred storage format.

5. BIOCHEMISTRY OF PROBIOTIC CHEESES

Apart from the health benefits, the overall sensory, chemical and physical properties of cheese must be maintained or improved when probiotic bacteria are incorporated. In general, probiotic bacteria do not affect the gross composition of the probiotic cheeses (Bergamini et al., 2005, 2006; Buriti et al., 2005; Daigle et al., 1999; Dinakar and Mistry, 1994; Gobbetti et al., 1998; Ong et al., 2006, 2007; Özer et al., 2009; Yilmaztekin et al., 2004). However, the biochemical and sensory properties of a probiotic cheese may show variation depending on the probiotic species/strain used in the manufacture. Proteolysis is the major biochemical event occuring in cheese during ripening and characteristic properties of a cheese are determined largely by type and/or concentration of proteolysis products. Therefore, factors affecting the proteolytic activity of probiotic bacteria (such as ripening temperature, relative humidity, antagonism with starter culture etc.) directly affect the cheese quality as well. The presence of non-starter lactic acid bacteria (NSLAB) may also limit the growth and biochemical activities of probiotics since they compete with probiotic bacteria for nutrients. In general, the primary phase of proteolysis is affected by probiotic bacteria at fairly limited degrees (Özer and Kırmacı, 2009; Özer et al, 2008; Ong et al., 2006), since primary proteolysis is mainly achieved by coagulants (*i.e.* chymosine, plasmin) and cell-wall enveloped proteases (Sousa et al., 2001). Kasımoğlu et al. (2004) showed that the level of water soluble nitrogen in white brined Turkish cheese produced with *Lb. acidophilus* 593N increased continuously during ripening period of 90 days. Similar results were obtained by Özer et al. (2008) who studied the proteolytic profile of white brined Turkish cheese manufactured using microencapsulated *Lb. acidophilus* LA-5 and *Bifidobacterium* BB-12. Varying results have been reported on development of proteolysis in probiotic Cheddar cheese in the literature. Gardiner et al (1998) and Bergamini et al. (2006) demonstrated that the proteolysis improved at limited levels in Cheddar cheese made with probiotic bacteria as adjunct cultures. On contrary, Ong and Shah (2009) showed that proteolysis in probiotic Cheddar cheese was accelerated at high ripening temperature (4 °C *vs.* 8 °C) and probiotic adjunct cultures (*B. longum* 1941, *B. animalis* ssp. *lactis* B94, *Lb. casei* 279, *Lb. casei* L26, *Lb. acidophilus* 4962, *Lb. acidophilus* L10) contributed the development of proteolysis at high levels. Similarly, a noticeable increase in the free aminoacids levels of the semi-hard probiotic cheese with *Lb. acidophilus* was reported by Bergamini et al. (2009a). The same authors also showed that while two-step fermentation improved peptidolytic activity of *Lb.acidophilus* in probiotic semi-hard cheese, this did not affect the peptidolytic capacity of *Lb. ca*sei. Bergamini et al. (2009b) investigated the proteolytic capacities of three probiotic adjunct cultures (*Lb. acidophilus*, *Lb. paracasei* and *B. lactis*) in semi-hard probiotic cheeses. While *B. lactis* showed no effect on proteolysis, *Lb. paracasei* showed limited impact on proteolysis. On contrary, *Lb. acidophilus* influenced the secondary proteolysis significantly (Bergamini et al., 2006) that was even more pronounced when it was added to cheese-milk after pre-incubation in an enriched milk fat substrate (Bergamini et al., 2009b). Isolation of bacteria from traditional cheese matrices and use them as starter or adjunct cultures are common practices in today's cheese production (Cogan et al., 2007; Johnson and Lucey, 2006). The selection of strains belonging to the genus *Lactobacillus* as food additives intended to improve cheese quality or to provide probiotic status is encouraged by the fact that lactobacilli are mostly considered GRAS microorganisms (Bernardeau et al., 2008; Milesi et al., 2009). Contribution of probiotic lactobacilli to proteolysis in cheese relies mainly on their peptidolytic potential. Some probiotic strains of lactobacilli are also able to change the primary proteolysis in cheese (*e.g.* Cheddar cheese) manufactured without starter culture (Lane and Fox, 1996). Formation of water soluble peptides and free amino acids as well as type of amino acids are the parameters that provide information about the proteolytic capacity of probiotic or potentially probiotic lactobacilli (Bergamini et al., 2006; di Cagno et al., 2003; Ong et al., 2007). Milesi et al. (2009) found that *Lb. rhamnosus* isolated from different food habitats had strong peptidolytic activity in semi-hard or soft cheeses. On contrary, *Lb. casei* 190 and *Lb. plantarum* 191 showed rather weak proteolytic activities in the same cheese medium. Authors also demonstrated that *Lb. rhamnosus* triggered the post-acidification in the cheeses, resulted in loss of quality in the final products. As a new approach, probiotic strains can be added into rennet paste instead of addition in cheese milk. Santillo and Albenzio (2008) investigated the influence of *Lb. acidophilus* LA-5, *B. lactis* BB-12 and *B. longum* BB-46 added into rennet paste on the proteolysis of Pecorino cheese. The cheese made from rennet paste containing mixture of *Bifidobacterium* spp. had the highest levels of α_s-casein degradation products, non-casein nitrogen fractions and water soluble nitrogen fractions, and this method could be used to accelerate cheese ripening. The effect of *Bifidobacterium* spp. on the degradation of β-casein is limited but *Lb. rhamnosus* LC705 and *Lb. paracasei* ssp. *paracasei* DC 412 accelerated the degradation of this casein fraction as well as α_s-casein in Kefralotyri cheese made from goat's milk (Kalavrouzioti et al., 2005). With increase in the ripening period, the contribution of probiotic bacteria to the proteolysis becomes more remarkable; however, in cheese varieties with rather shorter ripening period (*e.g.* cream cheese) proteolysis is also accelerated to a considerable level (Song et al., 2001). *Lb. helveticus* are described with their high and broad intracellular peptidolytic activities and owing to this property, the strains of this bacteria are widely used in probiotic cheese-making. Jensen et al. (2008) showed that the degree of casein degradation by *Lb. helveticus* was strain-dependent and the level of cell lysis was limited in cheese matrix compared with MRS broth. Proteolysis in probiotic cheese may be accelerated by using encapsulated recombinant aminopeptidase. Azarnia et al. (2008) found that encapsulated recombinant aminopeptidase (PepN) from *Lb. rhamnosus* accelerated the proteolysis and eventually shortened ripening period to a great extent.

The proteolytic potential of probiotic bacteria is also affected by the ripening conditions. According to Gomes et al. (1998b), changing in the relative humidity (from 85% to 95%) and ripening temperature (from 5 °C to 10 °C) led to variations in the proteolytic profile of the caprine cheese, and when relative humidity was adjusted to 95% at 10 °C, the ripening period of the probiotic cheese may be reduced up to 25 days.

Lipolysis is another biochemical event that affects the sensory and physical quality of probiotic cheeses (Fox et al., 2000). Although, the lipolytic and esterolytic activities of probiotic bacteria are, in general, limited (Özer et al., 2009), some probiotic strains may contribute to lipolysis at considerable levels. Kalavrouzioti et al. (2005) reported that the lipolysis developed fastly in Kefalotyri cheese made with *Lb. paracasei* ssp. *paracasei* DC 412 and *Lb. rhamnosus* L705. As with proteolysis, the ripening temperature affected the level of free fatty acids in caprine cheese; however, relative humidity was found to be ineffective on lipolysis (Gomes et al., 1998b). Özer et al. (2009) investigated the lipolytic capacity of microencapsulated *Lb. acidophilus* LA-5 and *Bifidobacterium* BB-12 in white brined Turkish cheese. Authors demonstrated that the level of free fatty acids was remarkably low in the cheese containing probiotic culture in free form. On contrary, in the cheeses made with probiotic bacteria microencapsulated by emulsion or extrusion technique, lipolysis developed more remarkably (*see* Figures 3a-c). In contrast, Gobbetti et al. (1998) found that *B. bifidum* showed a limited activity on long-chain free fatty acids (FFAs) in Crescenza cheese. Other researchers (Corbo et al., 2001) also demonstrated that incorporation of *Bifidobacterium* spp. into the hard or semi-hard Italian cheeses (*e.g.* Canastrato Pugliese cheese) resulted in increases in the concentrations of butyric ($C_{4:0}$), caproic ($C_{6:0}$), capric ($C_{10:0}$) and oleic ($C_{18:1}$) acids. The use of lamb rennet paste containing probiotics (*B. longum, B. lactis* or *Lb. acidophilus*) was reported to cause a lipase activity 2-fold greater than traditional lamb rennet paste in Pecorino cheese (Santillo et al., 2009). Lamb rennet containing *Lb. acidophilus* produced more total free fatty acids than that containing bifidobacteria or traditional rennet paste. The loss of free fatty acids was also limited in the cheeses made by probiotic containing rennet paste. This technology may offer a solution for the production of probiotic cheese characterized with lipolytic aroma and flavour, as well as reduction in ripening period of cheese. Fatty acids in milk or cheese may act as a growth promoter or inhibitor for *Bifidobacterium* spp. (Bolyston et al., 2004). While lauric and mrystic acids, accounting for 3.6% and 10.5% of the fatty acids in the milk triacylglycerols, respectively, inhibit the growth of bifidobacteria, butyric, palmitic, and stearic acids, which accounts for 8.5%, 23.5% and 10.0% of the fatty acids in the milk triacylglycerols, respectively, promote the growth of the bifidobacteria. The role of free fatty acids liberated during ripening of cheese on the growth of bifidobacteria should be studied in detail.

Fermentation of lactose by NSLAB produces some organic acid by-products such as formic acid and acetic acid (McSweeney and Fox, 2004). Excess of these compounds adversaly affects the flavour balance of cheese (Ong and Shah, 2009). Appropriate ripening temperatures are required to maintain the balanced growth of these bacteria to achieve the optimum cheese quality. The type and concentration of organic acids produced by probiotic bacteria depend on the strain and species used. *Lb. casei*, for example, can produce acetic acid as their metabolic end product (Ong and Shah, 2009).

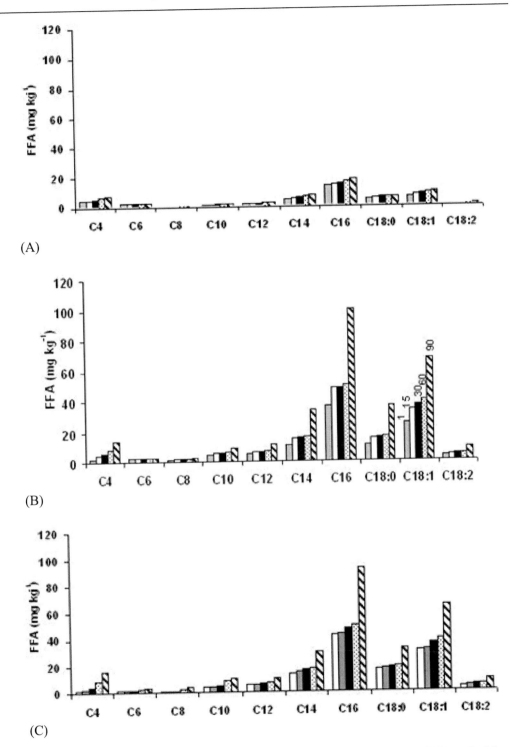

Figure 3. Free fatty acids levels of white brined cheese made from microencapsulated *Lb. acidophilus* La-5 and *B. animalis* BB-12. a) Cheese with added probiotics in unprotected state, b) Cheese with added probiotics microencapsulated by extrusion technique, c) Cheese with added probiotics microencapsulated by emulsion technique.

Acetic and lactic acid production by *Bifidobacterium* spp. relies on fructose-6-phosphate shunt pathway, yielding 3 mol of acetic acid and 2 mol of lactic acid per mol of glucose (Scardovi and Trotavelli, 1965). At small concentrations, acetic acid contributes to cheese flavour in a positive manner; however, excessive accumulation of acetic acid causes off-flavours in cheese (Grattepanche et al., 2008). Since free aminoacids may act as a precursor for the production of acetic acid (Ong et al., 2006), the increase in the level of free amino acids in probiotic cheeses likely have higher level of acetic acid. Ong and Shah (2009) investigated the organic acid profiles of six different probiotic Cheddar cheeses made from *Bifidobacterium longum* 1941, *Lactobacillus casei* 279, *Lactobacillus acidophilus* 4962, *Bifidobacterium animalis* ssp. *lactis* LAFTI®B94, *Lb. casei* LAFTI®L26 and *Lb. acidophilus* LAFTI®L10 as adjunct cultures. Lactic, acetic, butyric and citric acids were found to be the major organic acids. The concentrations of lactic, acetic and butyric acids increased throughout ripening. Probiotic bacteria used in the manufacture of cheese did not influence the concentrations of citric, succinic and propionic acids. Although it is strain- and pH-dependent, the rate of lactic acid production from lactose by *Bifidobacterium* spp. is high. Li et al. (2006) reported that the lactic acid production efficiacy and lactose conversion rate by *B. longum* at pH 5.5-6.5 were 85% and 100%, respectively. If *Lb. rhamnosus* is used in combination with *Str. thermophilus* in Minas Frescal cheese whey, the fermentation of whey is extended (Almeida et al., 2008). On contrary, the combination of *B. animalis* ssp. *lactis* and *Str. thermophilus* produces more promising results regarding functional fermented whey beverages production.

Aroma and flavour are among the criteria determining the quality of cheese. The formation of cheese flavour is a result of very complex series of biochemical events. Both volatile and non-volatile compounds derived from proteolysis, lipolysis and glycolysis metabolisms contribute to the cheese flavour. The starter and non-starter bacteria are primarily responsible for the formation of well-balanced cheese flavour. Ripening conditions, milk type, manufacturing practices also interfere with the cheese flavour chemistry at varying degrees. Acetaldehyde, diacetyl, aceton, acetoin, butyric acid, 2-butanol, ethanol and propionic acid have been reported to be flavour compounds that are most abundant in many cheese varieties including Cheddar (Fox et al., 2000) and brined cheeses (Kılıç et al., 2009; Özer et al., 2009). In general, the contribution of probiotic bacteria to cheese flavour is limited compared with *Lactococcus* spp. (Champagne and Gardiner, 2005). Özer et al. (2009) reported that immobilized mixture of *Lb. acidophilus* LA-5 and *Bifidobacterium animalis* ssp. *lactis* BB-12 produced aceton, ethanol, diacetyl and acetaldehyde at remarkable levels in Turkish white brined cheese. Among the *Bifidobacterium* spp., *B. bifidum* strains are able to produce acetaldehyde at higher levels (Yuguchi et al., 1989). Similarly, *Lb. paracasei* ssp. *paracasei* is able to produce acetaldehyde via lactate metabolisms or oxidation of ethanol (McSweeney and Sousa, 2000). Diacetyl is produced by cheese flora through citrate metabolisms and $Cit^{(+)}$ *Lactococcus* strains in combination with *B. bifidum* in cheese production caused increases in both EtOH and diacetyl levels (Starrenburg and Hugenholtz, 1991). Cichosz et al. (2006) demonstrated that the highest sensory quality was obtained in probiotic Gouda cheeses produced with *Lb. casei*, *Lb. acidophilus* or *Lb. rhmanosus* and it contained the highest amount of butyric acid, high of propionic acid, and much less of acetone, ethanol and also of acetoin and diacetyl determined by solid phase microextraction method. On contrary, Sarantinopoulous et al. (2002) obtained high level of acetone in probiotic Feta cheese made with *Enterococcus faecium*. Similarly, *E. faecium* PR88 yielded high level of aroma compounds in probiotic Cheddar cheese (Gardiner et al., 1999). Cheese starters and probiotic adjuncts have shown to express several enzymes that contribute to flavour development in cheese (Yvon and Rijnen, 2001). The first step in these pathways is performed by aminotransferases which are able to catabolise branched-chain (Leu, Ile, Val), aromatic (Phe, Tyr, Trp) and sulphur-containing (Met) aminoacids (Thage et al., 2005). *Lactobacillus paracasei* ssp. *paracasei* CHCC 4256 was shown to have a high aminotransferase activity, yielding high concentrations of aroma compounds from branched-chain aminoacids and Asp in semi-hard probiotic cheese (Thage et al., 2005).

6. HEALTH ASPECTS OF PROBIOTIC CHEESE

Apart from beneficially affecting the health of consumers by maintaining or improving intestinal microflora, the probiotics can exert additional positive effects on human health and well-being such as the prevention of gastrointestinal disorders, alleviation of lactose intolerance symptoms, stimulation of the immune system, lowering of cholesterol level, enhancement of mineral absorption and vitamin production (Ziemer and Gibson 1998; Gomes and Malcata 1999; Shortt 1999). Animal models offer an opportunity to test therapeutic efficiency of probiotic bacteria and probiotic products. Modzelewska-Kapitula et al. (2010) investigated the effect of feeding diets containing white cheese manufactured with prebiotics and the potentially probiotic *Lb. plantarum* strain, on the gastrointestinal microflora of rats. After a 10-day feeding experiment, a significant reduction in the counts of anaerobic proteolytic bacteria spores was noted. As stated earlier, probiotic fresh cheese is a suitable vehicle for the oral administration of *B. bifidum*, *Lb. acidophilus* and *Lb. paracasei*. Medici et al. (2004) studied the influence of probiotic fresh cheese containing *B. bifidum*, *Lb. acidophilus* and *Lb. paracasei*, on the immune response system of mice. The authors observed a significant increase in the phagocytic activity of peritonela macrophages, in the number of IgA^+ producing cells and in the $CD4^+/CD8^+$ ratio in the small intestine after 5 days feeding. These results indicated that probiotic fresh cheese enables *B. bifidum*, *Lb. acidophilus* and *Lb. paracasei* to exert important immunomodulating effects in the gut. Phagocytic cells play a key role in protecting hosts against microbial infections (da Cruz et al., 2009). Similarly, macrophages is primarily responsible for the regulation of immune response system, as well as tissue repair mechanism. Ibrahim et al. (2010) investigated the effect of commercial probiotic Gouda cheese containing *Lb. rhamnosus* HN001 and *Lb. acidophilus* NCFM on the nutritional modulation of immune parameter in older volunteers (31 elderly people age range from 72 to 103). The volunteers were given probiotic cheese for 4-week, preceded by a period of 2-week consumption of probiotic free cheese and followed by a 4-week wash out period. Cytotoxicity of natural killer cells (NK) increased significantly upon consumption of probiotic cheese. A significant increase in phagocytosis observed was found to be independent from probiotics. Authors concluded that regular consumption of probiotic cheese would enhance parameters of innate immunity in elderly people, and it is supposed to be determined whether this enhancement correlates with a beneficial effect of the health of the elderly population.

The positive effect of cheese on the prevention of dental caries have long been known. During the last decade, the efficiacy of cheese containing probiotics on the reduction of microorganisms that are responsible for dental caries has attracted researchers' attention. Hatakka et al. (2007) tested the hypothesis that cheese containing *Lb. rhamnosus* GG ATCC 53103 (LGG), *Lb. rhamnosus* LC 705 and *Propionbacterium freudenreichii* ssp. *shermanii* JS can reduce the prevalence of oral *Candida*. According to the results of 16-week, randomized, double-blind, placebo-controlled study (with 276 elderly people), the prevelance of high saliva yeast count decreased by 32% in the group consumed probiotic cheeses, but this figure increased from 28% to 32% in the control group. It was concluded that cheese containing probiotic bacteria could be effective in controlling oral *Candida* and hyposalivation in the elderly. Similarly, Ahola et al. (2002, 2003) demonstrated that *Lb. rhamnosus* GG ATCC 53103 (LGG) and *Lb. rhamnosus* LC 705 may reduce high salivary *Streptococcus mutants* counts and effectively prevents dental caries in children.

Probiotics are able to form conjugated linoleic acid (CLA) from either free linoleic acid added to the medium or from linoleic acid released by microbial lipase which gives rise to additional health promoting effects in cheese (Abd El-Salam et al., 2010a). Cheese is good source of CLA with concentrations varying depending on the activity of starter microflora. Bello et al. (2008) reported that *Lb. paracasei* and *Lb. plantarum* isolated from traditional Italian cheeses were capable of producing CLA in MRS medium supplemented with linoleic acid. Lin (2003, 2006) demonstrated the high linoleic isomerase activity, an enzyme responsible for the production CLA, in *Lb. acidophilus* CCRC 14079. The ability of *Bifidobacterium* spp. to form CLA was strain specific (Coakley et al., 2003). While the CLA production by *B. breve*, *B. dentium*, *B. animalis* ssp. *lactis* was high, the capability of *B. adolescentis*, *B. infantis* and *B. angulatum* was at negligible levels (Abd El-Salam et al., 2010a). Most recently, Abd El-Salam et al. (2010b) developed a novel probiotic Ras cheese high in CLA content. The product was characterised by high and persistent counts (~10^8 cfu/g) of probiotic strains of *Lb. casei* and *Lb. acidophilus* up to 3 months of storage. No significant changes have been found in the chemical composition and ripening indices and oxidative stability of cheese fat between control and probiotic Ras cheese. Similar results were reported by Bzducha-Wrobel et al. (2009) who investigated the changes in the concentration of CLA in model cheese inoculated with *B. animalis* ssp. *lactis* and *Lb. acidophilus* and ripened at 14 °C for 8 weeks. Incorporation of probiotics into rennet paste used in the manufacture of probiotic cheese seems to be a reasonable alternative to incresae CLA level in cheese. Santillo et al. (2009) manufactured probiotic Pecorino cheese using lamb rennet paste containing *Lb. acidophilus* or a mixture of *B. lactis* and *B. longum* and monitored the changes in CLA concentrations throughout 60-day of ripening. Cheese containing *Lb.acidophilus* was characterized by the greatest levels of total conjugated linoleic acids (CLA) 9-cis, 11-trans CLA and 9-trans, 11-trans CLA, whereas cheese containing bifidobacteria displayed the highest levels of free CLA.

It is a well-established fact that Angiotensin I-converting enzyme (ACE; dipeptidyl carboxypeptidase I, E.C. 3.4.15.1.) regulates blood pressure and ACE inhibitors may exert an antihypertensive effect (Wang et al., 2010). ACE prefers substrates or inhibitors that contain mainly hydrophobic (aromatic or branched side chains) amino acid residues at the three C-terminal positions. Cheese has been well-characterized with its high ACE-I inhibitor peptides. The ACE-I inhibitor peptides level in cheese is determined by many factors including starter and non-starter strains, fermentation and ripening conditions etc. Up until now, extensive studies have been carried out on the isolation of ACE-I inhibitor peptides from fermented milks (Nakamura et al., 1995) and cheese (Addeo et al., 1992; Smacchi and Gobbetti, 1998; Apostolidis et al., 2007; Saito et al., 2000; Ryhanen et al., 2001; Gomez-Ruiz et al., 2002). Although, it is known that some probiotic strains are able to produce dipeptides and tripeptides showing ACE-I inhibitor activity in skimmilk or dairy products, only a few studies have been conducted on the release of ACE-I inhibitor peptide from probiotic cheeses (*see* Table 4) (Ong and Shah, 2008ab; Wang et al., 2010; Shuang et al., 2008). Wang et al. (2010) produced a new probiotic Cheddar cheese made with *Lb. casei* Zhang previously isolated from koumiss collected in Inner Mongolia. High ACE-inhibitory activities were obtained from the probiotic Cheddar cheeses (between 100% and 85.30%). The authors reported no reduction in the ACE-I inhibitory activity during extended ripening. The formation of bioactive peptides is closely related with level of degradation of casein fractions. Ong et al. (2008b) found that ACE-I inhibitory peptides corresponded to the α_{s1}-CN N-terminal peptides [(f 1-6), (f 1-7), (f 1-9), (f 24-32) and (f 102-110)] and β-CN N-terminal peptides [(f 47–52) and (f 193–209)]. In a recent study, Ong and Shah (2008a) demonstrated that increasing ripening temperature from 4 °C to 8 °C or 12 °C caused increases in ACE-I inhibitory effect in probiotic Cheddar cheese made with *Lb. helveticus* H100 or *Lb. acidophilus* L10, but ripening temperature was ineffective on the IC_{50} values of the cheeses.

7. ENUMERATION OF PROBIOTIC BACTERIA IN CHEESE

Differential enumeration of probiotic and starter bacteria often poses difficulties due to the presence of multiple species of lactic acid bacteria in cheese (van de Casteele et al., 2006). Up until now, several selective media have been developed for the enumeration of probiotic bacteria in dairy products. Majority of these methods are based on phenotypic differences of the lactic cultures in food systems. The reliability of phenotypic identification of lactic acid bacteria is often poor because certain species cannot be distinguished by phenotypic characteristics (Bolyston et al., 2004). Additionally, environmental conditions may affect phenotypic responses of probiotic bacteria as well (Schleifer et al., 1995).

MRS agar is widely used for the enumeration of *Bifidobacterium* spp. in dairy products, if this probiotic bacteria is the only live culture present (Blanchette et al., 1995). In mixed culture systems, the selective media should be supplemented with some compounds which may either stimulate the growth of bifidobacteria or inhibit the bacteria other than bifidobacteria (Bolyston et al., 2004). Among the growth promoters/inhibitors added into selective medium, NNLP (neomycin sulfate, nalidixic acid, lithium chloride, paromomycin sulfate), clindamycin, acetic acid and salicin are commonly used in the enumeration of *Bifidobacterium* spp. and *Lactobacillus* spp. van de Casteele et al. (2006) and Darukaradhya et al. (2006) evaluated the effectiveness of a number of selective media for the enumeration of probiotic bacteria in cheese (Table 5). Darukaradhya et al. (2006) demonstrated that Reinforced Clostridum Agar with bromcresol green and clindamycin (RCABC) and Reinforced Clostridium Agar with anilin blue and dicloxacillin (RCAAD) were selective for *Lb. acidophilus* and *Bifido*-bacterium spp. in Cheddar cheese, respectively.

Table 4. Angiotensin inhibitory peptides (ACE-I) produced by probiotic bacteria in cheese

Probiotic strain	ACE-I inhibitory peptide sequence	Ripening conditions	Cheese type	Source
Lb. helveticus 130B4	Ala-Ile-Pro-Lys-Lys-Asn-Gln-Asp [κ-CN (f 107-115)]	24 weeks at 12 °C	Cheddar	Shuang et al. (2008)
Lb.casei Zhang	ACE-I inhibiton levels: 100% (2.0% Lb. casei Zhang inoculation level) 85.3% (1.0% Lb. casei Zhang inoculation level) 91.4% (0.1% Lb. casei Zhang inoculation level)	24 weeks at 12 °C	Cheddar	Wang et al. (2010)
Lb. acidophilus L10 Lb. helveticus H100	Higher IC$_{50}$ values in 24 week-old cheeses made with Lb. helveticus H100 Higher ACE-I inhibition capacity in 24-week old cheese made with Lb. acidophilus L10	24 weeks at 4, 8 or 12 °C	Cheddar	Ong and Shah (2008a)
Lb. acidophilus LAFTI® L10	Ala-Arg-His-Pro-His-Pro-His [κ-CN (f 96-102)] Arg-Pro-Lys-His-Pro-Ile-Lys-His-Gln [α$_{s1}$-CN (f 1-9)] Arg-Pro-Lys-His-Pro-Ile-Lys [α$_{s1}$-CN (f 1-7)] Arg-Pro-Lys-His-Pro-Ile [α$_{s1}$-CN (f 1-6)] Phe-Val-Ala-Pro-Phe-Pro-Glu-Val-Phe [α$_{s1}$-CN (f 24-32)] Tyr-Gln-Glu-Pro-Val-Leu-Gly-Pro-Val-Arg-Gly-Pro-Phe-Pro-Ile-Val [β-CN (f 193-209)]	24 weeks at 4 °C to 8 °C	Cheddar	Ong and Shah (2008b)
Lb. casei LAFTI®L26	Arg-Pro-Lys-His-Pro-Ile-Lys-His-Gln [α$_{s1}$-CN (f 1-9)] Arg-Pro-Lys-His-Pro-Ile-Lys [α$_{s1}$-CN (f 1-7)] Arg-Pro-Lys-His-Pro-Ile [α$_{s1}$-CN (f 1-6)] Asp-Lys-Ile-His-Pro-Phe [β-CN (f 47-52)] Phe-Val-Ala-Pro-Phe-Pro-Glu-Val-Phe [α$_{s1}$-CN (f24-32)] Lys-Lys-Tyr-Lys-Val-Pro-Gln-Leu-Glu [α$_{s1}$-CN (f102-110)] Tyr-Gln-Glu-Pro-Val-Leu-Gly-Pro-Val-Arg-Gly-Pro-Phe-Pro-Ile-Val [β-CN (f193-209)]		Cheddar	Ong et al. (2007)

Table 5. Selective media used for the enumeration of probiotic bacteria in cheese. Based on: van de Casteele et al. (2006) and Darukaradhya et al (2006)

Culture collection	MRS	MRS pH 5.2	MRS-Salicin	RCABC	RCA	MRS-Ox-Bile	WCM	MRS-clindamycin	NA-Salicin	MRS-NNLP	MRS-LP	LC	AMC	RCAAD*	RCABV*	Rogosa	LBS	M17
B. breve CSCC 1900	+		-	-		+	+			+			+	+	-	+	+	-
B. bifidum CSCC 1903	+		+	-		+	+			+			+	+	-	+	+	-
B. infantis CSCC 1912	+		+	-		+	+			+			+	+	-	+	+	-
B. longum CSCC 5188	+		+	-		+	+			+			+	+	-	+	+	-
Lb.acidophilus CSCC2400	+		+	+	+	-	+			-			-	-	-	+	-	+
Lb.acidophilus CSCC2422	+		+	+	+	+	-			+			-	-	-	+	+	-
Lb.acidophilus LMG 9433	+	+						+	-	+	-	+						+
Lb.acidophilus LMG 11430	+	+						+	-	+	-	+						+

Culture	MRS	RCA	RCABS	RCAAD	RCAABV	WCM	AMC
Lb. rhamnosus CSCC 2625	+	-	-	+	-	+	+
Lb. rhamnosus LMG 18020	+	-	+	+	-	+	+
Lb. casei ssp. casei LMG6904	+	-	+	+	-	±	+
Lb. casei ssp. casei CSCC 2603	+	-	+	+	-	-	+	+
Lb. paracasei ssp. paracasei CSCC 5437	+	-	-	-	-	+	+	+
Commercial probiotic cultures							
La-145	+	+	+	+	±	±	
Lafti L10	+	+	+	±	±	±	±
LBA	+	+	+	±	-	±	+
LBC 80	+	+	+	+	+	±	+
LBC 81	±	±	±	±	±	+	+
LBC 82	±	+	+	±	±	+	+
Lafti L26	+	-	-	+	-	+
B-420	+	±	+	±	+	-	+	±
BL	±	+	+	±	+	+	±
LAFTI B94	+	-	+	+	-	-	+

± Weak growth, + Growth, - No growth,

MRS: de Mann, Rogosa, Sharpe agar, **RCA**: Reinforced Clostridium Agar, **RCABS**: Reinforced Clostridium Agar with bromcresol green and clindamycin, **RCAAD**: Reinforced Clostridium Agar with anilin blue and dicloxacillin, **WCM**: Wilkins Chalgren Mupirocin Agar, **AMC**: Arroyo, Martin and Cotton Agar, **RCAABV**: Reinforced Clostridium Agar with bromcersol green and vancomycin.

CSCC from culture collection of Australian Starter Culture Research Center Ltd., Werribee, Victoria, Australia; LAFTI L26, LAFTI L19, LAFTI B94 from DSM Food Specialities; LBA, LBC8, LBC81, LBC82, BL from Rhodia Food, La-145 B420 from Danisco/Wisby; LMG from culture collection of BCCM™LMG Bacteria colelction, Ghent University, Belgium.

According to Dave and Shah (1996), MRS-Salicin agar was selective for *Lb. acidophilus*. However, Darukaradhya et al. (2006) demonstrated that MRS-Salicin allowed the growth of some *Bifidobacteria* spp. and *Lb. paracasei* in non-starter lactic acid bacteria (NSLAB) in Cheddar cheese. Regarding the enumeration of *Lb. acidophilus* strains in mixed cultures, RCABC medium provided far better selectivity. The *Lb. acidophilus* colonies on RCABC medium were characterized with rough, irregular, convex, granular, dark bottle green in color and medium size (3 mm) (Darukaradhya et al., 2006). Again, the NA-Salicin medium previously described as a selective medium fo *Lb. acidophilus* (Lankaputhra and Shah, 1996) was shown to be ineffective in enumerating commerical strains of *Lb. acidophilus* La-145 (van de Casteele et al., 2006). MRS-clindamycin medium does not allow the growth of *Bifidobacterium* spp. in mixed cultures containing *Lb. acidophilus*. Therefore, this medium can be considered as the preferred medium for the selective enumeration of commerical *Lb. acidophilus* strains La-145 and Lafti L10. LC agar was found to offer good selectivity for *Lb. casei* in mixed cultures. On contrary, regarding the growth of *Lb. acidophilus* on LC agar, contraversial results have been reported. Shah (2000) and Ravula and Shah (1998) showed that *Lb. acidophilus* could not grow on LC medium; however, van de Casteele et al. (2006) reported that the growth of *Lb. acidophilus* was well supported on LC medium. Same authors confirmed that MRS-AC and NA-Salicin were suitable media for selective enumeration of *Lb. rhamnosus* and *Lb paracasei*, respectively.

Darukaradhya et al. (2006) compared 5 different selective medium for the enumeration of bifidobacteria including MRS-Ox-Bile, WCM, MRS-NNLP, AMC and RCAAD. The first three medium allowed the growth of some strains of *Lb. acidophilus* (i.e. strain 2400) in mixed culture systems. *Lb. acidophilus* did not grow on AMC medium; however, this medium stimulated the growth of starter and non-starter lactic acid bacteria in cheese. To conclude, the RCAAD agar was considered as the suitable medium for the recovery of *Bifidobacteria* spp. In contrast, van de Casteele et al. (2006) showed that MRS-NNLP agar was insufficient towards *Lb. acidophilus* and *Lb. rhamnosus* in cheese system.

Whichever the selective media is used, the phenotypic differentiation of probiotic bacteria from other bacteria present in complex microbial systems like cheese is often problematic. In recent years, molecular techniques based on determination of genetic diversity among the bacterial species and strains have been more widely used for the identification of probiotic bacteria in foods. However; these techniques that are far more reliable than conventional plating methods, are yet to be developed for routine quantification of probiotics.

REFERENCES

Abd El-Salam, M.H., El-Shafie, K., Sharaf, O.M., Effat, B.A., Assem, F., and El-Aassar, M. (2010a). Screening of some potentially probiotic lactic acid bacteria for their ability to synthesis conjugated linoleic acid. *International Journal of Dairy Technology*, 63, 62-69.

Abd El-Salam, M.H., Rhippen, A., Assem, F., El-Shafie, K., Tawfik, N.F., and El-Aassar, M. (2010b). Preparation and properties of probiotic cheese high in conjugated linoleic acid content. *International Journal of Dairy Technology*, 63, 1-10.

Abraham, S., Cachon, R., Colas, B., Feron, G., and De Coninck J. (2007). Eh and pH gradients in Camembert cheese during ripening: measurements using microelectrodes and correlations with texture. *International Dairy Journal*, 17, 954-960.

Addeo, F., Chianes, L., Salzano, A., Sacchi, R., Cappucio, U., Ferranti, P., and Malroni, A. (1992). Characterization of the 12% trichloracetic acid-insoluble oligopeptides of Parmigiano-Reggiano cheese. *Journal of Dairy Research*, 59, 401-411.

Ahola, A.J., Knnuttila-Yli, H., Soulamanien, T., Poussa, T., Ahlsrom, A., and Meurman, J.H. (2002). Short-term consumption of probiotic containing cheese and its effect on dental caries risk factors. *Archives of Oral Biology*, 47(11), 799-804.

Ahola, A., Korpela, R., Yli-Knuuttila, H., and Meurman, J.H. (2003). Probiotic cheese may reduce high salivary *Streptococcus mutans* counts. *Journal of Dental Research*, 82, 557-557.

Almeida, K.E., Tamime, A.Y., and Oliveira, M.N. (2008). Acidification rates of probiotic bacteria in Minas frescal cheese whey. *LWT-Food Science and Technology*, 41(2), 311-316.

Ananta, E., and Knorr, D. (2004). Evidence on the role of protein synthesis in the induction of heat tolerance of *Lactobacillus rhamnosus* GG by pressure pre-treatment, *International Journal of Food Microbiology*, 96, 307-313.

Anonymous. (2008). More cheese trends. *Dairy Foods*, 109(3), 76-77.

Anonymous. (2010a). Market reports. 1st September, 2010. Available from: www.marketsandmarkets.com/Market-Reports/probiotic-market-advanced-technologies-and-global-market-69.html

Anonymous. (2010b) Probiotic cheese: a problem child? 1st September, 2010. Available from: www.dbicmsa.org/documents/ probiotic%20cheese%20article.pDF.

Apostolidis, E., Kwon, Y.I., and Sheety, K. (2007). Inhibitory potential of herb, fruit, and fungal-enriched cheese against key enzymes linked to type 2 diabetes and hypertension. *Innovation in Food Science and Technology*, 8, 46-54.

Araujo, E.A., de Carvalho, A.F., Leandro, E.S., Furtado, M.N., and de Moraes, C.A. (2009). Production of cottage-like symbiotic cheese and study of probiotic cells survival when exposed to different stress levels. *Pesquisa Agropecuaria Tropical*, 39(2), 111-118.

Audet, P., Paquin, C., and Lacroix, C. (1989). Sugar utilization and acid production by free and entrapped cells of *Streptococcus salivarius* subsp *thermophilus*, *Lactobacillus delbrueckii* subsp. *bulgaricus*, and *Lactococcus lactis* subsp. *lactis* in a whey permeate medium. *Applied and Environmental Microbiology*, 55(1), 185-189.

Azarnia, S., Lee, B.H., Robert, N., and Champagne, C.P. (2008). Enhancement of proteolysis and flavours in Cheddar cheese using encapsulated recombinant aminopeptidase of *Lactobacillus rhamnosus* S93. Proceedings of 5th IDF Symposium on Cheese Ripening Symposium, IDF, 9-13 March, Bern, Switzerland, p. 66.

Bello, B.D., Giordano, M., Dolici, P., and Zeppa, G. (2008). Production of conjugated linoleic acid (CLA) by lactic acid bacteria isolated from Italian traditional cheeses. Proceedings of 5th IDF Symposium on Cheese Ripening Symposium, IDF, 9-13 March, Bern, Switzerland, p. 84.

Bergamini, C.V., Hynes, E.R., Quiberoni, A., Suarez, V.B., and Zalazar, C.A. (2005). Probiotic bacteria as adjunct starters: influence of the addition methodolgy on their survival in a semi-hard Argentinian cheese. *Food Research International*, 38(5), 597-604.

Bergamini, C.V., Hynes, E.R., and Zalazar, C.A . (2006). Influence of probiotic bacteria on the proteolysis profile of a semi-hard cheese. *International Dairy Journal*, 16(8), 856-866.

Bergamini, C., V., Hynes, E.R., Candioti, M.C., and Zalazar, C.A. (2009a). Multivariate analysis of proteolysis patterns differentiated the impact of six strains of probiotic bacteria on a semi-hard cheese. *Journal of Dairy Science*, 92(6), 2455-2467.

Bergamini, C.V., Hynes, E.R., Palma, S.B., Sabbag, N.G., and Zalazar, C.A. (2009b). Proteolytic activity of three probiotic strains in semi-hard cheese as single and mixed cultures: *Lactobacillus acidophilus, Lactobacillus paracasei* and *Bifidobacterium lactis*. *International Dairy Journal*, 19(8), 467-475.

Bergamini, C.V., Hynes, E., Meinardi, C., Suarez, V., Quiberoni, A., and Zalazar, C. (2010). Pategras cheese as a suitable carrier for six probiotic cultures. *Journal of Dairy Research*, 77(3), 265-272.

Bernardeau, M., Vernoux, J. P., Henri-Dubernet, S., and Guéguen, M. (2008). Safety assessment of dairy microorganisms: The *Lactobacillus* genus. *International Journal of Food Microbiology*, 126, 278–285

Blanchette, L., Roy, D., and Gauthier, S.F. (1995). Production of cultured cottage cheese dressing by bifidobacteria. *Journal of Dairy Science*, 78, 1421-1429.

Blanchette, L., Roy, D., Belanger, G., and Gauthier, S.F. (1996). Production of Cottage cheese using dressing fermented by bifidobacteria. *Journal of Food Science*, 79(1), 8-15.

Bolyston, T.D., Vinderola, C.G., Ghoddusi, H.B. and Reinheimer, J.A. (2004). Incorporation of bifidobacteria into cheeses: challenges and rewards. *International Dairy Journal*, 14, 375-387.

Buriti, F.C.A., Rocha, J.S., Assis, E.G., and Saad, S.M.I. (2005). Probiotic potential of Minas fresh cheese prepared with the addition of *Lactobacillus paracasei*. *LWT-Food Science and Technology*, 38(2), 173-180.

Buriti, F.C.A., Okazaki, T.Y., Alegro, J.H.A., and Saad, S.M.I. (2007). Effect of a probiotic mixed culture on texture profile and sensory performance of Minas fresh cheese in comparison with the traditional products. *Archivos Latinoamericanos De Nutricion*, 57, 179-185.

Burns, P., Patrignani, F., Serrazanetti, D., Vinderola, G.C., Reinheimer, J.A., Lanciotti, R., and Guerzoni, M.E. (2008). Probiotic Crescenza cheese containing *Lactobacillus casei* and *Lactobacillus acidophilus* manufactured with high-pressure homogenized milk. *Journal of Dairy Science*, 91(2), 500-512.

Bzducha-Wrobel, A., and Obiedzinski, M. (2009). Changes in CLA concentration in cheese models with the addition of *Bifidobacterium animalis* subsp *lactis* and *Lactobacillus acidophilus*. *Bromatologia i Chemia Toksykologiczna*, 42(3), 241-246.

Cardarelli, H.R., Saad, S.M.I., Gibson, G.R., and Vulevic, J. (2007). Functional *petit-suisse* cheese: measure of the prebiotic effect. *Anaerobe*, 13(5-6), 200-207.

Cardarelli, H.R., Buriti, F.C.A., Castro, I.A., and Saad, S.M.I. (2008). Inulin and oligofructose improve sensory quality and increase the probiotic viable count in potentially synbiotic *petit-suisse* cheese. *LWT-Food Science and Technology*, 41(6), 1037-1046.

Champagne, C.P., and Gardiner, N.J. (2005). Challenges in the addition of probiotic cultures to foods. *Critical Review in Food Science and Nutrition*, 45(1), 61-84.

Champagne, C. P., and Molgaard, H. (2008). Production of probiotic cultures and their addition in fermented foods. In E.R. Farnworth (Ed.), Handbook of Fermented Functional Foods (pp. 513-532), Boca Raton, USA: CRC Press.

Champagne, C.P. (2009). Some technological challenges in the addition of probiotic bacteria to foods. In D. Charalampopoulos, R. Rastall (Eds.), Prebiotics and Probiotics Science and Technology, (pp.761-804), New York, USA: Springer.

Choisy, C., Desmazeaud, M., Gripon, J.C., Lamberet, G., and Lenoir, J. (1997). La biochimie de l'affinage. In: A, Eck, and J.C., Gillis (Eds.), Le Fromage (pp. 86-161), Paris, France: Lavoisier Pres.

Cichosz, G., Borejszo, Z., Tomera, K., and Kornacki, M. (2006). Aroma compounds in gouda cheese produced with addition of probiotic strains. *Polish Journal of Natural Sciences*, 20(2), 987-997.

Coakley, M., Ross, R.P., Nordgren, M., Fitzgerald, G., Devery, R., and Stanton, C. (2003) Conjugated linoleic acid biosynthesis by human-derived *Bifidobacterium* species. *Journal of Applied Microbiology*, 94, 138-145.

Coeuret, V., Gueguen, M., and Vernoux, J.P. (2004). *In vitro* screening of potential probiotic activities of selected lactobacilli isolated from unpasteurized milk products for incorporation into soft cheese. *Journal of Dairy Research*, 71(4), 451-460.

Cogan, T. M., Beredsford, T. P., Steele, J., Broadbent, J., Shah, N. P., and Ustunol, Z. (2007). Advanced in starter cultures and cultured foods. *Journal of Dairy Science*, 90, 4005-4021.

Collado, M.C., and Sanz, Y. (2006). Method for direct selection of potentially probiotic *Bifidobacterium* strains from human faeces based on their acid-adaptation ability, *Journal of Microbiology Methods*, 66, 560-563.

Corbo, M.R., Albenzio, M., de Angelis, M., Sevi, A., and Gobbetti, M. (2001). Microbiological and biochemical properties of Canestrato Pugliese hard cheese supplemented with bifidobacteria. *Journal of Dairy Science*, 84, 551-561.

Crowley, L. (2008). Danisco meets growing South American demand for probiotics. 25th August, 2008. Available from: http://www.nutraingredients-usa.com/Industry/Danisco-meetsgrowing-South-American-demand-for-probiotics.

Dabiza, N.M.A., and Fathi, F.A. (2006). Characteristics and chemical composition of probiotic Ras cheese. *Deutsche Lebensmittel-Rundschau*, 102(12), 561-566.

Dabiza, N., and El-Deib, K. (2007). Biochemical evaluation and microbial quality of ras cheese supplemented with probiotic strains. *Polish Journal of Food and Nutrition Sciences*, 57(3), 295-300.

da Cruz, A.G., Buriti, F.C.A., Souza, C.H.B., Faria, J.A.F., and Saad, S.M.I. (2009). Probiotic cheese: health benefits, technological and stability aspects. *Trends in Food Science and Technology*, 20(8), 344-354, 2009.

Daigle, A., Roy, D., Belanger, G., and Vuillemard, J.C. (1999). Production of probiotic cheese (Cheddar-like cheese) using enriched cream fermented by *Bifidobacterium infantis*. *Journal of Dairy Science*, 82(6), 1081-1091.

Darukaradhya, J., Phillips, M., and Kailasapathy, K. (2006). Selective enumeration of *Lactobacillus acidophilus*, *Bifidobacterium* spp., starter lactic acid bacteria and non-starter lactic acid bacteria from Cheddar cheese. *International Dairy Journal*, 16, 439-445.

Dave, R.I., and Shah, N. (1996). Evaluation of media for selective enumeration of *Streptococcus thermophilus*, *L. delbrueckii* ssp. *bulgaricus*, *L. acidophilus*, and bifidobacteria. *Journal of Dairy Science*, 77, 1529-1536.

Dave, R.I., and Shah, N. (1997). Effectiveness of ascorbic acid as an oxygen scavenger in improving viability of probiotic bacteria in yogurts made with commercial starter cultures. *International Dairy Journal*, 7, 435-443.

Desmond, C., Ross, R.P., O'Callaghan, E., Fitzgerald, G.F., and Stanton, C. (2002). Improved survival of *Lactobacillus paracasei* NFBC 338 in spray dried powders containing gum acacia. *Journal of Applied Microbiology*, 93, 1003-1011.

di Cagno, R., de Angelis, M., Upadhyay, V. K., McSweeney, P. L. H., Minervini, F., and Gallo, G., (2003). Effect of proteinases of starter bacteria on the growth and proteolytic activity of *Lactobacillus plantarum* DPC2741. *International Dairy Journal*, 13, 145-157.

Dinakar, P., and Mistry, V.V. (1994). Growth and viability of *Bifidobacterium bifidum* in Cheddar cheese. *Journal of Dairy Science*, 77, 2854-2864.

Doleyres, Y., and Lacroix, C. (2005). Technologies with free and immobilised cells for probiotic bifidobacteria production and protection. *International Dairy Journal*, 15(10), 973-988.

El-Kholy, W.I., Effat, B.A., Tawfik, N.F., and Sharaf, O.M. (2006). Improving soft cheese quality using growth stimulator for *Bifidobacterium bifidum*. *Deutsche Lebensmittel-Rundschau*, 102(3), 101-109.

El-Zayat, A. I., and Osman, M. M. (2001). The use of probiotics in Tallaga cheese. *Egyptian Journal of Dairy Science*, 29, 99-106

FAO/WHO (2001). Evaluation of health and nutritional properties of probiotics in food including powder milk with live lactic acid bacteria. Report of a joint FAO/WHO expert consultation, Cordoba, Argentina. Available from: ftp://ftp.fao.org/ es/esn/food/ probioreport_en.pdf

Fletcher, A. (2006). Chr Hansen expands US dairy cultures production. 20th August, 2008. Available from: http://www.dairyreporter.com/Industry- markets/Chr-Hansen-expands-US-dairycultures-production.

Fox, P. F., Guinee, T. P., Cogan, T. M., and McSweeney, P. L. H. (2000). Fundamentals of Cheese Sciences., Maryland, NJ: Aspen Publication.

Fernandez, M.F., Delgado, T., Boris, S., Rodriguez, A., and Barbes, C. (2005). A washed-curd goat's cheese as a vehicle for delivery of a potential probiotic bacterium: *Lactobacillus delbrueckii* subsp *lactis* UO 004. *Journal of Food Protection*, 68(12), 2665-2671.

Fritzen-Freire, C.B., Mueller, C.M.O., Laurindo, J. B., and Prudencio, E.S. (2010). The influence of *Bifidobacterium* Bb-12 and lactic acid incorporation on the properties of Minas Frescal cheese. *Journal of Food Engineering*, 96(4), 621-627.

Gardiner, G., Ross, R.P., Collins, J.K., Fitzgerald, G., and Stanton, C. (1998). Development of a probiotic cheddar cheese containing human-derived *Lactobacillus paracasei* strains. *Applied and Environmental Microbiology*, 64(6), 2192-2199.

Gardiner, G.E., Ross, R.P., Wallace, J.M., Scanlan, F.P., Jagers, P.P.J.M., Fitzgerald, G.F., Collins, J.K., and Stanton, C. (1999). Influence of a probiotic adjunct culture of *Enterococcus faecium* on the quality of cheddar cheese. *Journal of Agricultural and Food Chemistry*, 47(12), 4907-4916.

Ghoddushi, H.B., and Robinson, R.K. (1996). The test of time. *Dary Industries International*, 61(7), 25-28.

Gibson, G.R., and Williams, C.M. (2000). Functional Foods: Concept to Product. Cambridge, UK: Woodhead Publishing.

Gobbetti, M., Corsetti, A., Smacchi, E., de Angelis, M., and Rossi, J. (1997). Microbiology and chemistry of Pecorino Umbro cheese during ripening. *Italian Food Science*, 2, 111-126.

Gobbetti, M., Corsetti, A., Smacchi, E., Zocchetti, A., and de Angelis, M. (1998). Production of Crescenza cheese by incorporation of bifidobacteria. *Journal of Dairy Science*, 81, 37-47.

Goderska, K., Zybals, M., and Czarnecki, Z. (2003). Characterization of microcapsulated *Lactobacillus rhamnosus* LR7 strain. *Polish Journal of Food and Nutrition*, 12, 237-238.

Godward, G. (2000). Studies on enhancing the viability and survival of probiotic bacteria in dairy foods through strain selection and microencapsulation. MSc. thesis, University of Western Sydney, Australia.

Godward, G., and Kailasapathy, K. (2003). Viability and survival of free and encapsulated probiotic bacteria in Cheddar cheese. *Milchwissenschaft*, 58 (11-12), 624-627.

Gomes, A.M.P., Malcata, F.X., Klaver, F.A.M., and Grande, H.J. (1995). Incorporation and survival of *Bifidobacterium* sp. strain Bo and *Lactobacillus acidophilus* strain Ki in a cheese product. *Netherlands Milk and Dairy Journal*, 49(2-3), 71-95.

Gomes, A.M.P., and Malcata, F.X. (1998). Development of probiotic cheese manufactured from goat milk: Response surface analysis via technological manipulation. *Journal of Dairy Science*, 81(6), 1492-1507.

Gomes, A.M.P., Vieira, M.M., and Malcata, F.X. (1998a). Survival of probiotic microbial strains in a cheese matrix during ripening: Simulation of rates of salt diffusion and microorganism survival. *Journal of Food Engineering*, 36(3), 281-301.

Gomes, A.M.P., Silva, M.L.P.C., and Malcata, F.X. (1998b). Caprine cheese with probiotic strains: the effects of ripening temperature and relative humidity on proteolysis and lipolysis. *Zeitschrift für Lebensmittel-Untersuchung und-Forschung*, 207(5), 386-394.

Gomes A.M.P., and Malcata F.X. (1999). *Bifidobacterium* ssp. and *Lactobacillus acidophilus*: biological, biochemical, technological and therapeutical properties relevant for use as probiotics. *Trends in Food Science and Technology*, 10, 139-157.

Gomez-Ruiz, J.A., Ramos, M., and Recio, I. (2002). Angiotensin-I-converting enzyme-inhibitory activity of peptides isolated from Manchego cheeses manufactured with dfifferent starter cultures. *International Dairy Journal*, 14, 1075-1080.

Grattepanche, F., Miescher-Schwenninger, S., Meile, L., and Lacroix, C. (2008). Recent developments in cheese cultures with protective and probiotic functionalities. *Dairy Science and Technology*, 88(4-5), 421-444.

Gürakan, C.G., Cebeci, A., and Özer, B. (2010). Functional dairy beverages: microbiology and technology. In: F. Yıldız (Ed.), Development and Manufacture of Yogurt and Other Functional Dairy Products (pp. 165-196), Boca Raton, USA: CRC Press.

Gürsoy, O., and Kınık, O. (2010). Incorporation of adjunct cultures of *Enterococcus faecium*, *Lactobacillus paracasei* subsp *paracasei* and *Bifidobacterium bifidum* into white cheese. *Journal of Food Agriculture and Environment*, 8(2), 107-112.

Hamilton-Miller, J.M., Shah, S., and Smith, C.T. (1996). Probiotic remedies are not what they seem. *British Medical Journal*, 312, 55-56.

Hamilton-Miller, J.M., and Shah, S. (2002). Deficiencies in microbiological quality and labelling of probiotic supplements. *International Journal of Food Microbiology*, 72, 175-176

Hatakka, K., Ahola, A.J., Yli-Knuuttila, H., Richardson, M., Poussa, T., Meurman, J.H., andKorpela, R. (2007). Probiotics reduce the prevalence of oral *Candida* in the elderly-a randomized controlled trial. *Journal of Dental Research*, 86 (2), 125-130.

Hayes, W.W., Feijoo, S.C., and Martin, J.H. (1996). Effect of lactulose and oligosaccharides on survival of *Bifidobacterium longum* in Edam cheese. *Journal of Dairy Science*, 79(suppl. 1), 118.

Heller, K.J., Bockelmann, W., Schrezenmeir, J., and deVrese, M. (2003). Cheese and its potential as a probiotic food. In: E.R. Farnworth (Ed.), Handbook of Fermented Functional Foods (pp. 203-225). Boca Raton, USA: CRC Press.

Heller, L. (2008). Probiotics grow on innovation, Datamonitor. 30th August, 2009. Available from:http://www.meatprocess.com/Product-Categories/Ingredients-and-additives/ Probioticsgrow-on-innovation-Datamonitor.

Hoier, E., Janzen, T., Henriksen, C.M., Rattray, F., Brockmann, E., and Johansen, E. (1999). The production, application and action of lactic cheese starter cultures. In: B.A. Law (Ed.), Technology of Cheesemaking (pp. 99-131), Boca Raton, USA: CRC Press.

Ibrahim, F., Ruvio, S., Granlund, L., Salminen, S., Viitanen, M., and Ouwehand, A.C. (2010). Probiotics and immunosenescence: cheese as a carrier. *FEMS Immunologicaland Medical Microbiology*, 59, 53-59.

Jankowski, T., Zielinska, M., and Wysakowska, A. (1997). Encapsulation of lactic acid bacteria with alginate/starch capsules. *Biotechnology Techniques*, 11, 493-497.

Jarvenpaa, S., Tahvonen, R.L., Ouwehand, A.C., Sandell, M., Jarvenpaa, E., and Salminen, S. (2007). A probiotic, *Lactobacillus fermentum* ME-3, has antioxidative capacity in soft cheese spreads with different fats. *Journal of Dairy Science*, 90(7), 3171-3177.

Jatila, H., and Matilainen, K. (2008). Probiotic cheese quality. Proceedings of 5th IDF Symposium on Cheese Ripening Symposium, IDF, 9-13 March, Bern, Switzerland, p. 86.

Jensen, M.P., Slot, J., and Ardö, Y. (2008). Caseinolytic activity of *Lactobacillus helveticus* studied in a cheee model. Proceedings of 5th IDF Symposium on Cheese Ripening Symposium, IDF, 9-13 March, Bern, Switzerland, p.34.

Johnson, M. E., and Lucey, J. A. (2006). Major technological advances and trends in cheese. *Journal of Dairy Science*, 89, 1174-1178.

Kailasapathy, K. (2002). Microencapsulation of probiotic bacteria: technology and potential applications. *Current Issues in Intestinal Microbiology*, 3, 39-48.

Kailasapathy, K., and Masondole, L. (2005). Survival of free and microencapsulated *Lactobacillus acidophilus* and *Bifidobacterium lactis* and their effect on texture of feta cheese. *Australian Journal of Dairy Technology*, 60(3), 252-258.

Kalavrouzioti, I., Hatzikamari, M., Litopoulou-Tzanetaki, E., and Tzanetakis, N. (2005). Production of hard cheese from caprine milk by the use of two types of probiotic cultures as adjuncts. *International Journal of Dairy Technology*, 58(1), 30-38.

Kasımoğlu, A., Göncüoğlu, M., and Akgün, S. (2004). Probiotic white cheese with *Lactobacillus acidophilus*. *International Dairy Journal*, 14(12), 1067-1073.

Kearney, L., Upton, M., and McLaughlin, A. (1990). Enhancing the viability of *Lactobacillus plantarum* inoculum by immobilizing the cells in calcium-alginate beads incorporating cryoprotectants. *Applied and Environmental Microbiology*, 56, 3112-3116.

Kebary, K.M.K., Hussein, S.A., and Badawi, R.M. (1998). Improving viability of *Bifidobacteria* and their effect on frozen ice milk. *Egyptian Journal of Dairy Science*, 26, 319-337.

Kılıç, G.B., Kuleaşan, H., Eralp, I., and Karahan, A.G. (2009). Manufacture of Turkish Beyaz cheese added with probiotic strains. *LWT-Food Science and Technology*, 42(5), 1003-1008.

Kourkoutas, Y., Bosnea, L., Taboukos, S., Baras, C., Lambrou, D., and Kanellaki, M. (2006). Probiotic cheese production using *Lactobacillus casei* cells immobilized on fruit pieces. *Journal of Dairy Science*, 89(5), 1439-1451.

Krasaekoopt, W., Bhandari, B., and Deeth, H. (2003). Evaluation of encapsulation techniques of probiotic yogurt. *International Dairy Journal*, 13, 3-13.

Lane, C. N., and Fox, P. F. (1996). Contribution of starter and adjunct lactobacilli to proteolysis in Cheddar cheese during ripening. *International Dairy Journal*, 6, 715–728.

Lankaputhra, W.E.V., and Shah, N.P. (1996). A simple method for selective enumeration of *Lactobacillus acidophilus* in yogurt supplemented with *L. acidophilus* and *Bifidobacterium* spp. *Milchwissenschaft*, 51(8), 446-451.

Lee, K.Y., and Heo, T.R. (2000). Survival of *Bifidobacterium longum* immobilized in calcium alginate beads in simulated gastric juices and bile salt solution. *Applied and Environmental Microbiology*, 66, 869-873.

Li, Y., Shahbazi, A., and Coulibaly, S. (2006). Lactic acid production from cheese whey by *Bifidobacterium longum*. *Transactions of the ASABE*, 49(4), 1263-1267.

Lin, T.Y. (2003). Influence of lactic cultures, linoleic acid and fructo-oligosaccharides on conjugated linoleic acid concentration in non-fat set yogurt. *Australian Journal of Dairy Technology*, 58, 11-14.

Lin, T.Y. (2006). Conjugated linoleic acid production by cells and enzyme extract of *Lactobacillus delbrueckii* ssp. *bulgaricus* with additions of different fatty acid. *Food Chemistry*, 94 437-441.

Madureira, A.R., Giao, M.S., Pintado, M.E., Gomes, A.M.P., Freitas, A.C., and Malcata, F.X. (2005). Incorporation and survival of probiotic bacteria in whey cheese matrices. *Journal of Food Science*, 70(3), M160-M165.

Madureira, A.R., Soares, J.C., Pintado, M.E., Gomes, A.P., Freitas, A.C., and Malcata, F.X. (2008). Sweet whey cheese matrices inoculated with the probiotic strain *Lactobacillus paracasei* LAFTI®L26. *Dairy Science and Technology*, 88(6), 649-665.

Makelainen, H., Fossten, S., Olli, K., Granlund, L., Rautonen, N., and Ouwehand, A.C. (2009).

Probiotic lactobacillli in a semi-soft cheese survive in the simulated human gastrointestinal tract. *International Dairy Journal*, 19(11), 675-683.

Marcatti, B., Habitante, A.M.Q.B., Sobral, P.J.A., and Favaro-Trindade, C.S. (2009). Minas-type fresh cheese developed from buffalo milk with addition of *L. acidophilus*. *Scientia Agricola*, 66(4), 481-485.

Masuda, T., Yamanari, R., and Itoh, T. (2005). The trial for production of fresh cheese incorporated probiotic *Lactobacillus acidophilus* group lactic acid bacteria. *Milchwissenschaft*, 60(2), 167-171.

Matijasic, B.B. (2008). Application of probiotic Lactobacillus gasseri K7 in cheese production. Proceedings of 5th IDF Symposium on Cheese Ripening Symposium, IDF, 9-13 March, Bern, Switzerland, p. 21.

Maus, J.E., and Ingham, S.C. (2003). Employement of stressful conditions during culture production to enhance subsequent cold-and acid tolerance of bifidobacteria. *Journal of Applied Microbiology*, 95(1), 146-154.

Mc Brearty, S., Ross, R.P., Fitzgerald, G.F., Collins, J.K., Wallace, J.M., and Stanton, C. (2001). Influence of two commercially available bifidobacteria cultures on Cheddar cheese quality. *International Dairy Journal*, 11, 599-610.

McSweeney, P.L.H., and Sousa, M.J. (2000). Biochemical pathways for the production of flavour compounds in cheese during ripening: a review. *Lait*, 80, 293–324

McSweeney, P.L.H., and Fox, P.F. (2004). Metabolism of residual lactose and of lactate and citrate. In P.F. Fox, P.L.H. McSweeney, T.M., Cogan, and T.P. Guinee (Eds.), Cheese: Chemistry, Physics and Microbiology, Vol 1: General Aspects, (pp. 361-372), 3rd edition, Lpondon, Elsevier.

Medici, M., Vinderola, C.G., and Perdigon, G. (2004). Gut mucosal immunomodulation by probiotic fresh cheese. *International Dairy Journal*, 14(7), 611-618.

Milesi, M.M., Vinderola, G., Sabbag, N., Meinardi, C.A., and Hynes, E. (2009). Influence on cheese proteolysis and sensory characteristics of non-starter lactobacilli strains with probiotic potential. *Food Research International*, 42(8), 1186-1196.

Miller, C.W., Nguyen, M.H., Rooney, M., and Kailasapathy, K. (2002). The influence of packaging materials on the dissolved oxygen content of probiotic yogurt. *Packaging Technology and Science*, 15, 133-138.

Mintel. (2009). Study on the functional food in the USA. 1st August, 2010. Available from www. mintel.com

Misra, A.K., and Kuila, R.K. (1990). Cultural and biochemical activities of *Bifidobacterium bifidum*. *Milchwissenschaft*, 45, 155-158.

Modler, H.W., McKeller, R.C., and Yaguchi, M. (1990). Bifidobacteria and bifidogenic factors. *Canadian Institute of Food Science and Technology Journal*, 23, 29-41.

Modzelewska-Kapitula, M., Klebukowska, L., and Kornacki, K. (2007). Influence of inulin and potentially probiotic *Lactobacillus plantarum* strain on microbiological quality and sensory properties of soft cheese. *Polish Journal of Food and Nutrition Sciences*, 57(2), 143-146.

Modzelewska-Kapitula, M., Klobukowski, J., Klebukowska, L., and Wisniewska-Pantak, D. (2010). The influence of feding diets containing white cheese, produced with prebiotics and the potentially probiotic *Lactobacillus plantarum* strain, on the gastrointestinal microflora of rats. *Czech Journal of Food Science*, 28(2), 139-145.

Moreno, Y., Collado, M.C., Ferrus, M.A., Cobo, J.M., Hernandez, E., and Hernandez, M. (2006). Viability assessment of lactic acid bacteria in commercial dairy products stored at 4 °C using LIVE /DEAD® BacLight™ staining and conventional plate counts. *International Journal of Food Science and Technology*, 41, 275–280.

Nakamura, Y., Yamamoto, H., Sakai, K., Okuba, A., Yamzaki, S., and Takano, T. (1995). Purification and characterization of angiotensin I-converting enzyme inhibitors from sour milk. *Journal of Dairy Science*, 78, 777-783.

Okonogi, S., Ono, J., Kudo, T., Hiramatsu, A., and Teraguchi, S. (1984). *Streptococcus thermophilus* strain a high oxygen consuming ability used for protecting anaerobic microorganisms. Japanese patent, J59085288-A.

Ong, L., Henriksson, A., and Shah, N.P. (2006). Development of probiotic Cheddar cheese containing *Lactobacillus acidophilus, Lb. casei, Lb. paracasei* and *Bifidobacterium* spp. and the influence of these bacteria on proteolytic patterns and production of organic acid. *International Dairy Journal*, 16(5), 446-456.

Ong, L., Henriksson, A., Shah, N. (2007). Angiotensin converting enzyme-inhibitory activity in Cheddar cheeses made with the addition of probiotic *Lactobacillus casei* sp. *Lait*, 87(2), 149-166.

Ong, L., and Shah, N.P. (2008a). Influence of probiotic *Lactobacillus acidophilus* and. *L. helveticus* on proteolysis, organic acid profiles, and ACE-inhibitoryactivity of Cheddar cheeses ripened at 4, 8 and 12 °C. *Journal of Food Science*, 73(3), M111-M120.

Ong, L., and Shah, N.P. (2008b). Release and identification of angiotensin-converting enzyme-inhibitory peptides as influenced by ripening temperatures and probiotic adjuncts in Cheddar cheeses. *LWT-Food Science and Technology*, 41, 1555-1566.

Ong, L., and Shah, N.P. (2009). Probiotic Cheddar cheese: influence of ripening temperatures on survival of probiotic microorganisms, cheese composition and organic acid profiles. *LWT-Food Science and Technology*, 42(7), 1260-1268.

O'Riordan, K.O., and Fitzgerald, G.F. (1998). Evaluation of bifidobacteria for the production of antimicrobial compounds and assessment of performance in cottage cheese at refrigerated temperature. *Journal of Applied Microbiology*, 85, 103-114.

Ortega, O., Real, E., Garcia, H., Casals, C., and Gonzales, J. (2005).Cream cheese with soya milk and probiotics. *Alimentaria*, 42, 363, 72-75.

Özer, D., Akın, S., and Özer B.H. 2005. Effect of inulin and lactulose on survival of *L.acidopilus* LA-5 and *B.bifidum* BB-02 in acidophilus-bifidus yoghurt. *Food Science and Technology International*, 11(1), 19-24.

Özer, B., Uzun, Y.S., and Kırmacı, H.A. (2008). Effect of microencapsulation on viability of *Lactobacillus acidophilus* LA-5 and *Bifidobacterium bifidum* BB-12 during Kasar cheese ripening. *International Journal of Dairy Technology*, 61(3), 237-244.

Özer, B., and Kırmacı, H.A. (2009). Development of proteolysis in white-brined cheese: role of microencapsulated *Lactobacillus acidophilus* LA-5 and *Bifidobacterium bifidum* BB-12 used as adjunct cultures. *Milchwissenschaft*, 64(3), 295-299.

Özer, B., Kırmacı, H.A., Şenel, E., Atamer, M., and Hayaloğlu, A. (2009). Improving the viability of *Bifidobacterium bifidum* BB-12 and *Lactobacillus acidophilus* LA-5 in white-brined cheese by microencapsulation. *International Dairy Journal*, 19(1), 22-29.

Özer, B., and Kırmacı, H.A. (2010). Functional milks and dairy beverages. *International Journal of Dairy Technology*, 63, 1-15.

Perko, B., Bogovič Matijašić, B., and Rogelj, I. (2002). Production of probiotic cheese with addition of *Lactobacillus gasseri* LF221(Rif^r) and K7(Rif^r). Research reports of the Biotechnical Faculty University of Ljubljana, *Agriculture (Zootechny)*, 80(1), 61-70.

Phillips, M., Kailasapathy, K., and Tran, L. (2006). Viability of commercial probiotic cultures (*L.acidophilus, Bifidobacterium* sp., *L. casei, L. paracasei* and *L. rhamnosus*) in cheddar cheese. *International Journal of Food Microbiology*, 108(2), 276-280.

Picot, A., and Lacroix, C. (2004). Encapsulation of bifidobacteria in whey protein-based microcapsules and survival in simulated gastrointestinal conditions and in yoghurt. *International Dairy Journal*, 14, 505–515.

Pisano, M.B., Casula, M., Corda, A., Fadda, M.E., Deplano, M., and Cosentino, S. (2008). *In vitro* probiotic characteristics of *Lactobacillus* strains isolated from Fiore Sardo cheese. *Italian Journal of Food Science*, 20(4), 505-516

Prevost, H., and Divies, C. (1988). Continuous pre-fermentation of milk by entrapped yoghurt bacteria. I. Development of the process. *Milchwissenschaft*, 43(10), 621-625.

Ravula, R.R., and Shah, N.P. (1998). Selective enumeration of Lactobacillus casei from yoghurts and fermented milk drinks. *Biotechnology Techniques*, 12(11), 819-822.

Ross, R.P., Fitzgerald, G., Collins, K., and Stanton, C. (2002). Cheese delivering biocultures : probiotic cheese. *Australian Journal of Dairy Technology*, 57(2), 71-78.

Ross, R.P., Desmond, C., Fitzgerald, G.F., and Stanton, C. (2005). Overcoming the technological hurdles in the development of probiotic foods. *Journal of Applied Microbiology*, 98, 1410-1417.

Roy, D. (2005). Technological aspects related to the use of bifidobacteria in dairy products. *Lait*, 85(1-2), 39-56.

Roy, D., Mainville, I., and Mondou, F. (1997). Selective enumeration and survival of bifidobacteria in fresh cheese. *International Dairy Journal*, 7(12), 785-793.

Ryhanen, E.L., Pihlanto-Leppala, A., and Pahkala, E. (2001). A new type of ripened, low-fat cheese with bioactive properties. *International Dairy Journal*, 11(4-7), 441-447.

Saarela, M., Rantala, M., Hallamaa, K., Nohynek, L, Virkajarvi, I., and Mattö, J. (2004). Stationary-phase acid and heat treatments for improvement of the viability of probiotic lactobacilli and bifidobacteria. *Journal of Applied Microbiology*, 96(6), 1205-1214.

Saito, T., Nakamura, T., Kitazawa, H., Kawai,Y., and Itoh, T. (2000). Isolation and structural analysis of antihypertensive peptides that exist naturally in Gouda cheese. *Journal of Dairy Science*, 83, 1434-1440.

Samona, A., and Robinson, R.K. (1991). Enumeration of bifidobacteia in dairy products. *Journal of the Society of Dairy Technology*, 44, 64-66.

Samona, A., and Robinson, R.K. (1994). Effects of yogurt cultures on the survival of bifidobacteria in fermented milks. *Journal of the Society of Dairy Technology*, 47, 58-60.

Santillo, A., and Albenzio, M. (2008). Influence of lamb rennet paste containing probiotic on proteolysis and rheological properties of Pecorino cheese. *Journal of Dairy Science*, 91(5), 1733-1742.

Santillo, A., Albenzio, M., Quinto, M., Caroprese, M., Marino, R., and Sevi, A. (2009). Probiotic in lamb rennet paste enhances rennet lipolytic activity, and conjugated linoleic acid and linoleicacid content in Pecorino cheese. *Journal of Dairy Science*, 92(4), 1330-1337.

Sanz, Y. (2007). Ecological and functional implications of the acid-adaptation ability of *Bifidobacterium*: a way of selecting improved probiotic strains. *International Dairy Journal*, 17(11), 1284-1289.

Sarantinopoulos, P., Kalantzopoulos, G., and Tsakalidou, E. (2002). Effect of *Enterococcus faecium* on microbiological, physicochemical and sensory characteristics of Greek Feta cheese. *International Journal of Food Microbiology*, 76, 93-105.

Sarkar, S. (2010). Approaches for enhancing the viability of probiotics: a review. *British Food Journal*, 112(4), 329-349.

Scardovi, V., and Trotavelli, L. D. (1965). The fructose-6-phosphate shunt as a peculiar pattern of hexose degradation in the genus Bifidobacterium. *Analytical Microbiology Enzymology*, 15, 19–27.

Schleifer, K.H., Eharmann, M., Beimhofr, E., Brockmann, E., Ludwig, W., and Amann, R. (1995). Application of molecular methods for the classification and identification of lactic acid bacteria. *International Dairy Journal*, 5, 1081-1094.

Shah, N. (2000). Probiotic bacteria: Selective enumeration and survival in dairy foods. *Journal of Dairy Science*, 83, 894-907.

Sharp, M.D., McMahon, D.J., and Broadbent, J.R. (2008). Comparative evaluation of yogurt and low-fat Cheddar cheese as delivery media for probiotic *Lactobacillus casei*. *Journal of Food Science*, 73(7), M375-M377.

Sheu, T.Y., and Marshall, R.T. (1993). Microencapsulation of lactobacilli in calcium alginate gels. *Journal of Food Science*, 54(3), 557-561.

Shortt, C. (1999). The probiotic century: historical and current perspectives. *Trends in Food Science and Technology*, 10, 411-417.

Shuang, Q., Tsuda, H., and Myamoto, T. (2008). Angiotensin I-converting enzyme inhibitory peptides in skim milk fermented with *Lactobacillus helveticus* 130B4 from camel milk in Inner Mongolia, China. *Journal of Science of Food and Agriculture*, 88, 2688-2692.

Smacchi, E., and Gobbetti, M. (1998). Peptides from several Italian cheeses inhibitory to proteolytic enzymes of lactic acid bacteria, *Psdeudomonas flourescens* ATCC 948 and to the angiotensin I-converting enzyme. *Enzyme Microbiology and Technology*, 22, 687-694.

Song, E. H., Won, B. R., and Yoon, Y.H. (2001). Production of probiotic cream cheese by utilizing *Lactobacillus helveticus* CU 631. *Journal of Animal Science and Technology*, 43(6), 919-930.

Songisepp, E., Kullisaar, T., Hutt, P., Elias, P., Brilene, T., Zilmer, M., and Mikelsaar, M. (2004). A new probiotic cheese with antioxidative and antimicrobial activity. *Journal of Dairy Science*, 87(7), 2017-2023.

Sousa, M.J., Ardö, Y., and McSweeney, P.L.H. (2001). Advances in the study of proteolysis during cheese ripening. *International Dairy Journal*, 11(4-7), 327-345.

Souza, C.H.B., Buriti, F.C.A., Behrens, J.H., and Saad, SM.I. (2008). Sensory evaluation of probiotic Minas fresh cheese with *Lactobacillus acidophilus* added solely or in co-culture with a thermophilic starter culture. *International Journal of Food Science and Technology*, 43(5), 871-877.

Souza, C.H.B., and Saad, S.M.I. (2009). Viability of *Lactobacillus acidophilus* La-5 added solely or in co-culture with a yogurt starter culture and implications on physico-chemical and related properties of Minas fresh cheese during storage. *LWT-Food Science and Technology*, 42(2), 633-640.

Stanton, C., Gardiner, G., Lynch, P.B., Collins, J.K., Fitzgerald, G. and Ross, R.P. (1998). Probiotic cheese. *International Dairy Journal*, 8(5-6), 491-496.

Stanton, C., Desmond, C., Coakley, M., Collin, J.K:, Fitzgerald, G. and Ross, R. (2003). Challanges facing development of probiotic-containing functional foods. In: E.R.Farnworth (Ed.), Handbook of Fermented Functional Foods (pp. 27-58), Boca Raton, USA: CRC Press.

Starling, S. (2009). Kraft: probiotic cheeses a disappointment. 6th March, 2010. Available from:http://www.nutraingradients-usa.com/Industry/Kraft-probiotic-cheese-is-a-disappointment.

Starrenburg, M. J. C., and Hugenholtz, J. (1991). Citrate fermentation by *Lactococcus* and *Leuconostoc* spp. *Applied and Environmental Microbiology*, 57, 3535-3540.

Steenson, L., Klaenhammer, R., and Swaisgood, H.E. (1987). Calcium alginate-immobilized cultures of lactic streptococci are protected from bacteriophages. *Journal of Dairy Science*, 70(6), 1121-1127.

Suarez-Solis, V., Cardoso, F., Nunez de Villavicencio, M., Fernandez, M., and Fragoso, L. (2002). Probiotic fresh cheese. *Alimentaria*, 39(333), 83-86.

Sung, H.H. (1997). Enhancing survival of lactic acid bacteria in ice cream by natural encapsulation. *Dissertation Abstracts International*, 13(9), 5407.

Talwalkar, A.L., and Kailasapathy, K.A. (2004). A review of oxygen toxicity in probiotic yogurts: influence on the survival of probiotic bacteria and protective techniques. *Comprehensive Reviews in Food Science and Safety*, 3(3), 117-124.

Talwalkar A.L., Miller, C.W., Kailasapathy, K., and Nguyen, M.H. (2004). Effect of packaging materials and dissolved oxygen on the survival of probiotic bacteria in yoghurt. *Journal of Food Science and Technology*, 39(6), 605-611.

Temmerman, R., Pot, B., Huys, G. and Swings, J. (2002). Identification and antibiotic susceptibility of bacterial isolates from probiotic products. *International Journal of Food Microbiology*, 81, 1-10.

Thage, B.V., Broe, M.L., Petersen, M.H., Petersen, M.A., Bennedsen, M., and Ardö, Y. (2005). Aroma development in semi-hard reduced-fat cheese inoculated with Lactobacillus paracasei strains with different aminotransferase profiles. *International Dairy Journal*, 15(6-9), 795-805.

Tharmaraj, N., and Shah, N.P. (2009). Antimicrobial effects of probiotic bacteria against selected species of yeasts and moulds in cheese-based dips. *International Journal of Food Science and Technology*, 44(10), 1916-1926.

van de Casteele, S., Ruyssen, T., Vanheuverzwijn, T., and van Assche, P. (2003). Production of Gouda cheese and Camembert with probiotic cultures: The suitability of some commercial probiotic cultures to be implemented in cheese. *Communications in Agricultural and Applied Biological Sciences*, 68(2B), 539-542

van de Casteele, S., Vanheuverzwijn, T., Ruyssen, T., van Assche, P., Swings, J., and Huys, G. (2006). Evaluation of culture nedia for selective enumeration of probiotic strains of lactobacilli and bifidobacteria in combination with yogurt or cheese starters. *International Dairy Journal*, 16, 1470-1476.

van den Tempel, T., Gundersen, J.K., and Nielsen, M.S. (2002). The microdistribution of oxygen in Danablu cheese measured by a microsensor during ripening. *International Journal of Food Microbiology*, 75, 157-161.

Vinderola, C.G., Prosello, W., Ghiberto, D., and Reinheimer, J.A. (2000). Viability of probiotic (*Bifidobacterium*, *Lactobacillus acidophilus* and *Lactobacillus casei*) and nonprobiotic microflora in Argentinian Fresco cheese. *Journal of Dairy Science*, 83(9), 1905-1911.

Vinderola, C.G., Costa, G.A., Regenhardt, S., and Reinheimer, J.A. (2002a). Influence of compounds associated with fermented dairy products on the growth of lactic acid starter and probiotic bacteia. *International Dairy Journal*, 12, 579-589.

Vinderola, C.G., Mocchiutti, P., and Reinheimer, J.A. (2002b). Interactions among lactic acid starter and probiotic bacteria used for fermented dairy products. *Journal of Dairy Science*, 85, 721-729.

Vinderola, G., Prosello, W., Molinari, F., Ghiberto, D., and Reinheimer, J. (2009). Growth of *Lactobacillus paracasei* A13 in Argentinian probiotic cheese and its impact on the characteristics of the product. *International Journal of Food Microbiology*, 135(2), 171-174.

Wang, H.K., Dong, C., Chen, Y.F., Cui, L.M., and Zhang, H.P. (2010). A new probiotic Cheddar cheese with high ACE-inhibitory activity and gamma-aminobutyric acid content produced with koumiss-derived *Lactobacillus casei* Zhang. *Food Technology and Biotechnology*, 48(1), 62-70.

Yilmaztekin, M., Özer, B.H., and Atasoy, F. (2004). Survival of *Lactobacillus acidophilus* LA-5 and *Bifidobacterium bifidum* BB-02 in white-brined cheese. *International Journal of Food Sciences and Nutrition*, 55(1), 53-60.

Yuguchi, H., Hiramatsu, A., Doi, K., and Idachi, O.S. (1989). Studies on the flavour of yoghurt fermented with *Bifidobacteria*: significance of volatile components and organic acids in the sensory acceptance of yoghurt. *Japaneese Journal of Zootechnical Sciences*, 60, 734-741.

Yvon, M., and Rijnen, L. (2001). Cheese flavour formation by amino acid catabolism. *International Dairy Journal*, 11(4-7), 185-201.

Zehntner, U. (2008). Behaviour of the probiotic strain *Lactobacillus gasseri* K7 in ripened semi-hard cheese. *Agrarforschung*, 15(4), 194-197.

Ziarno, M., Dorota, Z., and Bzducha-Wrobel, A. (2010). Study on dynamics of microflora growth in probiotic rennet cheese models. *Polish Journal of Food and Nutrition Sciences*, 60(2), 127-131.

Ziemer C.J., and Gibson G.R. (1998). An overview of probiotics, prebiotics and synbiotics in the functional food concept: perspectives and future strategies. *International Dairy Journal*, 8, 473-479.

In: Cheese: Types, Nutrition and Consumption
Editor: Richard D. Foster, pp. 43-70

ISBN 978-1-61209-828-9
© 2011 Nova Science Publishers, Inc.

Chapter 2

THE RELATIONSHIP BETWEEN GENETIC AND TECHNOLOGICAL ASPECTS AND CHEESE QUALITY

M. Fresno[*] and S. Álvarez

Unidad de Producción Animal Pastos y Forrajes. Instituto Canario de Investigaciones Agrarias. Apdo. nº 60. 38200 La Laguna, S/C de Tenerife, Spain

ABSTRACT

Cheese quality is dependent on its physiochemical composition and sensory properties. These factors are influenced by milk composition, which, in turn, depends on the structure of the feed ingested by the dairy animals. However, technological and genetic aspects can also interact and can often mask the effect of diet in addition to being an important source of quality variation. Studies investigating the role of genetic factors (species and breed) in cheese quality frequently take place looking at differences between cheeses made with a local breed's milk and those elaborated with milk from international breeds. In addition, the autochthonous genotypes are usually linked to labelled products and normally have higher concentration of certain milk components, such as protein and casein. The relationship between genotype and quality is mainly linked to changes in milk quality that modify the physicochemical composition of cheeses that affect the nutritional value of the product. Furthermore, technological parameters also influence changes of cheese quality. The two traditional cheese-making practices, type of rennet and smoking process, can play an important role in cheese quality in two different ways: to recover traditional characteristics of Protected Denomination of Origin cheeses or other labelled products, and to impart different organoleptic properties to new products. These cheese-making practices can be useful commercial tools for cheese producers to identify and differentiate their products in current global market. The type of rennet used has an important influence in milk clotting and cheese quality. Artisan rennet (kids or lambs) pastes and traditional vegetable coagulants, especially different species of the *Cynara* genus, affect fat, protein fraction and sensory profile. Smoking, together with drying and salting, is one of the oldest food preservation techniques. Smoke has an

---

[*] Email: mfresno@icia.es.

antioxidant and bacteriostatic action; it also dries the rind of the cheeses and contributes to their conservation. In modern food technology, smoking is no longer considered as food preservation practice and the primary purpose of this technique is to give the product a characteristic taste, texture and appearance. Where smoked products are concerned, the most important feature of consumer choice is distinctiveness in the sensory properties. The purpose of the present chapter is to analyze how genetic aspects and some technological practices (type of rennet and smoking process) affect cheese quality.

Keywords: cheese quality, breed, rennet, smoking process.

INTRODUCTION

Quality is a complex concept; there is a primary perception that is "safety" (hygienic quality) - it is obvious that no cheeses can be a risk for human health. There is another point of view regarding the "nutritional or dietary quality" of cheeses; its estimated cheese chemical composition and bioavailability. There is another definition of quality that is "sensory attributes" and it is related with satisfaction and gastronomic cheese properties. Nonetheless, where consumer's preferences are concerned, the most important factor is usually the price, although the label, packaging and marketing strategies plays a more important role than some other considerations.

The physicochemical composition, microbiological and sensory properties of cheese depend on many factors (Table 1) which influence the quality of cheeses through the composition and technological behaviour of the milk. However, cheese making aspects and storage processing (refrigeration, raw or pasteurized milk, coagulation enzymes and coagulation parameters, addition of different products, moulding, drainage, salting, ripening, smoking, etc.) can also interact and often mask the effect of milk quality. Frequently on-site experience has led to the conclusion that many aspects are interacting, although it is only under experimental conditions that it is possible to analyze the effect of any particular feature by itself.

There are very well known, all over the world, type of cheeses with some characteristics well defined (Cheddar, Gouda, Edam, etc.) and regional specific products that can be classified in two groups (Roest and Menghi, 2000):

- Products that serve small nice markets. They are highly exclusive and are appreciated by connoisseurs who are willing to pay high prices for them; these cheeses often do not reach beyond their local market.
- Products that covering significant shares of the relevant market. These products, although produced in delimited area, supplies a national market and they are frequently exported.

Table 1.

Factors Affecting Milk Quality
Factors linked to animal:
• Genetic aspects: species, breed and individual considerations
• Lactating stage: milk quantity and quality varies from offspring to the end of lactating period
• Offspring season: date of kidding has an indirect effect on milk quality because weather conditions affects pasture and forage quality
• Number of animals born
• Health status of females
Factors linked to management and environment:
• Animal feeding that has an important effect in milk quantity and quality (fat and protein)
• Milking routines
• Environmental factors as weather that has an evident effect on pasture and forage quality

Protected Designation of Origin (PDO), Protected Geographical Indication (PGI) and Traditional Speciality Guaranteed (TSG) are European geographical regimes to protect the names of regional foods and eliminate the unfair competition and misleading of consumers by non-genuine products.

The objective of this paper is to describe the effect of genetic, type of rennet and smoking process on cheese quality. Further to the comment at the end of the paper published by Verdier-Metz et al. (1998), it is very important not to forget that the results obtained for a specific cheese are only directly applicable to this particular cheese and under the experimental conditions employed. Before adopting for other products the findings must be confirmed through strict research.

The final purpose of the present paper is to show how the breed and some technological practices (type of rennet and smoking process) can be important tools for the definition and differentiation of traditional and labelled cheeses and can even contribute to the production of new types of cheeses. There are many traditional cheese varieties that can have an important niche in this difficult and global market as long as they are well defined and their characteristic attributes shown.

GENETIC ASPECT

All factors affecting milk quality should also influence cheese making and the characteristics of the cheese, although the effect of genetic factors in milk is still not fully elucidated (Coulom et al., 2004). There are many studies concerning cows' milk that show genetic factors involved in milk composition, their technological properties and their repercussion in cheese quality and yield (Macheboeuf et al., 1993; Verdier-Metz et al., 1998; White et al., 2001; Auldist et al., 2002, 2004; Coulon et al., 2004; Todaro et al., 2004; Casandro et al., 2005; Malacarne et al., 2006). However, in scientific literature, references regarding influence of goat breeds in cheese quality are limited (Ronningen, 1965; Skjevdahl, 1979; Pizzillo et al.,1992, 1996, 2005; Fresno et al., 2001; Coulom et al., 2004; Kumar and Kansar, 2005) and those on ovine species even more so (Coulom et al., 2004). Furthermore, many of the references that involved different genotypes included more than one aspect, so it is difficult to show the isolated effect of the breed. Many recent research are focusing on the effect of animal genetics on lactoprotein polymorphisms and their repercussion on milk suitability for cheese making and cheese quality (chemical and sensorial). Nevertheless, the conjugated linoleic acid (CLA) content in milk depends on the type of feed provided to the animals, recent studies involved other factors such as breed (Kelsey et al., 2003; Kewalramani et al., 2003; Kumar and Kansar, 2005; Tsiplakon et al., 2006).

In many studies the comparisons are made between a local breed, usually linked to a labelled product, and conventional dairy cattle (Friesian or Holstein), whereas other research evaluates these international breeds compared with dual purpose breeds (Figure 1) Local or dual purpose breeds, normally have a higher concentration of most milk components, especially protein and casein (Macheboeuf et al., 1993; Auldist et al., 2002, 2004; Coulon et al., 2004; Todaro et al., 2004; Casandro et al., 2005; Knowles et al, 2006; Malacarne et al., 2006); although other surveys have not shown significant differences between breeds (Verdier-Metz et al., 1998). The different chemical components of milk determined a greater suitability for coagulation properties and cheese yield. Most of this effect can be related to differences in casein content among breeds and to casein genetic polymorphism; particularly the frequency of de κ-B variant (Coulom et al., 2004). Milk coagulating properties are also strongly correlated to milk acidity parameters (Macheboeuf et al., 1993; Ikoneen et al., 2004), so it is necessary to take into account the genotype influence. Verdier-Metz et al. (1998) showed that higher milk pH from Tarentaise cows induced longer clotting time and Malacarne et al. (2006) found better rennet coagulation properties related to higher values of titratable acidity milk from Italian Brown cows. The differences in coagulation are not all explained by κ casein variants and acidity values, these are probably due to other milk characteristics, such as the micellar structure or the proportion of α_s-caseins or β-caseins (Verdier-Metz et al., 1998), that are affected by breed and also within breed (Coulom et al., 2004).

The physicochemical characteristics are influenced by breed, but higher percentages of fat or protein in milk do not always lead to cheeses with a superior level of these chemical compounds. Under the same conditions, Modicana cows produced milk richer in fat and protein than Friesian cows, but cheese obtained with the milk from this local breed had more fat but less protein than others made with Friesian milk (Todaro et al., 2004).

Many of the variations in cheese characteristics are due to the differences in milk composition and when milk is not standardized, the effect of breed in cheese chemical composition is more evident. Additionally, cheese yield differences disappeared when milk was standardised to a constant solid ratio (Auldist et al., 2004). However, not all differences are explained by cheese composition; breed had shown a significant effect in some textural, colour and sensorial properties in cheeses with non statistical differences in gross chemical values, especially taste intensity that was more intense in local breeds than in Holstein cows (Verdier-Metz et al., 1998; Coulom et al., 2004).

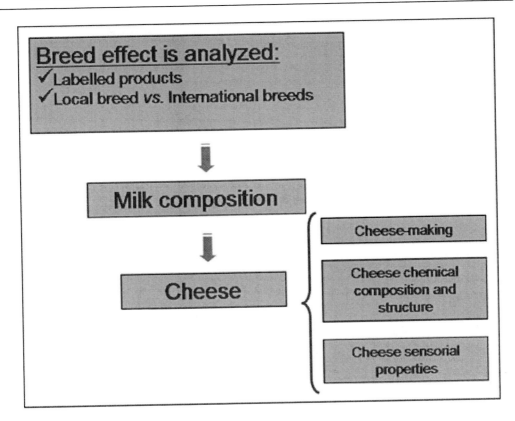

Figure 1.

Fat yield and composition used to be more affected by feeding practices and the influence of technological factors are very low (Chilliard et al., 2006), but there are also differences in the fatty acid profile between breeds (White et al., 2001; Auldist et al., 2004; Coulom et al., 2004; Chilliard et al., 2006). In other trials, volatile cheese compounds were not affected by genotype (Verdier-Metz et al., 1998).

Indigenous Italian sheeps' milk showed significant differences in fatty acid profile between breeds, Altamurana showed a higher content of C4:0, C12:0 and C14:0 than Sarda and higher content of C4:0, C14:0, and C16:0 than Gentile di Puglia (Signorelli et al., 2008). Other authors in experimental conditions (Barbosa et al., 2003; Mihaylova et al., 2004; Tsiplakou et al., 2006; Signorelli et al., 2010) did not find a breed effect on sheep milk fat CLA content. Tsiplakou et al. (2006) and Signorelli et al. (2010) have reported a large variation in milk fat content of CLA among individuals.

Coagulation parameters did not differ significantly between Manchega and Guirra sheep breed (Jaramillo et al., 2008). Lightness (L) and hardness of cheese has been affected by sheep breed, Castellana, Churra and Assaf, while consumers' panel had no different sensory preference between cheeses made with milk from both breeds (Lurueña-Martinez et al., 2010).

Many years ago, Ronningen (1965) showed that the characteristic "goat" flavour was linked to animal breed and that cheeses made with Norwegian goat milk showed a stronger taste than others made with Saanen goat milk (Skjevdal, 1979).

Gross milk composition of the Nubian goat breed in Egypt was significantly higher (in fat, total protein, casein and total solids) than that of the Alpine goat. This variation affected cheese yield, but did not change cheese composition and sensorial scores, only oleic acid and total unsaturated fatty acids were affected with higher scores for Alpine milk (Soryal et al., 2005). In India, Alpine Beetal's milk had higher CLA than Saanen Beetal's milk (Kumar and Kansar, 2005).

A complete study (Pizzillo et al., 2005) was undertaken with four Italian goat genotypes (Girgentana, Siriana, Maltese and Local). Breed was shown to affect milk composition in pH, fat and protein/fat ratio, and while whey composition was dependent on dry matter and protein/fat ratio. When whey was transformed into ricotta cheese more differences were found: fat, dry matter, lactose and protein/fat ratio. Local breed ricotta cheeses had higher percentage of saturated acids and less monounsaturated acids, while polyunsaturated concentration was higher in Girgentana> Local> Siriana=Maltese. Breed had a limited influence in textural and colour properties. Sensorial characteristics of cheeses were affected by breed; cheeses made with Siriana goats' milk had higher score for "goat taste" and greater granulosity. Also under experimental conditions, Dahlem Cashemere milk had higher values for dry matter, total protein and casein and superior cheese making properties compared with German White goats breed (Thomann et al., 2008).

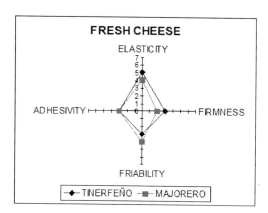
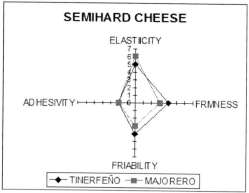
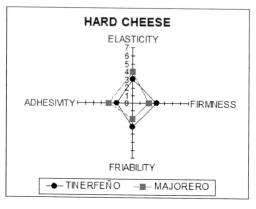

From: Fresno et al. (2001).

Figure 2. Breed effect on sensorial characteristics of goat cheeses.

Table 2. Effects of ripening and breed on physicochemical and sensorial characteristics

	breed(b)		ripening time(r)				Level of significance		
	Majorera	Palmera	2d	30d	60d	RSD	b	r	b x r
			LSM						
pH	5.77	6.15	6.51^c	5.25^a	6.12^b	0.12	0.001	0.001	0.001
Moisture (%)	42.54	44.95	47.50^c	44.67^b	39.07^a	0.68	0.001	0.001	0.001
Protein (%)	22.01	20.67	19.58^a	22.27^b	22.18^b	0.32	0.005	0.001	0.066
Fat (%)	26.77	23.64	20.21^a	24.82^b	30.58^c	0.81	0.001	0.001	0.001
Fat (% TS)	46.27	42.72	38.56^a	44.76^b	50.16^c	0.91	0.001	0.001	0.001
Roughness	1.67	1.68	1.26^a	1.88^b	1.88^b	0.60	0.854	0.001	0.001
Moisture	3.33	2.69	4.75^c	2.51^b	1.77^a	0.21	0.001	0.001	0.001
Elasticity	3.65	2.70	5.50^b	2.02^a	2.00^a	0.28	0.001	0.001	0.001
Firmness	2.52	3.70	3.01^b	2.13^a	4.20^c	0.19	0.001	0.001	0.001
Friability	2.67	3.31	2.45^b	2.00^a	4.53^c	0.21	0.001	0.001	0.001
Adhesivity	2.32	2.87	1.96^a	2.55^b	3.28^c	0.11	0.001	0.001	0.713
Solubility	4.17	3.47	3.21^a	5.59^b	3.78^a	0.26	0.457	0.001	0.001
Granulosity	1.39	2.22	1.88^b	1.28^a	2.25^b	0.11	0.001	0.001	0.064
Sweetness	0.00	0.17	0.25^b	0.00^a	0.00^a	0.04	0.004	0.001	0.001
Bitterness	0.00	1.46	0.00^a	0.52^b	1.66^c	0.20	0.001	0.001	0.001
Acidity	2.33	2.70	2.13^a	3.08^b	2.33^a	0.09	0.002	0.001	0.124
Pungent	0.17	1.46	0.00^a	0.52^b	1.92^c	0.21	0.001	0.001	0.001
Astringent	0.33	0.68	0.25^a	0.52^{ab}	0.74^b	0.08	0.001	0.001	0.001
Residual taste	3.89	3.71	1.86^a	4.61^b	4.94^b	0.25	0.206	0.001	0.001
Taste persistence	4.11	3.74	2.42^a	4.46^b	4.90^b	0.22	0.040	0.001	0.001
Odour intensity	3.14	3.79	2.21^a	3.67^b	4.51^c	0.17	0.001	0.001	0.001
Flavour intensity	3.08	4.00	2.13^a	3.71^b	4.79^c	0.20	0.001	0.001	0.001

From: Álvarez et al. 2007.
LSM: Least square mean.
RSD: Residual standard deviation.
a-c Within a row, means marked with different superscripts differ significantly (p<0.05).

Table 3. Effects of ripening and breed on fatty acid composition

	breed(b)		ripening time(r)				Level of significance		
	Majorera	Palmera	2d	30d	60d	RSD	b	r	b x r
			LSM						
C4	0.64	0.74	0.69[ab]	0.59[a]	0.80[b]	0.04	0.118	0.036	0.036
C6	2.34	2.58	2.43[ab]	2.25[a]	2.69[b]	0.06	0.014	0.003	0.124
C8	3.19	3.60	3.42[b]	3.16[a]	3.60[b]	0.06	0.001	0.001	0.080
C10	12.94	13.58	13.31[b]	12.51[a]	13.95[b]	0.18	0.017	0.001	0.034
C10:1	0.45	0.46	0.44	0.45	0.47	0.01	0.632	0.290	0.027
C12	6.55	6.10	6.15	6.22	6.61	0.09	0.002	0.050	0.029
C14	11.56	11.57	11.52	11.47	11.70	0.07	0.963	0.324	0.066
C15	1.10	0.79	0.90[a]	1.03[b]	0.91[a]	0.03	0.001	0.003	0.947
C16	32.72	32.85	32.83	32.45	33.08	0.16	0.633	0.197	0.004
C16:1	1.17	1.20	1.19	1.14	1.23	0.04	0.691	0.569	0.237
C18	5.19	6.02	5.60	6.09	5.13	0.19	0.013	0.056	0.025
C18:1	18.03	17.54	17.88[b]	18.82[b]	16.65[a]	0.25	0.140	0.001	0.003
C18:2	3.11	2.27	2.72[ab]	2.84[b]	2.51[a]	0.10	0.001	0.045	0.007
C18:3	0.36	0.30	0.35[b]	0.35[b]	0.28[a]	0.01	0.009	0.006	0.110
CLA	0.57	0.35	0.51[b]	0.53[b]	0.35[a]	0.03	0.001	0.001	0.018
C20	0.02	0.02	0.02	0.03	0.01	0.01	0.797	0.512	0.661
C20:4	0.08	0.05	0.06	0.08	0.05	0.01	0.174	0.649	0.173

From: Álvarez et al. 2007.
LSM: Least square mean.
RSD: Residual standard deviation.
[a-c] Within a row, means marked with different superscripts differ significantly ($p<0.05$).

Other authors (Fresno et al., 2001) found significant differences between Majorera and Tinerfeña goats milk; chemical composition only affected soft cheese, although sensory properties showed many differences between soft, semi-hard and hard cheeses (Figure 2). Majorero and Palmero cheese are labelled products with Protected Denomination of Origin, elaborated in Spain, linked to local breeds: Majorera and Palmera goat's breeds respectively. Cheeses made with Majorera milk presented better values for fat and protein; genotype had medium effect on fatty acid profile while sensorial features had many differences, as it is shown in Tables 2 and 3 (Álvarez et al., 2008). In these labelled cheeses, breed has a significant effect on milk and cheese mineral composition and both breeds have interesting minerals concentration for human nutrition (Díaz et al., 2008): Palmero cheeses were richer in Ca, P and Mg with lower concentrations of Na and Cu; no differences where observed in K, Fe, Zn and Se concentrations.

All this research demonstrating the significance of a breed in cheese yield and quality are of special importance concerning branded products, including market strategies. Their success can be seen with the initiative of a producer group of Parmigiano-Reggiano cheese who created a new niche market for cheese produced only with milk from Reggiana cows which commands a price that is about 50% higher than the normal product (Roest and Menghi, 2000). Many local breeds would not be in danger of extinction if a Protected Designation of Origin (PDO) or a Protected Geographical Indication (PGI) included, as part of their specification requirements, that only a particular autochthonous genotype should be involved. Examples are shown in some goat breeds as the cases of the Canary goat's breeds Majorera and Palmera with *Queso Majorero PDO* and *Queso Palmero PDO*, and the Portuguese goat breed Serrana Transmontana with *Queijo de cabra transmontana PDO*. Other sheep's breeds are linked to labelled cheeses: *Queso Manchego*, Machega sheep breed, *Queso Roquefort*, Lacaune breed; *Queso Idiazabal*, Latxa and Carranzana breed; *Queso Zamorano*, Castellana and Churra breeds; *Queso La Serena*, Merina Breed, *Queso Roncal*, Latxa and Rasa breeds, etc.

Different studies have demonstrated that is not possible to isolate all the factors that contribute to a specific characteristic of a cheese: animal species and breed, animal feeding and other management practices, raw or pasteurized milk as well as the type of cheese making process including ripening conditions (Le Jaouen et al., 2001), because the quality of the final product is the result of all these interactions.

As a final thought, all these regional specific cheeses linked to a breed and a geographical area can be considered as products of rural development; it is always necessary to remember that behind them there is a great effort and know-how of farmers and cheesemakers. In the other extreme, the consumers demand high specificity, exclusivity and a better definition of the product.

RENNET EFFECT

Milk coagulation enzymes play and important role in cheese quality. Nowadays different types of products are available with different origin and variability in proteases:

- Animal rennet. These coagulants can be artisan animal rennet from the fourth stomach of wearing ruminants (abomasa of calf, lamb, kid) or commercial (industrial) animal rennet that can be extracted from ruminants stomach or from chicken and pigs.
- Vegetable rennet that can be artisan or commercial.
- Microbial with proteases from *M. miehei* or *M. pusillus*.
- Recombinant from genetically modified microorganism with cDNA for calf chymosin.

In the past, cheese-makers have used rennet paste preparations for curdling milk that were produced by macerating the stomachs from suckling ruminants according to the local uses. Nowadays most of the cheeses are made with commercial rennet and these artisan pastes are used only in some ovine and caprine raw milk cheeses (Bustamante et al., 2000; Irigoyen et al., 2000; Fresno et al., 2006; Addis et al., 2008), mainly in Italy (Provolone, Pecorino Romano and Pecorino Sardo), Spain (Idiazábal, Roncal, Palmero, Gomero) and Greece (Kefalotyri, Feta). Other traditional clotting agent is vegetable rennet (Sanjuan et al., 2002) used in Spain (Torta del Casar, Serena, Pedroches and Queso de Flor de Guía) and Portugal (Serra d'Estrela and Serpa).

A highly complex system of enzymes is present in artisan rennet depending on the age and diet at slaughtering, paste preparation and slaughtering conditions (Addis et al., 2008), even there is an important effect of species (calf, lamb, kid). In the young suckling abomasa, full of milk, the proteolytic enzyme present is chymosin and from the oral tissues there is also present a pregastric enzyme with lipolitic activity. In older animals fed with hay, pasture or concentrate the predominant proteolytic enzyme is the pepsin and from abomasal mucosa there are gastric lipases with lipolitic activity. Many authors agree that rennet pastes prepared from suckling animals slaughtered sudden after suckling has a significant higher lipase activity, from pregastric enzymes, than that prepared from animals with empty stomachs (Bustamante et al., 2000; Addis et al., 2005a; Addis et al., 2008).

Table 4. Evolution of artisan rennet use in traditional Canarian cheeses

Palmero cheese PDO	1992 96% artisan 1% commercial 3% both	2001 93.6% artisan 6.4% commercial	2007 16% artisan 58% commercial 26% both	2010 14% artisan 60% commercial 26 % both
Gomero cheese	1992 100% artisan	2003 76% artisan	2005 60% artisan	2010 20% artisan
Majorero cheese PDO	1992 56% artisan 27% commercial 16% both		2007 100% commercial	2010 100% commercial

The most important reasons for changing from natural rennet coagulants (animal or vegetable) to commercial products (such as commercial animal rennet, vegetable aqueous rennet, microbial origin rennet and recombinant chymosin) are related to microbial safety and the needs of standardized cheeses. An enquiry of Canary Islands (Spain) cheeses (Table 4) is a good example of how the use of this artisan rennet has changed in recent years. Safety or hygienic quality of natural rennet pastes from kids or lambs abomasa is one of the reasons to forbid the use of these coagulants, although no pathogen like *Salmonella spp*, *S. Aureus* or *Listeria monocytogenes* was found in artisan rennet samples (Etayo et al., 2006, Moschoupoulou et al., 2008; Fresno et al., 2010).

Cheese makers have an important tool with all these types of coagulants and all of them can be useful depending on the type of cheese:

a) Industrial cheeses without any PDO or PGI: milk normalization and pasteurization allows the standardization of cheese making process and the final chemical and sensorial characteristics. Milk coagulation should be made with standard rennet (animal, vegetable, microbiological or recombinant from genetically modified microorganism) and culture starters. Over the past few decades recombinant chymosin has been widely used and some of the research completed did not find differences in rheological or sensorial characteristics of the cheeses (Núñez et al., 1992).

b) Industrial or semi-industrial cheeses included in a quality label (PDO or PGI): in these cases cheese must comply with the specification requirements. For these products it should be necessary to obtain rennet pastes and strain starter cultures from the traditional cheeses in order to reproduce the characteristics of the protected cheeses. Much research has been conducted on these topics with reference to Majorero PDO goat cheese (Requena et al., 1992; Calvo and Fontecha, 2004; Calvo et al., 2007; Castillo et al., 2007). Other research had been carried out by Hernández et al. (2001 and 2009) concerning the use of commercial lipases to obtain the characteristic "natural rennet paste" flavour of Idiazábal PDO sheep cheese. It is necessary to take into account that, before being used by cheesemakers, research results must be validated by the official tester panel of the Regulatory Council of the Protected Origin Denomination or Geographical Indication.

c) Traditional raw handmade cheeses, with PDO or PGI: in these cases traditional rennet (animal or vegetable) should be employed and no starter culture should be added. Rennet pastes must be prepared by traditional methods; it is recommended that a test is performed for total milk coagulation activity and microbiological analysis. During parturition period(s) abomasas can be collected, prepared and conserved, so they will be used throughout the year. For each PDO cheese some research support will be necessary to determine the lipolytic and proteolytic activity throughout storage and the conditions of conservation (Bustamante et al., 2000; Virto et al., 2003; Moschoupoulou et al., 2008). Other aspects to control include the age at slaughtering, the diet of suckling animals, the paste preparation and the slaughtering conditions (Pireda and Addis, 2003; Addis et al., 2005 a,b; Sandillo et al., 2005; Addis et al., 2008).

There has been some research conducted comparing rennet pastes with commercial ones:

Effects in Fat Fraction

Traditional rennet pastes, compared with commercial animal rennet, increased the concentration of total free fatty acids, but also showed a significantly higher percentage of short-chain free fatty acids in Idiazabal cheese with natural lamb rennet pastes (Larráyoz et al., 1999; Bustamante et al., 2000; Virto et al., 2003); in Majorero cheese made with artisan kids rennet (Fontecha et al., 2006); in Feta cheese made with artisan kids and lambs rennet (Moatsou et al., 2004; Georgala et al., 2005); in Fiore Sardo cheese and Pecorino Romano Cheese made with artisan lamb rennet paste (Addis et al., 2005a; Pirisi et al., 2007).

Effects in Protein Fraction

In Canestato Pugliese and Idiazabal cheeses (Santoro and Faccia, 1998; Bustamante et al., 2003) showed that lamb rennet was as proteolitic as bovine rennet. Other results showed higher levels of proteolysis in Idiazabal cheese (Vicente et al., 2000), Roncal cheese (Irigoyen et al., 2002) and Murcia al Vino cheese (Ferrandini, 2006); Candreli et al. (1997) found that traditionally prepared kid rennet pastes gave significantly lower levels of soluble nitrogen. Addis et al (2005a) compared two traditional lamb rennet pastes with commercial rennet paste and they did not find differences in proteolysis indices due the rennet type. The casein fraction was affected by the type of rennet in Roncal cheese (Irigoyen et al., 2000) and Idiazábal cheese (Bustamante et al., 2003) and were not affected in other experiments involving other Idiazábal cheeses (Vicente et al., 2000). Lamb rennet showed a greater proteolytic activity against α_s casein, especially α_{s1} casein, than calf rennet (Irigoyen et al., 2002). The rennet type did not affect the degradation of β- casein (Trujillo et al., 2000). Vicente et al. (2001) found significant differences in total and individual concentrations of free amino acids, while Bustamante et al. (2003) only found evidence of variations in a few free amino acids. These differences in the results can be due to differences in the raw ovine milk composition and the cheese manufacturing plant. Variations may also be due to the rennet characteristics (the use of rennet with different portions of chymosin and pepsin affect significantly the protein degradation) and total milk clotting activity added to vats, the analysis method, factors involved (ripening time, season etc.), the size sample and also statistical analysis.

Effects in Sensory Evaluation

The increase of lipolysis origin cheeses with higher intensity scores for strong sensorial attributes with the characteristics of pungent and "natural rennet" flavour or "pecorino" or goat taste (Woo and Lindsay, 1984; Candreli et al., 1997; Bustamante et al., 2000; Virto et al., 2003; Georgala et al., 2005). In Idiazábal cheese, odour and flavour descriptors were affected (except acid flavour descriptor), but not sensory texture parameters (Virto et al., 2003). In goat cheeses, colour and instrumental texture was affected by type of rennet; cheeses made with natural kid's rennet paste were harder, more elastic, breakable and darker than those made with commercial rennet (Fresno et al., 2006). The use of natural lamb rennet paste on goat's Murcia al Vino cheese determined significant changes in texture: great firmness associated with lower moisture content (Ferrandini, 2006). Four different rennet, usually used by cheese makers, were tested (kid's rennet, commercial animal rennet, microbial rennet and recombinant chymosin) by Fresno et al. (2009): type of rennet had significant effect in texture and flavour profile. Fungus rennet cheeses were more sour, pungent and bitter, while recombinant chymosin cheeses were more pungent. Cheeses made with natural's kids were the highest valuated by expert and consumer panels, followed by those made with commercial natural rennet. Another study conducted by the same research team (Fresno et al, 2010) analyzing 70 kid's abomasa that were manipulated from no selected animals (from 10 to 60 days live) concluded that all rennet samples were under EU limits (R CE 1441/2007) for cheese microbiological parameters. In this research two types of rennet pastes were prepared: stomach with milk suckled by the kids (TR, traditional artisan rennet) and empty stomach refilled with raw milk (AR, adapted artisan rennet). Cheeses where elaborated with raw milk and the type of rennet was the only variation factor (TR, AR and CR, commercial recombinant chymosin). Seven expert judges determined the cheeses sensory profile, while preference tests were performed with experts, semiexperts and consumers. Cheeses texture was not affected by rennet type. Results are showed in Table 5, cheeses made with traditional rennet pastes presented higher odour and flavour intensities. Both expert and consumers preferred cheeses manufactured with these artisan rennet pastes.

Table 5. Rennet effect on odour, flavour and taste sensory profile of goat cheeses

Odour, Flavour and Taste Sensory profile	Intensity
Global odour intensity and persistency	PSM > PRM = CR ***
Global flavour intensity, pungent in odour and flavour and rancid odour	PSM > PRM > CR ***
Sweet	PRM > CR ***
Pungent in taste	PSM > PRM > CR ***
Bitter	CR > PSM ***
Milky odour	PRM > PSM > CR ***
Rennet odour and flavour, lactic odour and rancid flavour	PSM > PRM ***
Traditional odour, flavour and taste	PSM > PRM > CR ***
Butter in odour and flavour	CR ***
Fermented fruits in odour and flavour	CR ***

From Fresno et al. 2010.
Kids Rennet paste with suckling milk (PSM); Kids Rennet paste cleaned and refilled with raw milk (PRM); Commercial Chymax® rennet as control (CR).
*** Significant differences p< 0.001.

In some other traditional cheeses milk is clotted with vegetable rennet, dry flowers, (in the past wild flowers and now wild or cultivated) of thistles (*Cynara spp*, mainly *Cynara Cardunculus*, *Cynara humilis* and *Cynara scolymus*) but also other vegetable species such as papaya (*Carica papaya*), pineaple (*Ananas comosum*), fig-tree (*Ficus carica*), *Solanum dobium*, *Opuntia ficus indica*, *Diffenbachia maculate*, and spices from *Eurphorbia*, like *E. serrata*. These products contribute to the specific characteristics of some local cheeses. There are some studies that demonstrate the effects of this coagulant in chemical composition of cheeses but sensory studies are limited. No effect in basic chemical composition had been found in different cheeses as it was reported in the following studies: Portuguese sheep milk cheeses (Sousa and Malcata, 1997); Flor de Guía, a Spanish cheese from mixed milk from the Canary Islands (Álvarez et al., 2001); sheep milk cheese made in Australia (Shao Jian et al., 2003); Los Pedroches, a Spanish cheese made with ewes' milk (Tejada and Fernández Salguero, 2003); goat cheese (Pino et al., 2009) or cow cheese (Agboola et al., 2009). However, some differences were reported by Sanjuán et al (2002) in another study about Los Pedroches cheese and Nuñez et al (1991) about La Serena cheese.

Most authors (Galan et al., 2008; Tejada et al., 2008; Pino et al., 2009) suggest that there is greater proteolysis, with qualitative differences in protein fractions, in vegetable rennet (cyprosin) than in animal rennet (chymosin). Fatty acids profile was not modified significantly by the type of coagulant. Cheeses made with cardoon used to be creamier, softer and with differences in bitterness (Álvarez et al., 2001; Agboola et al., 2009). Sensory texture was affected by rennet type, Figure 3 shows that cheeses made with vegetable rennet (*Cynara cardunculus*) were more adhesive but less firm and friable than other made with animal rennet and a mixture of animal and vegetable rennet (Álvarez et al., 2001).

Other research have been carried out concerning the comparison of different species of *Cynara spp* in cheese characteristics (Viroque et al., 2000) and about the characterization of different cardoon, wild or cultivated (Viroque and Gómez, 2005) and their uses in cheese making.

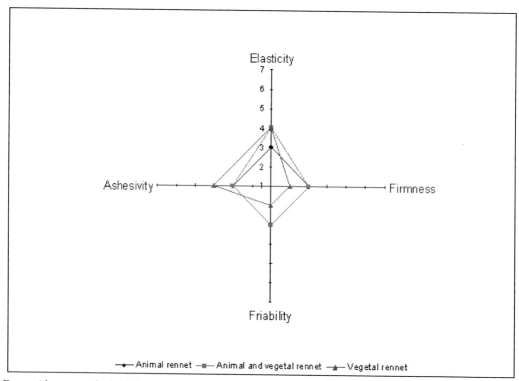

From: Alvarez et al., (2001).

Figure 3. Rennet effect on sensorial texture characteristics of cheeses.

As a final consideration, the choice of rennet should depend on the desired characteristics of the cheese. Traditional coagulants contribute to a genuine texture, taste and flavour. New rennet in branded products must be well validated by the official panels of the protected cheeses before they are introduced in cheese making.

Table 6. Relation of some international smoked cheeses

America	Venezuelan Cheeses	Venezuela	Different Vegetable Matter
	"Rofumo"	EEUU	Walnut
	"Maple Smoked Cheddar"	Canada	Maple
Europe	"Blarney Castle cheese"	Ireland	Oak
	"Bruder Basil"	Germany	Beech
	"Smoked Rambol"	France	Walnut
	"Provolone Affumicato"	Italy	Apple tree
	"Sherwood Smoked Cheddar"	England	
	"Damski", "Smoked Kurpianca"	Poland	
	"Smoked Gouda"	Holland	Walnut
	San Simón DOP	Spain	Birch-tree
	Quesucos de Liébana DOP	Spain	Juniper
	Idiazábal DOP	Spain	Hawthorn and beech tree
	Urbía	Spain	Beech tree
	Palmero DOP	Spain	Shell of almond or Dry nopal or Pine (needles and wood)
	Herreño	Spain	Fig wood and Dry nopal
	Gomero	Spain	Rock rose and Heather
	Queso de Teno and Queso de Anaga	Spain	Different aromatic plants
Australia	"Smoked Rommey"	Australia	Elm

SMOKE EFFECT

Smoking, together with drying and salting, is one of the oldest food preservation techniques (Barylko-Pikelna, 1977). Smoke has an antioxidant and bacteriostatic action; it also dries the rind of the cheeses and contributes to their conservation (Ahmad, 1993). In modern food technology smoking is no longer considered as food preservation practice and the primary purpose of this technique is to give the product a characteristic taste, texture and appearance. Where smoked products are concerned, the most important feature of consumer choice is the distinctiveness in the sensory properties (Mohler, 1980). Table 6 shows a relation of some international smoked cheeses.

In the past (Fresno et al., 2004), and also in some current cheeses (Drozdz, 2001), smoking was produced on a shelf hanging above the fire in the shepherd's hut. Later, with the introduction of electric or gas kitchens, cheese makers used mini kilns or smoking chambers and the smoke was generated with different woods or vegetable products from the region. Some cheese factories use modern smokehouses that use different smoke generators such as friction smoke and wet smoke generators.

Smoked foods are sometimes suspected of containing contaminants as polycyclic aromatic hydrocarbons (PAHs), harmful to human health (Guillén et al., 1997); for this reason the food industry has started to use smoke flavourings (Guillén et al., 2000), although some European countries, as Spain, forbid the use of this type of smoke cheeses.

The contamination of cheese with PAH in smoking process depends on many factors (Anastasio et al., 2004; Guillén et al., 2007; Fresno et al., 2007b; Guillén et al., 2011) such as:

- Smoking technology: smokehouse, smoke flavouring, smoke in open fire, etc.
- Vegetable matters used for smoking generation
- Smoke temperature
- Oxygen content
- Duration of smoking practice
- Type of cheese: chemical composition, age of cheese at smoking, etc.
- Portion of the cheese analyzed: rind or interior zone of the cheese
- The position of cheese within the smokehouse

Total PHAs concentration ratio in some smoked cheeses varies between 29.21-739.55 µg/kg for soft Palmero PDO cheese made with raw goat milk (Guillén et al., 2007), 367.53-1037.23 µg/kg for ripen cow pasteurized milk cheese, 194.65 µg/kg for fresh goat raw milk cheese and 36.31-175.44 µg/kg for ripen raw sheep milk cheese (Guillén et al., 2004a). For mixed milk cheeses (soft Herreño cheese made with pasteurized milk from goat, cow and sheep) the variation is higher: 423.39-1915.16 µg/kg (Guillén et al., 2011).

Heavy PAH benzo(a)pyrene has been classified as carcinogenic to humans by the International Agency for Research on Cancer (IARC, 2010) and restrictive concentration has been marked for smoked cheeses as it is shown in Spanish regulation (Real Decreto 1113/2006, de 29 de septiembre) with a maximum of 10 µg/kg in the rind of ripen smoked cheeses. Benzo(a)pyrene concentration varies in different smoked cheeses between non detected and 3.8 µg/kg (Riha et al., 1992; García Falcon et al., 1999; Michalski and Germuska, 2003; Pagliuca et al., 2003; Anastasio et al., 2004; Guillén y Sopelana, 2004;

Guillén et al., 2007; Naccari et al., 2008; Suchanová et al., 2008; Guillén et al., 2011), although higher results in some smoked cheese samples (4.1 – 7.8 µg/kg) were reported by Bosset et al. (1998) and Michalski and Germuska (2003). It is necessary to note a higher contamination in the rind than inside the cheeses and the rind is not usually consumed.

Smoking techniques play an important role in the development of new products (Mc Ilveen and Vallely, 1996 a,b; Bárcenas et al., 1998); smoke flavourings are frequently used as novel flavours for products not previously smoked (Ojeda et al., 2002). Comparison between natural and liquid smoked cheeses had been completed (Atasever et al., 2003).

Many traditional cheeses are currently smoked, or used to be smoked; the vegetable matter, temperature and moisture of the smoke together with the physicochemical characteristics of the cheese are the main factors that can modify the quality of these type of cheeses.

Vegetable matter used for smoking has a significant effect in the volatile components of cheeses and can be of interest as marker compounds for the identification of the different cheeses (Guillén et al., 2004a; Guillén et al., 2005). In traditional Palmero PDO cheese smoked with needles of canary pine (*Pinus canariensis*), more than 320 components that play an important role in the flavour were detected (Guillén et al., 2004b). This cheese is the only PDO cheese that has regulated the use of different smoking materials in its making practice: dry needles and dry wood of canary pine (*Pinus canariensis*), dry segmented prickly pear cactus (*Opuntia ficus indica*) and shell of almonds (*Prunus dulcis*).

Under experimental conditions, smoking materials did not have a significant effect on pH or total fat, protein and dry extract (Álvarez et al., 2005). During the smoking process there is an increase of lipids and proteins in the cheese rind, (Ahmad, 1993) while moisture decreases (Álvarez et al., 2005).

Smoking has an important effect in instrumental colour and texture and especially in sensorial properties of cheeses. Surface colour is one of the most important characteristic affecting the consumer acceptance of smoked cheese (Riha and Wendorff, 1993a). Colour is related with pH and moisture of cheeses, temperature and time of smoking process (Möhler, 1980, Riha and Wendorff, 1993b) and the vegetable matter used for smoking (Ruiter, 1979). Canarian experimental cheeses smoked with six several materials showed differences in rind colour (Fresno et al., 2007b), these changes were detected by instrumental analysis and also were appreciated by a consumer panel (Fresno et al., 2007a). Table 7 shows the effect of ripening (cheeses smoked 4 and 10 days after making) and the material used for smoked in cheese external colour. External Lightness was higher for the cheeses smoked with pine needles. Differences were found in Croma values, the most intensive colour were detected for cheeses being smoked with almond shell and pine wood and products smoked with heather wood and pine needle were the least. In relation to ripening time, smoking moment only present significant differences in lightness values. Cheeses smoked four days after elaboration were lighter than chesses smoked 10 days after.

Smoke also produces changes in textural properties of cheeses (Álvarez et al., 2007); higher smoke temperature origins softer and melted cheeses (Mc Ilveen and Vallely 1996a). Instrumental texture has been also affected by ripening time and material used for smoked (Fresno et al., 2007b). Table 8 presents the mean values for textural characteristics on compression test for cheeses smoked at two different ripening time and smoked with six different vegetal materials. Cheese aging at smoking had higher effect on textural characteristics.

Table 7. Effect of smoking materials on surface cheese colour

	Ripening time (R)*		Smoking type (S)**							Effects			
	1	2	1	2	3	4	5	6	RSD	R	S	RxS	L.P.C.I
			LSM										
Lightness	79.94	75.58	76.65^{ab}	75.88^{ab}	77.92^{ab}	79.44^{ab}	82.37^b	74.37^a	0.80	0.003	0.024	0.354	---
Croma	28.09	29.27	31.66^b	26.47^{ab}	27.68^{ab}	29.14^{ab}	25.27^a	31.86^b	0.55	0.198	0.000	0.291	-0.661
H. Angle	85.81	85.46	84.84	84.32	85.72	87.39	88.22	83.33	0.54	0.743	0.091	0.679	0.751

From: Fresno et al., 2007b
* 1: smoked 4 days after elaboration; 2: smoked 10 days after elaboration
** 1: almond shell; 2: *Erica arborea*; 3: *Cistus monspeliensis*; 4: *Opuntia ficus indica*; 5: *Pinus canariensis* needles; 6: *Pinus canariensis* wood
LSM: Least square mean. RSD: Residual standard deviation.
L.P.C.I.: Lightness Pearson Correlation index

Table 8. Effect of smoking materials on compression textural characteristics

	Ripening time (R)*		Smoking type (S)**							Effects		
	1	2	1	2	3	4	5	6	RSD	R	S	RxS
			LSM									
Fracturability	22.34	40.74	20.11	27.64	24.87	31.75	21.70	33.17	3.30	0.002	0.073	0.030
Hardness	41.46	55.12	59.89	52.87	48.09	47.55	37.08	44.28	3.40	0.017	0.264	0.006
Cohesiveness	0.21	0.22	0.21^{abc}	0.20^{ab}	0.18^a	0.23^{bc}	0.23^{bc}	0.24^c	0.01	0.970	0.000	0.006
Adhesiveness	0.69	0.71	0.54	0.84	1.05	0.70	0.45	0.63	0.73	0.884	0.235	0.922
Elasticity	54.79	51.55	54.22	51.57	51.03	52.92	54.06	55.21	0.56	0.004	0.193	0.907

From: Fresno et al., 2007b
* 1: smoked 4 days after elaboration; 2: smoked 10 days after elaboration
** 1: almond shell (*Prunus dulcis*); 2: Heather wood (*Erica arborea*); 3: Rock rose (*Cistus spp*); 4: Dry nopal (*Opuntia ficus indica*); 5: Pine needles (*Pinus canariensis*); 6: Pine wood (*Pinus canariensis*)
LSM: Least square mean. RSD: Residual standard deviation.

Cheeses smoked later (10 days after elaboration) presented higher values for hardness ($p<0.05$) and fracturability ($p<0.01$) but were less elastic ($p<0.01$). Only cohesiveness was affected by the smoke type used, cheeses smoked with pine wood were the most cohesive while the ones smoked with rose rock wood were the least. Cheese chemical composition was not affected by the material used in the smoking process. This type of changes could be related with a higher smoke temperature.

The vegetable matter also has an effect in sensorial analysis. The odour and taste of cheese is affected by the smoking process, not only due to the volatile compounds of the smoke but also because the different reactions between the smoke and the cheese chemical components; these differences were observed by trained panels and consumers (Fresno et al., 2007b). The comparison of the effect of smoking material as a technical factor in the cheese production of Palmero PDO cheeses revealed significant sensory differences. Sensory analysis is a very useful and effective tool in differentiating and defining these cheeses; cheeses smoked with four different products can be classified in different groups as can be seen in Figure 4 for the texture sensory profile and Fig 5 for the odour, flavour and taste profile.

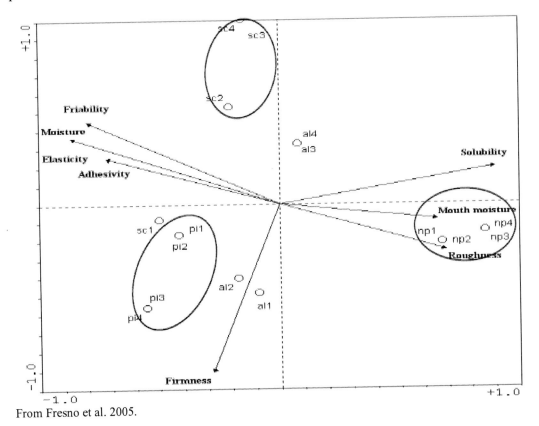

From Fresno et al. 2005.

Figure 4. PCA of the texture sensory characteristics of cheeses smoked with: al, shell of almond; pi, pine wood; sc, segment cacti (dry nopal); np, needle of pine.

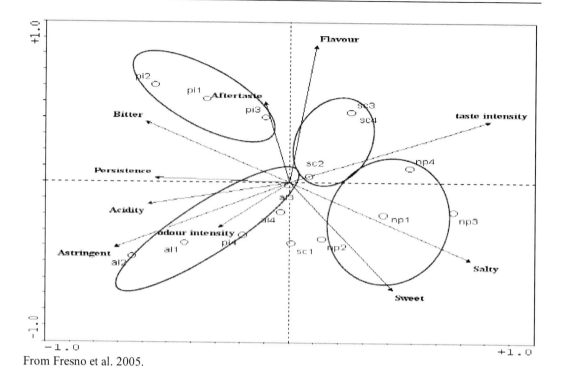

From Fresno et al. 2005.

Figure 5. PCA of the odour and flavour sensory characteristics of cheeses smoked with: al, shell of almond; pi, pine wood; sc, segment cacti (dry nopal); np, needle of pine.

As a conclusion, traditional smoking process in cheese generates low concentration of heavy carcinogenic PAHs, although further studies should be carried out because food contamination should be as minimum as possible. The possibilities of smoking cheeses and all the variation of different sources can be used to characterize the traditional smoked cheeses and the different sensorial properties which could help them to improve their market position. The use of local materials for smoking can help to link this product to the place in which they are made. New cheeses with different flavours can be developed using traditional smoking practices or smoke flavouring in countries where they are allowed.

ACKNOWLEDGMENTS

Authors would like to thank Ms Heather R. Briggs MSc for reviewing the English grammar for the paper.

REFERENCES

Addis, M., Pireda, G., Pes, M., Salvo, R. di, Scintu, M., Pirisi, A. 2005a. Effect of the use of three different lamb paste rennet on lipolysis of PDO Pecorino Romano cheese. *International Dairy Journal*, 15 (6/9), 563-569.

Addis, M., Pirisi, A., di Salvo, R., Podda, F., Pireda, G. 2005b. The influence of enzymatic composition of lamb rennet paste on some properties of experimentally produced PDO Fiore Sardo cheese. *International Dairy Journal*, 15 (12), 1271-1278.

Addis, M., Pireda, G. Pirisi, A. 2008. The use of lamb rennet paste in traditional sheep milk production. *Small Ruminat Research*, 79, 2-10.

Agboola, S.O., Chan, H.H., Zhao, J., Rehman, A. 2009. Can the use of Australian cardoon (*Cynara cardunculus*) coagulant overcome the quality problems associated with cheese made with ultrafiltered milk? *Food Science and Technology*, 42 (8), 1352-1359.

Ahmad, J. 1993. Smoked foods, Encyclopaedia of Food Science, Food Technology and Nutrition, Academic Press, Vol. 6., Londres, (Reino Unido).

Álvarez, S., Fresno, M., González, C., González, L.A., Darmanin, N., Sosa, J.M., Suárez, L., Estévez, F.J. 2001. Efecto del tipo de cuajo en la calidad organoléptica de los quesos de las medianías del noreste de Gran Canaria. In: proceedings of I Formaggi D'alpeggio e Loro Tracciabilitá, Bella, Italy, 146-158.

Álvarez S., Argüello A., Rodríguez V., Ruiz M. E., Castro N, Fresno M., 2005. Utilización de diferentes materiales para ahumar como elemento diferenciador de los quesos artesanos. Memorias del VI Simposio Iberoamericano sobre la conservación de los recursos zoogenéticos locales y el desarrollo rural sostenible. ISBN: 970-9825-00-3. Chiapas, México, 335-337.

Álvarez S., Fresno M., Rodríguez V., Ruiz M. E. 2007. Evaluación sensorial de la textura de quesos canarios ahumados con diferentes materiales. *Archivos de Zootecnia*, 216 (1), 705-711

Álvarez, S., Méndez, P., Darmanin, N., Briggs, M.R., Fresno, M. 2008. Breed effect on raw milk goat cheese quality. *International Dairy Federation Bulletin*, 0801/Part 4, 278-280.

Anastasio, A., Mercogliano, R., Vollano, L., Pepe, T., Cortesi, M.L. 2004. Levels of benzo(a)pyrene (BaP) in "mozzarella di bufala campana" cheese smoked according to different procedures. *Journal of Agricultural and food Chemistry*, 52, 4452-4455.

Atasever, M., Ucar, G., Keles, A., Köse, Z. 2003. The effects of natural smoke and liquid smoke applications on the quality factors of Kashar cheese, *Turkish Journal of Veterinary and Animal Science*, 27, 781-787 (Abstract).

Audist, M., Mullins, C., O'Brien, B., O'Kennedy, B.T., Guinee, T. 2002. Effect of breed on milk coagulation properties. *Milchwissenschaft*, 57, (3), 140-143.

Auldist, M., Johnston, K., White, N., Fitzsimons, W., Boland, M. 2004. A comparison of the composition, coagulation characteristics and cheesemaking capacity of milk from Friesian and Jersey dairy cows. *Journal of Dairy Research*, 71, 51-57.

Barbosa, E., Oliveira, C., Casal, S., Soares, L., Vale, A.P., Lopes, J., Brito, N.V. 2003. Quantification and variability of conjugated linoleic acids levels in sheep milk of two Portuguese breeds. *EJEAFCHE*, 2, 493-497.

Bárcenas, P., Pérez-Elortondo, F.J., Salmerón, J., Albisu, M. 1998. Recalled preference of Spanish consumers for smoked food. *Nutrition and Food Science*, 6, 338-342.

Barylko-Pikelna, N. 1977. Contribution of smoked compounds to sensory, bacteriostatic and antioxidative effects in smoked food. *Pure and Applied Chemistry*, 49, 1667-1671.

Bosset, J.O., Bütikofer, U., Dafflon, O., Koch, H., Scheurer-Simonet, L., Sieber, R. 1998. Teneur en hydrocarbures aromatiques polycycliques de fromages avec et sans flaveur de fumée. *Science des Aliments*, 18, 347-359.

Bustamante, M., Chávarri, F., Santiesteban, A., Ceballos, G., Herández, I., Mígueles, J. M., Aramburu, I., Barrón, L.J.R., Virto, M., de Renovales, M. 2000. Coagulating and lipolytic activities of artisanal lamb rennet pastes, *Journal Dairy Research*, 67, 393-402.

Bustamante, M.A., Virto, M., Aramburu, M., Barrón, L.J.R., Pérez- Elortondo, F.J., Albisu, M., de Renobales, M. 2003. Lamb rennet paste in ovine cheese (Idiazabal) manufacture. Proteolysis and relationship between analytical and sensory parameters. *International Dairy Journal*, 13, 547-557.

Candrelli, M., Rubino, R., Masoero, R., Clementi., E., Monrone, G., Pizillo, M., Nicastro, D. 1997. Effect of kids rennet production technology on its microbiological characteristics and on the chemical composition of Semicoto goat cheese. *Scienza et Tecnica Lattiero Casearia*, 48 (4), 343-360.

Calvo, M.V., Fontecha, J. 2004. Purification and characterization of a pregastric esterase from a hygienized ked rennet paste. *Journal Dairy Science*, 87, 1132-1142.

Calvo, M.V., Castillo, I., Díaz-Barcos V., Requena, T., Fontecha, J., 2007, Effect of a hygienized rennet paste and a defined strain starter on proteolysis, texture and sensory properties of semi-hard goat cheese, *Food Chemistry*, 102, 917-924.

Castillo, I., Calvo, M.V., Alonso, L., Juárez, M., Fontecha, J. 2007. Changes in lipolysis and volatile fraction of a goat cheese manufactured employing a hygienized rennet paste and a defined strain starter. *Food Chemistry,* 100, 590-598.

Casandro, M., Provinelli, M., Marcomin, D., Gallo, L., Carnier, P., Zotto, R., Valorz, C., Brittante, G. 2005. Breed effect on milk coagulation and cheese quality parameters of dairy cattle. In: Indicators of milk and beef quality, 313-319, Editors: Hocquete, J.F., Gigli, S.

Chilliard, Y., Rouel, J., Ferlay, A., Bernard, L., Gaborit, P., Raynal-Ljutovac, K., Lauret, A.,Leroux, C., 2006, Optimising goat's milk and cheese fatty acid composition, In: Improving the content of foods, 281-312 (Abstract), Editors: Williams, C. Buttriss, J.

Coulon, J.B., Delacroix-Buchet, A., Martín, B., Pirisi, A. 2004. Relationships between ruminant management and sensory characteristics of cheeses: a review. *Lait*, 84, 221-241.

Díaz, C., Rodríguez, E., Pérez, S., Álvarez, S., Fresno, M. 2008. La composición mineral de la leche y los quesos de cabra: efecto de la raza. IX Simposio Iberoamericano sobre la Conservación y utilización de los Recursos Genéticos Animales. ISBN 978-987-9455-73-9. Ed. Delgado Bermejo, 447-479.

Drozdz, A. 2001. Quality of the Polish traditional mountain sheep cheese "Oscypek". *Options Méditerraneénnes Serie A*, 46, 111-114.

Etayo, I., Pérez-Elortondo, F.J., Gil, P.F., Albisu, M., Virto, M., Conde, S., Rodríguez Barrón, L.J., Nájera, A.I., Gómez Hidalgo, M.E., Delgado, C., Guerra, A.; de Renobales, M. 2006. Hygienic quality, lipolysis and sensory properties of Spanish Protected Designation of Origin ewe´s cheeses milk manufactured with lamb rennet pastes. Lait 86, 415-434.

Ferrandini, E. 2006. Elaboración de queso de Murcia al Vino con cuajo natural en pasta. Tesis doctoral. Universidad de Murcia, Facultad de Veterinaria. 196 pp.

Fresno, M., Álvarez, S., Darmanin, N., Menendez, P., Capote, J., Romero del Castillo, R. 2001. La race des chévres comme element de differentiation des fromages tradicionnels des Canaries. In: Proceedings of I Formaggi d'alpeggio e loro Tracciabilitá, Bella, Italy, 178-199.

Fresno, M., Álvarez, S., Darmanin, N., Méndez, P., Fernández, E., Guillén, M.D. 2004. La industria quesera en la isla de El Hierro: Pasado, presente y futuro. *Alimentación, Equipos y Tecnología*, 192, 69-73.

Fresno, M., Pino, V., Álvarez, S.,Darmanin, N., Fernández, M., Guillén, M.D. 2005. Effects of the smoking materials used in the sensory characterization of the Palmero (PDO) cheeses. *Options Méditerranéennes Serie A*, 67, 195-199.

Fresno, M., Álvarez. S., Rodríguez, V., Castro, N. Argüello, A. 2006. Evaluation of the effect of rennet type on the texture and colour of goats' cheese. *Journal Applied of Animal Research*, 30, 157-160.

Fresno M., Rodríguez V., Ruiz M. E., Álvarez S. 2007a. Preferencia de los consumidores según el material de ahumado utilizado en la elaboración de los quesos. *Archivos de Zootecnia*, 216 (1), 713-717.

Fresno, M., Ruiz, M.E., Argüello, A., Castro, N., Álvarez. S. 2007b. Effects of smoking on surface colour and texture of traditional goat cheeses. *Journal Applied of Animal Research*, 6(3), 310-313.

Fresno M., Álvarez S., Darmanin N., González L. A., Rodríguez T., Camacho E. 2009. Recuperación de los cuajos tradicionales: comparación del efecto de cuatro coagulantes en las características sensoriales de quesos de cabra de pasta prensada. X Simposio Iberoamericano sobre la Conservación y Utilización de Recursos Zoogenéticos ISBN nº 978-958-8095-57-8. Ed: Álvarez Franco L.A. and Muñoz Flores J.E. Colombia, 625-628.

Fresno M., Álvarez S., Díaz E., Rodríguez B., Darmanin N., Domínguez O., Esperanza M. E. 2010. Diferenciación de quesos artesanos: utilización de cuajo natural de cabrito: tradicional y adaptado XI Simposio Iberoamericano sobre la Conservación y Utilización de Recursos Zoogenéticos. Ed: Roberto Germano, Laura Leandro, Geovergue Rodrigues. ISSN: 2179-1961. Joao Pessoa-Editora da UFPB, Instituto Nacional do Semiárido, Brazil, 68-71

Fontecha, J., Castillo, I., Blasco, L., Alonso, L., Juárez, M. 2006. Effect of artisanal kid rennet paste on lipolysis in semi-hard goat cheese, *Food Chemistry*, 98, 253-259.

Galán, E., Prados, E., Pino, A., Tejada, L., Fernández –Salguero, J. 2008. Influence of different amounts of vegetable coagulant from cardoon *Cynara cardunculus* and calf rennet on the proteolysis and sensory characteristic of cheese made with sheep milk. *International Dairy Journal*, 18(1), 93-98.

García Falcón, M.S., González Amigo, S., Lage Yusty, M.A. Simal Lozano, J., 1999, Determination of benzo(a)pyrene in some Spanish commercial smoked products by HPLC-FL. *Food Additive and Contaminants*, 16, (1) 9-14.

Georgala, A., Moschopoulou, E., Aktypis, A., Massouras, T., Zoidou, E., Kandarakis, I., Anifantakis, E. 2005. Evolution of lipolysis during the ripening of traditional Feta cheese. *Food Chemistry*, 93,73-80.

Guillén, M.D., Sopelana, P., Partearroyo, M.A. 1997. Food as a resource of polycyclic aromatic carcinogens. *Review of Environmental and Health*, 12, 133-146.

Guillén, M.D., Sopelana, P., Partearroyo, M.A.. 2000. Occurrence of polycyclic aromatic hydrocarbons in smoke flavouring. *Polycyclic Aromatic Compounds*, 21, 215-229.

Guillén, M.D., Ibargoitia, M.L., Sopelana, P., Palencia, G. 2004a. Components detected by headspace-solid phase microextraction in artesanal fresh goat's cheese smoked using dry prickly pear (*Opuntia ficus indica*). *Lait*, 84, 385-397.

Guillén, M.D., Ibargoitia, M.L., Sopelana, P., Palencia, G., Fresno, M. 2004b. Components Detected by Means of Solid-Phase Microextraction and Gas Chromatography/Mass Spectrometry in the Headspace of Artisan Fresh Goat Cheese Smoke by Traditional Methods. *Journal of Dairy Science*, 83, 284-299.

Guillén, M.D., Sopelana, P. 2004. Occurrence of Polycyclic Aromatic Hydrocarbons in Smoked Cheese. *Journal of Dairy Science*, 87, 556-564.

Guillén, M.D., Palencia, G., Sopelana, P., Ibargoitia, M.L., Fresno, M. 2005. Prospective study on the presence of polycyclic aromatic hydrocarbons in Herreño cheese. In proceedings of IntraFood- Effosst Conference, 415-418.

Guillén, M. D., Palencia G., Ibargoitia M. L., Sopelana, P. 2007. Occurrence of polycyclic aromatic hydrocarbons in artisanal Palmero cheese smoked with two types of vegetable matter. *J. Dairy Sci.* 90, 2717-2725.

Guillén, M.D., Palencia, G., Ibargoitia, M.L., Fresno, M.,Sopelana, P., 2011 (in press). Contamination of cheese by PAHs in tradicional smoking. Influence of the position in the smokehouse on the contamination level of smoked cheese. *J. Dairy, Sci*TBC 1-12 doi:10.3168/jds 2010-3647.

Hernández, I., Virto, M., Ceballos, G., Santiesteban,A., Pérez-Elortondo F.J., Albisu, M., Barrón, L.J.R., de Renobales, M. 2001. Development of characteristic flavour in Idiazábal cheese adding commercial lipases. *Food Flavours and Chemistry*, 274, 151-159.

Hernández, I., Barrón, L.J.R.,Virto, Pérez-Elortondo F.J., Flanagan, F.J., Rozas, C., Nájera, A.I., M., Albisu, M., Vicente, M.S., de Renobales, M. 2009. Lipolysis, proteolysis and sensory properties of ewe's raw milk cheese (Idiazabal) made with lipase additions. *Food Chemistry*, 116 (1), 158-166.

IARC. 2010. Some non-heterocyclic polycyclic aromatic hydrocarbons and some related exposures. In IARC Monographs on the evaluation of the carcinogenic risk of chemicals to humans. Vol. 92. IARC, Lyon, France.

Ikonen, T., Morri, S., Tyriseva, AM., Ruottinen, O., Ojala, M. 2004. Genetic and phenotypic correlation properties, milk production traits, somatic cell count, casein content and pH of milk. *Journal of Dairy Science*, 87, 458-467.

Irigoyen, A., Izco, J.M., Ibáñez, F.C., Torre, P. 2000. Evaluation of the effect of rennet type on casein proteolysis in an ovine milk cheese by means of capillary electrophoresis, *Journal of Chromatography*, 881, 59-67.

Irigoyen, A., Izco, J.M., Ibáñez, F.C.,Torre, P. 2002. Influence of calf or lamb rennet on the physico chemical proteolytic and sensory characteristics of an ewe's milk cheeses. *International Dairy Journal*, 13, 547-557.

Jaramillo, D.P., Zamora, A., Guamis, G., Rodríguez, M., Trujillo, A.J. 2008. Cheesemaking aptitude of two Spanish dairy ewe breeds: Changes during lactation and relationship between physico -chemical and technological properties. *Small Ruminant Research*, 78: 48-55.

Kelsey, J.A., Corl, B.A., Collier, R.J., Bauman, D.E. 2003. The effect of breed, parity, and stage of lactation on conjugated linoleic acid (CLA) in milk fat from dairy cows. *Journal Dairy Science*, 86, (8), 2588-2597.

Kewalramani, N., Harjit Kaur, T.R. 2003. Factors affecting conjugated linoleic acid content of milk-a review. *Animal Nutrition and Feed Technology*, 3, (2), 91-105.

Knowles, S.O., Grace, N.D., Knight, T.W., McNabb, W.C., Lee, J. 2006. Reasons and means for manipulating the micronutrient composition of milk from grazing dairy cattle. *Animal Feed Science and Technology*, 131, 154-167.

Kumar, J.S., Kansar, V.K. 2005. Effects of breed and parity of animals, stage of lactation and processing of milk on the content of conjugated linoleic acid in dairy products. *Milchwissenschaft* 60, 370-372.

Le Jaouen, J.C., Dubeuf, J.P., Rubino, R. 2001. Le système de production dans le cahier des charges des fromages caprins et ovins AOP de l'Union Européenne. *Options Méditerranéennes Serie A*, 46, 81-92.

Larráyoz, P., Martínez, M.T., Barrón, L.J.R., Torre, P., Barcina, Y. 1999. The evolution of free fatty acids during ripening Idiazábal cheese: influence of rennet type. *European Food Research Technology*, 210, 9-12.

Lurueña-Martinez, M.A., Revilla, I., Severiano-Pérez, P., Vivar-Quintana, A.M. 2010. The influence of breed on the organoleptic characteristics of Zamorano sheep's raw milk cheese and its assessment by instrumental analysis. *International Journal of Dairy Technology*, 63, 216-223.

Macheboeuf, D., Coulon, J. B., D'Hour, P. 1993. Effect of breed, protein genetic variants and feeding on cows' milk coagulation properties. *Journal of Dairy Research*, 60, 43-54.

Malacarne, M., Summer, A., Fossa, E., Formaggioni, P., Franceschi, P., Pecorari, M., Mariani, P. 2006. Composition, coagulation properties and Parmigiano-Reggiano cheese yield of Italian Brown and Italian Friesian herd milk. *Journal of Dairy Research*, 73, 171-177.

Mcllveeen, H., Vallely, C. 1996a. The development and acceptability of a smoked processed cheese. *British Food Journal*, 98/8, 17-23.

Mcllveeen, H., Vallely, C. 1996b. Something's smoking in the development kitchen. *Nutrition and Food Science*, 6, 34-38.

Michalski, R., and R. Germuska. 2003. The content of benzo(a)pyrene in Slovakian smoked cheese. *Pol. J. Food Nutr. Sci.* 12, 33-37.

Mihaylova G., Gerchev, G., Moeckel, P., Jahreis, G. 2004. Comparative study on fatty acid content in milk of Tsigay and Karakachan sheep. *Bulg. J. Vet. Med.* 7, 181-187.

Moatsou, G., Moschopoulou, E., Georgala, A., Zoidou, E., Kandarakis, I., Kaminarides, S., Anifantakis, E. 2004. Effect of artisanal liquid rennet from kids and lambs abomasa on characteristics of Feta cheese. *Food Chemistry*, 88 (4), 517-525.

Möhler, K. 1980. El Ahumado. Ed. Acribia. Zaragoza. 74 pp.

Moschopoulou, E., Onoufriou, E., Kandarakis, I. 2009. Effect of diet and abomasums parts on enzymic properties of liquid lam rennet. *Italian Journal of food Science*, 21 (1), 73-80.

Naccari, C., M. Cristani, P. Licata, F. Giofre, and D. Trombetta. 2008. Levels of benzo(a)pyrene and benz(a) anthracene in smoked "Provola" cheese from Calabria (Italy). *Food Addit. Contam. Part B*, 1, 78-84.

Nuñez, M., Fernández del Pozo, B., Rodríguez Marín, M.A., Gaya, P., Medina, M. 1991. Effect of animal and vegetable rennet on the chemical, microbiological, rherological and sensory characteristics of La Serena cheese. *Journal of Dairy Research*, 58, 511-519.

Nuñez, M., Medina, M., Gaya, P., Guillén, A.M., Rodríguez Marín, A. 1992. Effect of recombinant chymosin on ewe's milk coagulation and Manchego cheese characteristics. *Journal of Dairy Research*, 59 (1), 81-87.

Ojeda, M., Bárcenas, P., Pérez-Elortondo, F.J., Albisu, M., Guillén, M.D. 2002. Chemical references in sensory analysis of smoke flavourings. *Food Chemistry*, 78, 433-442.

Pagliuca, G., Gazzotti, T., Zironi, E., Serrazanetti, G.P., Mollica, D., Rosmini, R. 2003. Determination of high molecular mass polycyclic aromatic hydrocarbons in a typical Italian smoked cheese by HPLC-FL. *Journal of Agricultural and food Chemistry*, 51, 5111-5115.

Pino, A., Prados, F., Galan, E., McSweeney, P.L.H. Fernández -Salguero, J. 2009. Proteolysis during the ripening of goats' milk cheese made with plant coagulant or calf rennet. *Food research International*, 42 (3), 324-330.

Pireda, G., Addis, M. 2003. The lamb rennet paste used in ewe's milk cheeses manufactured in Sardinia. *Scienza e Tecnica Lattiero- Casearia*, 54 (4), 225-235.

Pirisi, A., Pinna, G., Addis, M., Pireda, G., Mauriello, R., de Pascale S., Caira, S., Mamone, G., Ferranti, P., Addeo, F., Chianese, L. 2007. Relationship between enzymatic composition of lamb rennet pastes and proteolytic and lipolitic pattern and texture of PDO Fiore Sardo ovine cheese. *International Dairy Journal*, 17, 143-156.

Pizzillo, M., Cogliandro, E., Tripaldi, C. 1992. Caratteristiche del latte delle principali razze ellevate e fattori che vi influiscono, In: Proceedings of the Conference on Milk and Cheese of Goats, Bella, Italy, 5-31.

Pizzillo, M., Rubino, R., Cogliandro, E., Fedele, V., Chianese, L., Dáuria, R. 1996. Effect of breed, casein polymorphism and feeding system on casein number of individual goat milk. *Scienza e Tecnica Lattiero-Casearia*, 47, 315-330.

Pizzillo, M., Claps, S., Cifuni, G.F., Fedele, V., Rubino, R. 2005. Effect of goat breed on the sensory, chemical and nutritional characteristics of ricotta cheese. *Livestock Production Science*, 94, 33-40.

Real Decreto 1113/2006, de 29 de septiembre, por el que se aprueban las normas de calidad para quesos y quesos fundidos. B.O.E. 239, 6.10.2006: 34717-34720.

Riha, W. E., W. L. Wendorff, and S. Rank. 1992. Benzo(a)pyrene content of smoked and smoked-flavoured cheese products sold in Wisconsin. *J. Food Prot.* 55, 636-638.

Riha, W.E., Wendorff, W.L., 1993a, Evaluation of color in smoked cheese by sensory and objective methods, *Journal of Dairy Science*, 76, 1491-1497.

Riha, W.E., Wendorff, W.L. 1993b. Influence of processing conditions on surface color of liquid smoke treated cheeses. *Cultured Dairy Products-Journal*, 28(4), 4-9.

Roest, K., Menghi, A. 2000. Reconsidering Traditional Food: The Case of Parmigiano Reggiano Cheese. European Society for Rural Sociology nº 4, 390-451.

Ronningen, K. 1965. Causes of variation in the flavour intensity of goat milk. *Acta Agriculturae Scandinavica*, 15, 301-343.

Ruiter, A. 1979. Color of Smoked foods. *Food Techonology*, 33, 54- 63.

Requena, T., de la Fuente, M.A., Fernández de Palencia, P., Juárez, M., Peláez, C. 1992. Evaluation of a specific starter for the production of semi-hard goat's milk cheese. *Lait*, 72, 437-448.

Sandillo, A., D'Angelo, F., Caproprese, M., Marino, R., Albenzio, M. 2005. Influence of diet and lamb slaughtering age on the coagulating properties of rennet paste. *Italian Journal of Animal Science*, 4(2), 336-338.

Sanjuán, E., Millán, R., Saavedra, P., Carmona, M. A., Gómez, R., Fernández- Salguero, J. 2002. Influence of animal and vegetable rennet on the physicochemical characteristics of

Los Pedroches cheese during ripening. *Food Chemistry*, 78, 281-289. Santoro, M., Faccia, M. 1998. Influence of mould size and rennet on proteolysis and composition of Canestrato pugiliese cheese. *Italian Journal of Food Science*, 10(3), 217-228.

Shao Jian, Ch., Agboola, S., Zhao J.A. 2003. Use of Australian cardoon extract in the manufacture of ovine milk cheese; a comparison with commercial rennet preparations. *International Journal of Food Science and Technology*, 38(7), 799-807.

Signorelli, F., Contarini, G., Annicchiarico, G., Napolitano, F., Orrù, L., Catillo, G., Haenlein, G.F.W., Moioli, B. 2008. Breed differences in sheep milk fatty acid profiles: Opportunities for sustainable use of animal genetic resources. *Small Ruminant Research*, 78, 24-31

Skjevdal, T. 1979. Flavour of goat's milk: a review of studies on the sources of its variation. *Livestock Production Science*, 6, 397-405.

Soryal, K., Beyene, F.A., Zeng, S., Bash, B., Tesfai, K. 2005. Effect of goat breed and milk composition on yield, sensory quality, fatty acid concentration of soft cheese during lactation. *Small Ruminant Research*, 58, 275-281.

Sousa. M.,J., Malcata, F.X. 1997. Comparison of plant and animal rennet in terms of microbiological, chemical and proteolysis characteristics of ovine cheese. *Journal of Agricultural and Food Chemistry*, 45, 74-81.

Suchanová, M., J. Hajslová, M. Tomaniová, V. Kocourek, and L. Babicka. 2008. Polycyclic aromatic hydrocarbons in smoked cheese. *J. Sci. Food Agric.* 88, 1307-1317.

Tejada, L., Fernández- Salguero J. 2003. Chemical and microbiological characteristics of ewe's milk cheese (Los Pedroches) made with a powdered vegetable coagulant or calf rennet. *Italian Journal of Food Science*, 15(1), 125-131, Abstract.

Tejada, L., Abellan, A., Prados, F., Cayuela, J.M. 2008. Composition and characteristics of Murcia al Vino cheese made with calf rennet and plant coagulant. *International Journal of Dairy Science*, 61 (2), 119-125.

Thomann, S., Brechenmacher, A., Hinrichs, J. 2008. Strategy to evaluate cheesemaking properties of milk from different goat breeds. *Small Ruminant Research*, 74, 172-178.

Todaro, M., Arrabito, P., Celiberti, T., Gagliano, B., Gambuzza, M.R., Giansiracusa, E., Guastella, S., Terra, K., la Presti, L., lo Matarazzo, M., Sortino, C., Sortino, E. 2004. Effect of the bovine breed on milk and "Ragusano" cheese composition. *Scienza e tecnica Lattiero-Casearia*, 55(55), 403-412.

Trujillo, A., Guamis, B., Lencina, J., López M.B. 2000. Proteolytic activity of some milk clotting enzymes on ovine casein. *Food Chemistry*, 71, 449-457.

Tsiplakon, E., Mountzouris, K.C., Zervas, G. 2006. The effect of breed, stage of lactation and parity on sheep milk fat CLA content under the same feeding practices. *Livestock Science*, 105, 162-167.

Verdier-Metz, I., Coulon, J.B., Pradel, P., Viallons, C., Berdagué, J.L. 1998. Effect of forage conservation (hay or silage) and cow breed on the coagulation properties of milks and on the characteristics of ripened cheeses. *Journal of Dairy Research*, 65, 9-21.

Vicente, M.S., Ibáñez, F.C., Barcina, Y., Barrón, L.J.R. 2000. Casein breakdown during ripening of Idiazábal cheese: influence of starter and rennet type. *Journal of the Science of Food and Agriculture*, 81(2), 210-215.

Vicente, M.S., Ibáñez, F.C., Barcina, Y., Barrón L.J.R. 2001. Changes in the free acid content during ripening of Idiazábal cheese; influence of starter and rennet type. *Food Chemistry*, 72, 309-317.

Viroque, M., Gómez, R., Sánchez, E., Mata, C., Tejada, L., Fernández- Salguero, J. 2000. Chemical, microbiological characteristics of ewe's milk cheeses manufactured with extracts from flowers of *Cynara cardunculus* and *Cynara humilis* as coagulants. *Journal of Agriculture and Food Chemistry*, 48, (2), 451-456.

Viroque, M., Gómez, R., 2005, Coagulantes vegetales empleados en la fabricación de quesos tradicionales: caracterización de algunas variedades. *Alimentación Equipos y Tecnología*, 203, 48-55.

Virto, M. Chávarri, F., Bustamante M., Barrón, L .J. R., Aramburu, I., Vicente, M. S., Pérez-Elortondo, F. J., de Renovales, M. 2003. Lamb rennet paste in ovine cheese manufacture: lypolysis and flavour, *International Dairy Journal*. 13, 391-399.

White, S.L., Bertrand, J.A., Wade, M.R., Washburn, S.P., Green, T., Jenkins, T.C. 2001. Comparison of fatty acid content of milk from Jersey and Holstein cows consuming pasture or a total mixed ration. *Journal of Dairy Science*, 84, 2295-2301.

Woo, A. H., Lindsay, R.C. 1984. Concentration of mayor free fatty acids flavour development in Italian cheese varieties. *Journal of Dairy Science*, 67(5), 960-968.

In: Cheese: Types, Nutrition and Consumption
Editor: Richard D. Foster, pp. 71-88

ISBN 978-1-61209-828-9
© 2011 Nova Science Publishers, Inc.

Chapter 3

AUTHENTICATION OF LOCAL CHEESES: A GLOBAL PERSPECTIVE

Ahmet Koluman, Rind Kürşat Aktaş and Abdullah Dikici
National Food Reference Laboratory, Ankara, Republic of Turkey

ABSTRACT

Globalization of food sources triggered a demand and public tendency for organic foods and local products. This demand caused a massive application for patenting the local products. With this perspective, authentication studies for all food products have been started globally. Like all food other types cheese has become one of the major subject for authentication process. Authentication includes patenting and under the defined names are: Protected Designation of Origin (PDO) and Protected Geographical Origin (PGO). "Geographical indications (GI)" is also a term for proving the authentication with geographical parameters. European Union (EU) has started to use the patenting approach at their local products on 12 June 1996 with "Commission Regulation (EC) No 1107/96" of the registration of geographical indications and designations of origin under the procedure laid down in "Article 17 of Council Regulation (EEC) No 2081/92". This regulation leads to PDO and PGO patenting of different food products including cheese. Some samples for patenting of authentic cheeses can be listed as; Beacon Fell traditional Lancashire cheese (PDO), Bonchester cheese (PDO), Buxton blue (PDO), Dorset Blue cheese (GI), Dovedale cheese (PDO), Exmoor Blue cheese (PGO), Single Gloucester (PDO), Staffordshire Cheese (PDO), Swaledale cheese (PDO), Swaledale ewes' cheese (PDO), Teviotdale cheese (GI), Stilton - White cheese (PDO), Stilton - Blue cheese (PDO), West Country farmhouse Cheddar cheese (see Cheddar cheese) (PDO).

This chapter aims to summarize definitions of authentic and local products, PDO, PGO, and GI. On the other hand, it underlines the regulations for authentication, makes a comprehensive review for PDO, PGO and GI procedures and sustainability for authentic cheese production. Global supply and demand for authentic cheeses and labeling of these cheeses is also given under this chapter.

1. INTRODUCTION

During the last decade, the behavior of developed country citizens has been undergoing gradual change. The citizens now require not only much higher dietary, hygienic, and health standards in the products they buy, but also look for certification and reassurance of products' origins and production methods. 'Quality' has become the watchword and showstopper in some cases. This elevated consumer awareness is reflected in the demand for products with individual characteristics, due to specific production methods, composition or origin. Increased freedom of movement of goods has certainly helped to make a much wider variety of products from all over the Europe available, creating a need for better consumer information (Jordana, 2000).

Two regulations were adopted in 1992, namely regulation (EEC) No 2081/92 on the production of geographical indications and designations of origin for agricultural products and foodstuffs, and Regulation (EEC) No 2082/92 on certificates of specific character for agricultural products and foodstuffs, reflecting the need to adapt to the changing attitudes of both producers and consumers. Additional regulations are designed for Protected Designation of Origin (PDO), Protected Geographical Indications (PGI) and authentication of foods (Anon, 2004).

This chapter aims to build comprehension about local products, traditional production, PDO, PGI, regulations in this area, authentication status of global cheeses, sustainability for authentic production, labeling process of these cheeses.

2. WHAT IS A LOCAL PRODUCT?

There are numerous definitions for local product. To identify them clearly, supply and demand curves and their correlation with needs and wants must be clarified. There is a strict competition between needs, wants and goods. Needs and wants define the character and the commodity of goods to be produced. The competitive market forces these products to be prominent among others by having distinctive characteristics to be chosen or to be endured. The most logical way to produce such goods is to make them reflect some territorial characteristics, special climatic conditions or advantages and privileges of the natural habituate in the production processes (Anon, 2004). The terms "local" and "traditional" usually goes arm in arm, in this concern it is inevitable to define traditional product seperately. According to Jordana (2000) "a traditional product is a representation of a group, it belongs in a definite space, and it is part of a culture that implies the cooperation of the individuals operating in that territory". This definition states that a traditional product has its own specialty due to the territory it has been produced or made, the eligible culture in that territory is somehow linked with the traditions. So it can be concluded that the definition of "traditional product" covers the term "local product".

Standardization between the batches will be crucial if the mentioned product is any kind of food. Since the raw material generally is an agricultural product, the quality depends on some outer factors such as climatic conditions and production techniques, which make the sustainability hard to be altered. While reflecting some cultural background, manufacturing the food in a defined territory where the variability of the outer factors mentioned above gets minimum, will provide desired sustainability. Thus, a local food can be described as food prepared by using resources, of a definite location including raw material, labor force and traditional background. In preparation of a traditional food, the only requirement is the traditional background. It is not essential to use local raw material or local labor force etc. (Larson 2007).

3. SOME TERMS FOR COMPREHENSION

3.1. Traditional Food

In a European context, there are two regulations in force with respect to traditional foods. Council regulation 2081/92 of 14 July 1992 (Anon, 1992a) which applies for the protection of geographical indications and designations of origin of agricultural products, and regulation 2082/92 of 14 of July 1992 (Anon, 1992b) on certificates of specific character of agricultural products and foodstuffs. Regulation 2081/92 has been successfully implemented in many European food, whilst very few food have been certified according to the regulation 2082/92 as 'Traditional Specialty Guaranteed'. One of the reasons for the 'gap' in the enforcement of the regulation is that, it does not convey adequate protection, neither to the producer nor food. Furthermore, it lacks a distinct definition of the concept 'traditional' resulting in an inability to ensure the exclusive registration of traditional foods. Only recently EU has acknowledged the importance of introducing a definition of the term 'traditional' into the regulation, which according to the proposal is 'Traditional means proven usage on the community market for a period at least equal to that generally ascribed to a human generation.'

3.1.1. Traditional Material

The raw material used in the past in identifiable geographical origins is still being used today, taking into account the cases where use of name was abandoned but was brought back again, and its characteristics are in accordance with currently in force specifications of European and national legislation.

3.1.2. Traditional Formulation

The formulation in terms of ingredients, which has been transmitted from generation to generation, even if the formulation was abandoned for a period but was brought back to use, is unique or differentiated from the formulation defined by legislation or templates of the wider food group in which the product is listed.

3.1.3. Traditional Type of Production and/or Processing

The production and/or processing of food that has been transmitted from generation to generation through unwritten tradition or other means and is applied until today, even if it has been occasionally abandoned in the past. Despite its adjustment to binding rules from national or European regulations on food hygiene or the incorporation of technological progress, its production and/or processing remains in line with methods used in the past.

3.2. PDO

Regulation (EEC) No 2081/92 distinguishes between two categories of protected names:

- Designations of origin and
- Geographical indications.

The distinction between the two categories depends on how closely the product is linked to the specific geographical area whose name it bears. The regulation also defines the concept of generic names, which cannot be protected.

The protected designation of origin is for products closely associated with the area whose name they bear. In order to become eligible to use a protected designation of origin (PDO), a product must meet two following conditions:

1) The quality or characteristics of the product must be essentially or exclusively due to the particular geographical environment of the place of origin; the geographical environment is taken to include inherent natural and human factors, such as climate, soil quality, and local know-how;
2) The production and processing of the raw materials, up to the stage of the finished product, must take place in the defined geographical area whose name the product bears.

Therefore, there must be an objective and a very close link between the features of the product and its geographical origin. The regulation provides for exceptions to the condition that the name of the product should designate the defined area from which the product comes, in particular that a non-geographical product name may be registered, provided that it is traditionally associated with a given geographical area. For example, the PDO '*Reblochon*' is based upon a traditional name, which designates a French cheese which is exclusively associated with its geographical area of production. Nevertheless, the regulation requires that all the other conditions must be fulfilled: the production area must be precisely defined; all stages of production, processing and preparation must take place in that area, and there must still be the close and objective link mentioned above between the features of the product and its place of origin. Moreover, certain geographical designations can be registered as protected designations of origin although the raw materials (i.e. live animals, meat, milk) of the product come from a geographical area larger than or different from the processing area. In this respect, the regulation provides for a limited period to register these names, in order to take into account some very specific situations previously covered by national laws. Examples include "*Prosciutto di Parma*" and "*Roquefort*."

3.3. PGO and GI

A geographical indication (GI) is "a sign, used on goods that have a specific geographical origin and possess qualities or a reputation that are due to that place of origin".

Products protected by geographical indications (GIs) must have qualities linked to their territory of origin. The character and strength of the quality/geographical link varies according to the natural and cultural history of the resources and their transformation processes, and the legal framework in which the GI develops. The increasing use of GIs worldwide reflects that economic stakes involved in the commercial use of geographical names are high, and that diverse stakeholders perceive in origin-labeled products a strategy that promotes rural development. GI protection involves recognizing a collective, exclusive right to the use in trade of a geographical name or symbol on an item or product. The GI-labeled product represents a public good because its intrinsic characteristics have patrimonial values that belong to nobody in particular: a reputation built collectively over generations. This is why GI management is delegated by the State and their patrimonial character justifies public intervention against misuse. GIs are usually geographical names but they can also be just symbols or icons, as long as they convey geographical information. Legally, the options for GI protection include defense against unfair competition (*e.g.* through litigation or fraud repression) and positive protection through registration under various forms (such as designations or appellations of origin, protected geographical indications or certification trademarks). Figure 1 presents a schematic overview of available GI protection schemes. Although the diversity of legal approaches to GI protection might suggest that it is a subject difficult to grasp, it has a basic, simple rationale: to provide producers with legal protection against "free riders" and give them the means through which to differentiate their product on the market. A broad definition of GIs helps to avoid cultural or geographical bias in a study that seeks to provide an overview of current trends in GI development worldwide (Larson 2007, Anon. 1993a, 1993b, 1996a, 1996b, 1997).

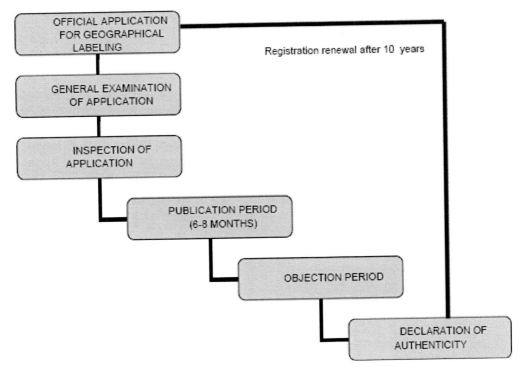

Figure 1.

The protected geographical indication (PGI) also designates products attached to the region whose name they bear; but the link is of a different nature than that between the product with a PDO and its geographical area or origin. To be eligible to use a protected geographical indication a product must meet condition that it must be produced in the geographical area whose name it bears. Unlike the protected designation of origin, it is sufficient that one of the stages of production has taken place in the defined area. For example, the raw materials used in production may have come from another region; there must also be a link between the product and the area, which gives its name. However, this feature does not need to be, as in the case of the protected designation of origin, essential or exclusive, and it allows a more flexible objective link. A specific quality, reputation or other characteristic be attributable to the geographical origin is sufficient (Larson 2007).

Under the rules for protected geographical indications, the link may consist simply in the reputation of the product, if it owes its reputation to its geographical origin. In this case, the actual characteristics of the product are not the determining factor for registration; it is enough for the name of the product to enjoy an individual reputation based specifically on its origin at the time the application for registration is lodged (Larson 2007).

These rules are based on the idea that a geographical indication deserves protection even though it cannot be proven that the product owes its special features to its region of origin. The indication may be very regarded, and be a necessary factor in building up and maintaining a following among customers. Based on the characteristics of their products, producers decide whether to apply for a PDO or a PGI (Larson 2007).

3.4. TSG

The purpose of this regulation is to take advantage of the typical features of products by granting a certificate of specific character. To be registered under these provisions, a product must have features that distinguish it from other products. First, it must have a 'specific character'. The exact definition of the "specific character" in the regulation is: 'the feature or set of features which distinguishes an agricultural product or foodstuff clearly from other similar products or foodstuffs, belonging to the same category'. For example, some these features could be listed as its taste, or the specific raw materials. Under the definition in the regulation, specific character does not consist in:

- A particular presentation (e.g. particularly luxurious or attractive packaging that no other
- product would have);
- A composition or mode of production simply meeting the requirements of mandatory rules or voluntary standards;
- A specific provenance or geographical origin;
- The results of applying technological innovation.

Under the regulation, traditional character is an essential additional element for the purposes of the certificate of specific character. In this context, traditional character means that the product is:

- Produced using traditional raw materials, or is characterized by a traditional composition; or by a mode of production and/or processing reflecting a traditional mode of production and/or processing.

Thus the regulation lays down two conditions for registration of a product name: the product must possess features that distinguish it from other products, and it must be a traditional product. Besides these two conditions relating to the product itself, the name must also satisfy certain requirements. It must either be specific in itself, i.e. it must be clearly distinguished from other names, and will often be untranslatable, (e.g. *Gueuze*) or express the specific character of the foodstuff (e.g. traditional farm-fresh turkey). If the name does not refer to features of the product, but is specific in itself, it should be traditional or be established by custom. Finally, the name may not include any geographical term covered by the regulation on the protection of geographical indications and designations of origin.

These definitions and conditions for registration clearly show the basic principle of this regulation:

- Differentiation from the mass, as a factor in competitiveness; in this case, differentiation relates, not to geographical origin, but to other specific features or 'character'. Only producers complying with the registered product specification may use the indication "traditional speciality guaranteed".

4. AUTHENTICATION PROCEDURES

This section sets out the procedures for the registration of protected geographical indications, protected designations of origin, and traditional specialties guaranteed as updated on 1 July 2004 (Larson 2007).

4.1. Registration of PGI and PDO Related to an Area Located in the Community

The Community registration procedure is the same for protected geographical indications and for protected designations of origin. The present section sets out the procedure as regards PGIs and PDOs related to an area located in the Community. The procedure as regards PGIs and PDOs related to areas outside the Community is explained in the following section.

4.1.1. Procedure at National Level

Registration is the outcome of a private voluntary initiative on the part of the producers concerned. The first step is to fill an application for registration.

4.1.1.1. The Applicant

The system is voluntary and open. Any producer located in the area and respecting the conditions of production specified in the product specification is entitled to use the registered name to market its product. Therefore, as a principle, applications are made in the name of producer groups. A 'group' means any association of farmers, producers and/or processors dealing with the same product. Other interested parties, for example consumers, may also participate in the group. Such groups prepare the application for registration of their products together. As an exception, according to Commission Regulation (EEC) No 2037/93 which lays down implementing rules for PDOs and PGIs, when there is only one person or company in the area producing the product bearing the name to be registered; the single producer may, in this case, apply for registration if no one else uses certain local manufacturing processes, and if the area defined is clearly different from neighboring areas, or if the product is different from other products. However, the specifications will be checked in order to ensure that they are not formulated in such a way that gives any of the producers a monopoly over the product. In fact, according to Regulation (EEC) No 2081/92, any producer who is established in the defined geographical zone may use the name as long as all the conditions of the specifications are fulfilled. The specifications must be transparent, clearly defined and made public. This must be ensured through the precise and thorough description of the given product and its method of production.

4.1.1.2. The Content of the Application

The application must state clearly whether the name is to be registered as a protected geographical indication or as a protected designation of origin. The application for registration of a name must include the following elements: the product specification providing information for each required element as laid out in Article 4 of Regulation (EEC) No 2081/92; all other supporting documents upon which the Member State decides that the application is complete. For example, such documents could include the results of surveys or literary works proving the reputation of a name or maps showing the particular natural elements of a geographical zone. Additional illustrative documents such as photos, menus, recipes or invoices can be useful.

A summary application should have two objectives:

1) This launches the procedure at Community level;
2) The summary is published in the Official Journal of the European Union in all the official languages of the EU, which allows any person demonstrating a legitimate economic interest to consult and object to the application. The specifications are of major importance to producers: they establish the conditions to be observed subsequently. From this point of view, producers make their own rules, and the discipline required is self-imposed. The specifications must include all the necessary information so that new producers in the geographical zone, for example, have these specifications at their disposal if they wish to start production of the specified product. These specifications should be provided by the concerned authorities or by the group of producers. New producers will also have to be sure that they comply with current national rules and that their products are submitted to the inspection mechanism appointed for the name. Moreover, the specifications are the main evidence in support of the application. It is in the interests of the producers to provide all the required and necessary information in order to enable the application to be properly assessed. Producers are free to formulate conditions as they see; the only constraint is that the specifications must show that the requirements of registration are fulfilled. Once formulated, the conditions are of course binding and constitute the

reference point for inspections. Only products that comply with the conditions are eligible to be marketed and sold under the protected designation of origin or the protected geographical indication. The specifications may, however, be changed later, taking into consideration in particular the development of scientific or technical knowledge or redefinition of the geographical zone: the regulation provides for a uniform community procedure for applying to the commission for such a change. The specifications are therefore determining factors both in obtaining registration and in imposing discipline on conditions of manufacture. It will always be well worth expending considerable efforts to draw up suitable specifications, and ensuring that they are specific and detailed enough to allow misuse of the registered name to be effectively prevented.

4.1.1.3. Main Elements of the Specification for PDOs and PGIs

Name

This section should include the name of a region, a specific place, or, in exceptional cases, a country (remark: in principle, names of countries cannot be registered; nevertheless, it is possible when the area of the country presents homogeneous characteristics as regards those factors that refer particular features on the product). In the case of a PDO, it can be a traditional name, not necessarily geographical, indicating an agricultural product or foodstuff originating exclusively from a specific region or defined geographical area.

In addition, a name may not be registered where:

- It conflicts with the name of a plant variety or an animal breed and as a result is likely to mislead the public as to the true origin of the product;
- In the light of a trademark's reputation and renown and the length of time it has been used, registration is liable to mislead the consumer to the true identity of the product.

Examples of possible confusion with plant varieties or animal breeds include the French cheese name "*Abondance*" that was registered as a protected designation of origin although it also designates a cattle breed. Nevertheless, it was considered that there could be no possible confusion between the cheese and the breed. In the case of the Portuguese designation "*Carnalentejana*", it was shown that the traditional designation used for the meat was the same as that used for the breed. But, as the breed "*Alentejana*" had always been produced exclusively in the geographical area concerned, it was considered that this would not confuse the consumer. This must in the first place be appreciated by the Member State concerned. Another interesting case, which could not give rise to confusion, is that of the Greek designation for olives "*Konservolia Stylidas*", because it is composed of the name of a variety, *Konservolia* and the name of the geographical area, *Stylida*. An example of possible conflict with trademarks concerns the geographical indication "*Bayerisches Bier*". Following notification of the application by the German authorities to register the name as a protected geographical indication, the Dutch and Danish authorities informed the Commission of the existence of trademarks used for beer, which include that name (the Dutch trademark "*Bavaria*" and the Danish trademark "*Høker Bajer*"). In the light of information available, it was, however, considered that registration of the name "*Bayerisches Bier*" was not liable to mislead the consumer as to the true identity of the product and the name was registered. Therefore the trademark and the geographical indication may coexist on the market.

Description

This section must include the raw materials to be used and, where appropriate, the principle:

a) Physical (shape, color, weight, etc.);
b) Chemical (minimum fat content, maximum water content, etc.);
c) Microbiological (type of bacteria present, etc.);
d) Biological (race, species, etc.);
e) And/or organoleptic (colour, taste, flavour, odour, etc.) characteristics of the product or
f) foodstuff.

The significance of this section is to put forward the specificity of the product. In other words, the specificity allows the objective differentiation of the product from other products of the same category through characteristics conferred on the product by its origin. A precise description is not only an essential element allowing producers to better respect the determined features of the product, but also a guideline for controls. It will help official inspection services from all Member States to better recognize the genuine product and to prevent fraud throughout the entire EU territory.

It is also important to indicate how the product can be presented. For example, the protected name could be reserved to the product being fresh or whole. If the name is allowed to designate the product in a further stage, for instance processed, cut, sliced, grated and/or packaged, this has to be specified as well as any specific conditions required. This will allow the applicant to determine at or until which point of transformation the product displays the characteristics of the name.

Geographical Area

This is the area in which the production and/or processing takes place, with evidence of production within the defined area. Generally, the limits of the area are naturally defined by natural and/or human factors which give the final product its particular characteristics.

In certain cases, the area will be defined by administrative borders. Supporting documents, such as maps, must be provided for this section.

Proof of Origin

This section refers to evidence that the agricultural product or foodstuff originates in the geographical area. This is related to the 'traceability' of a product, i.e. following the product's path from its area of production to its final destination. The specification must include the measures taken to ensure this traceability, for example register-keeping and specific controls. Illustrative documents such as flow-charts or tables showing all the steps of the process and control points could be helpfully provided.

Method of Production

The method outlined in this section must be explained in such a way so as to allow any producer within the region to produce the given product on the basis of the information given in the specification. This should include: method of obtaining the agricultural product or foodstuff; if appropriate, the authentic and unvarying local methods of production; in certain cases, information concerning the packaging, if the group making the request, determines and justifies that the packaging must be undertaken in the limited geographical area to safeguard quality, ensure 'traceability' or ensure control. If operations such as grating, slicing and/or packaging have to be undertaken in the geographical area, this provision must be justified in order to prove that it is necessary and proportionate to the objective of protection of the name in terms of safeguarding the quality and authenticity of the product (see judgments of the Court in Cases C-496/00 and C-108/01) on the condition that a cheese is grated and packaged in the region of production and the requirement for ham to be sliced and packaged in the region of production. A list of relevant cases is provided in the Annex.

Link

The explanation of the 'link' is the most important element of the product specification with regard to registration. The link must provide an explanation of why a product is linked to one area, and not another, i.e. how far the final product is affected by the characteristics of the region in which it is produced. For both PDOs and PGIs, demonstrating that a geographical area is specialized in a certain production is not enough in order to justify the link. In all cases, the effect of geographical environmental or other local conditions on the quality of the product should be emphasized.

Labeling

Specific labeling details relating to the indication PDO or PGI, whichever is applicable, or the equivalent traditional national indications should be laid out in this section. Conditions of labeling a product which uses PDO and/or PGI products as ingredients could also feature in this section if the producer group determines provisions in this respect. Nevertheless, such provisions should always be examined to see whether they are necessary and proportionate to the objective of protection of the name registered.

It is therefore possible for a producer group to set out a requirement that the protected name may not be used on the label of final products if a similar product to the PDO or the PGI is used at the same time in the composition of the final product. It would not be acceptable, however, to require that the final product be produced in the same geographical area as the PDO or PGI to be used. Nevertheless, the possibility exists to cite the registered name in the list of ingredients according to the rules of Directive 2000/13/EC of the European Parliament and of the Council on the approximation of the laws of the Member States relating to the labeling, presentation and advertising of foodstuffs.

The Community logo may only be used on the product covered by the registration. In other words it cannot be used on a product that only includes a PDO or PGI as an ingredient, or when the product is a mixture of different PDOs or PGIs.

4.1.1.4. The Authorities Concerned First: The Member State

As outlined above, the initiative for introducing an application for registration must come from a group of farmers, producers, processors and/or consumers. The application to register the name of a geographical area must then be sent, along with the specification of the product that is to bear the name, to the appropriate authorities in the Member State where that area is located. A list of relevant national authorities may be consulted on the commission's official website at : http://europa.eu.int/comm/agriculture/foodqual/quali1_en.htm.

The national authority checks the application, if the requirements of the regulation are found to be satisfied, and that registration of the name as a protected geographical indication or protected designation of origin is appropriate, the application is forwarded to the European Commission. If it is not found appropriate, applicants are informed of this negative outcome and the application process is discontinued. This highlights the importance of Member States ensuring a thorough examination of each application before transmitting it to the Commission, in order to ensure that all requirements are met.

Member States have to make sure that they transmit a complete application to the Commission, including all documents described in section 2.1.1. National rules may be established on preparation of the application, especially of the summary application. For example, it might be decided that a draft version should be prepared by the relevant authorities and then submitted for approval of the group of producers.

When the application is forwarded, the Member State may grant a transitional national protection period for the name, starting from the date of transmission of the application to the Commission until the date upon which a decision on registration under the regulation is taken, as laid out in Regulation (EEC) No 2081/92.

If a group of producers applies for the registration of a name that designates a border geographical area, or a traditional name connected to that geographical area situated in another country; the 16 national authorities must consult the relevant authorities of this country before transmitting the application to the Commission. These provisions is aimed at establishing whether a product is being produced elsewhere under the same name, on both sides of the border, as well as try to find an overall solution to the problem. One solution, for example, could consist of the establishment of a common specification and a joint application with a third country or Member State concerned. In this case, producers would be able to keep their rights to use the name, even if they represent a minority of producers located in a country different from that where the majority is located.

4.1.1.5. National Objections Procedure

Based on general rules of good administrative conduct, Member States have a national objections procedure. Before an application is forwarded to the European Commission, the relevant Member State authorities must examine the application thoroughly. Any legitimately concerned natural or legal person should normally be provided with the opportunity to object to an application for registration at national level. All such objections coming from the same Member State should be dealt with before submitting the application to the Commission 4. This is particularly important since objections coming from the same Member State cannot be examined during the procedure at Community level.

4.1.2. Procedure at Community Level

The appropriate forms and practical instructions can be requested from the Commission services, or downloaded from the Commission's official website at the following address: http://europa.eu.int/comm/ agriculture/foodqual/quali1 en.htm.

4.1.2.1. Examination by the Commission

The Commission examines the applications received. It has six months to verify, by means of a formal investigation, that the application comprises all the particulars required, and that the name qualifies for protection. If the Commission finds that the application is lacking in clarity and evidence, it may request supplementary information from the Member State. In this case, the timing is halted and the period of six months recommends at zero from the date the Member State's reply is received.

4.1.2.2. First Publication

If the Commission finds that the application meets the requirements for registration, it publishes the summary application in the Official Journal of the European Union. Within a six-month period from the date of publication, statements of objection can be transmitted to the Commission.

4.1.2.3. Objections Procedure

If a statement of objection is received, the objections procedure is also initiated. Statements of objection must be sent to the Commission by a Member State, although objections will usually originate with economic and business interests rather than with government departments. WTO members as well as recognized third countries may also send objections to an application. It is therefore up to the Member States to see that all interested parties are able to consult the applications published, and to notify the appropriate national authorities in good time of any objections they may have. Statements of objection generally come from manufacturers who use the designation for which protection is sought.

A statement of objection is may be under consideration only if it shows that the product does not meet the conditions required; or if it shows that the name is a generic name, and therefore not eligible for registration; or if it shows that registration of the name would jeopardize the existence of an entirely or partly identical name or of a mark, or the existence of products legally on the market for at least five years preceding the date of the publication provided for in Article 6(2) of the regulation.

When the Commission receives a statement of objection, it first examines its admissibility.

If the Commission finds that the objection is not eligible to take under consideration, it is rejected. The registration procedure continues as normal. Once the six-month period for objections has expired, the name will be accepted as "registered".

However, if the objection is eligible, the Commission passes the matter to the concerned Member States, with a request to them to reach a mutually acceptable solution, under the so-called 'amicable procedure', within three months. Once again, final decision is left up to the Member States whenever possible, so as to improve the chances of acceptable decisions. If the Member States cannot reach to an agreement, the Commission must make a decision within the framework of the Regulatory Committee.

The objections procedure thus ensures that names will not be unjustifiably protected. By allowing all interested parties to have their say, the procedure helps to guarantee a well-balanced decision.

4.1.2.4. Second Publication

If no statement of objection is received within six months of publication in the Official Journal or if the outcome of the objection procedure is a decision to register, the name is recorded by the Commission to the register of protected designations of origin and protected geographical indications. This list of registered names may be consulted in the 'food quality policy' section of the Commission's official website.

4.1.2.5. Rejection of Applications

If the Commission concludes that the name does not qualify for protection, it can decide, in accordance with the Regulatory Committee procedure (explained in section 3), to refuse the application. In that case, the name is not registered. If an agreement cannot be reached within the Committee itself; the Commission may then bring the case to the Council's attention, where a positive decision for registration may be taken only by unanimity if the Commission does not change its proposal.

4.1.2.6. Cancellation of Registration

Regulation (EEC) No 2081/92 provides information about the two cases of possible cancellation of the registration of a name. This would be possible at the request of a group or a natural or legal person concerned if the national authorities decide to forward the request to the Commission. Another case would be for well-founded reasons where compliance with the specifications laid down for an agricultural product or foodstuff bearing the protected name can no longer be ensured.

4.2. Registration of PGI and PDO Rto an Area Located Outside the Community

The regulation also provides for the registration of geographical indications and designations of origin related to areas located outside the Community. The applicable procedures are closely parallel to those applicable for the registration of PGIs and PDOs from within the Community. The present section will therefore set out only some specific aspects relevant to PGIs and PDOs relating to areas outside the Community. According to Article 12 (1) of Regulation (EEC) no. 2081/92, subject to international agreements, the Regulation may apply to an agricultural product or foodstuff from a third country provided that:

1) The third country is able to give guarantee identical or equivalent to those referred to in Article 4;
2) The third country concerned has inspection arrangements and a right to objection equivalent to those laid down in the Regulation;

3) The third country concerned is prepared to provide protection equivalent to those available in the Community to corresponding agricultural products for foodstuffs rooted from the Community.

In accordance with Article 12 (3) of Regulation (EEC) no. 2081/92, the Commission shall examine, at the request of the country concerned, and in accordance with the procedure laid down in Article 15 of the Regulation, whether these conditions are fulfilled.

However, the conditions in Article 12 (1) of Regulation (EEC) no. 2081/92 are without prejudice to international agreements. Relevant international agreements include the WTO Agreements, in particular the TRIPS Agreement. Since under the TRIPS Agreement, WTO Members are obliged to provide protection to geographical indications, the conditions set out in Article 12 (1) do not apply to WTO Members. Accordingly, an application for registration of a PGI or PDO relating to an area located in a WTO Member may be made without a prior Commission decision on the basis of Article 12 (3) of Regulation (EEC) no. 2081/92. Any application for the registration of a PGI or PDO relating to an area located in a WTO Member or a third country recognized in accordance with Article 12 (3) of Regulation (EEC) no. 2081/92 shall be sent to the authorities in the country in which the geographical area is located. The product specifications must be accompanied by the product specifications referred to in Article 4 of the Regulation. In accordance with Article 12a (2) of Regulation (EEC) no. 2081/92, if the third country referred to in paragraph 1 deems the requirements of this Regulation to be satisfied, it shall transmit the registration application to the Commission accompanied by:

1) A description of the legal provisions and the usage on the basis of which the designation of origin or the geographical indication is protected or established in the country,
2) A declaration that the inspection structures provided for in Article 10 are established on its territory, and
3) Other documents on which it has based its assessment on to.

The participation of the home country of the PGI or PDO is crucial for the proper conduct of the registration procedure. The evaluation of applications for the registration of PGIs or PDOs requires detailed knowledge of the conditions in the specific geographical area, which frequently only the home country will have. Moreover, the evaluation of whether a PGI or PDO is protected in its country of origin requires an examination of questions of law of the third country involved, which the country is best placed to carry out. The further procedure for the registration is set out in Article 12b of Regulation (EEC) no. 2081/92, which is closely parallel to Articles 6 and 7 of the Regulation. For details, reference can therefore 19 be made to Section 2.1 above. In accordance with Article 12b (2), any natural or legal person with a legitimate interest from a Member State, a WTO Member, or a third country recognized in accordance with Article 12 (3) of the Regulation may object to an application regarding the registration of a PDO/PGI from outside the EC. As regards the registration of PGIs or PDOs from within the Community, a similar right of objection is provided in Article 12d (1) for any natural or legal person with a legitimate interest which is resident or established in a WTO Member or a third country recognized in accordance with Article 12 (3) of the Regulation. As in the case of objections from individuals that are resident or established in a Member State;

the statement of objection must be transmitted by the third country where the individual is resident or established.

4.3. Registration of a TSG

The procedure for registering a certificate of specific character is very similar to that for protected geographical indications and protected designations of origin. Applications for a certificate of specific character must also be sent in the first instance to the competent authorities in the Member States. Once again, applicants must be producer groups. The application must be accompanied by specifications enabling compliance with the conditions for registration to be checked. The specifications must include at least:

The name to be registered ; a description of the method of production, including the nature and characteristics of the raw material and/or ingredients used and/or the method of preparation of the product, referring to its specific character; aspects allowing appraisal of traditional character; a description of the characteristics of the product giving its main physical, chemical, microbiological and/or organoleptic characteristics which relate to the specific character; the minimum requirements and inspection procedures to which the specific character is subject.

The main points of the specification have to be summarized in a summary application. If the Member State considers that these requirements are fulfilled, the application is forwarded to the Commission. The Commission translates the applications and forwards them to the other Member States. The summary application is then published at the Official Journal of the European Union, after which objections may be lodged. The objections procedure follows the same course as that described above for protected geographical indications and protected designations of origin. Once a final positive decision has been reached, the name is recorded to the register of certificates of specific character and is published along with the main points referred to above in the Official Journal of the European Union.

5. IMPORTANCE IN AUTHENTICATION OF CHEESES

Cheese is one of the major protein source (Ünlü et al. 2010). There are many varieties and many types of cheese. The technological aspect in manufacturing classifies these cheese types. Globalization of food sources and increasing import of food goodies has been leading a question of patenting and protecting the originality of food products. In last two decades of 20th century and awareness rising among people who consumes these foods became clearer. Additionally, the increasing trend in organic food demand has become more visible. People have more tendencies to consume organic produced food. In many countries organic food and authentic food, even they differ from each other significantly, are usually accepted as same things (Jordana 2000, Larson 2007). For a significant comprehension good manufacturing practices, organic product and authentic food terms are explained in previous sections.

6. AUTHENTICATION STATUS OF CHEESES

Table. Some examples for PDO and PGI cheeses

Name of the Cheese	Country	Declaration Date	Authentication Type
Gailtaler Almkäse	Austria	24.1.97	(PDO)
Tioler Bergkäse	Austria	13.6.97	(PDO)
Vorarlberger Alpkäse	Austria	13.6.97	(PDO)
Fromage de Herve	Belgium	2.7.96	(PDO)
Danablu	Denmark	21.6.96	(PGI)
Esrom	Denmark	21.6.96	(PGI)
Allgäuer Bergkäse	Germany	24.1.97	(PDO)
Odenwälder Frühstückskäse	Germany	25.11.97	(PDO)
Metsovone	Greece	21.6.96	(PDO)
San Michali	Greece	21.6.96	(PDO)
Cabrales	Spain	21.6.96	(PDO)
Idiazábal	Spain	21.6.96	(PDO)
Mahón	Spain	21.6.96	(PDO)
Roncal	Spain	21.6.96	(PDO)
Quesucos de Liébana	Spain	21.6.96	(PDO)
Queso de l'Alt Urgell y la Cerdanya	Spain	7.11.00	
Queso Majorero	Spain	20.2.99	(PDO)
Roquefort	France	21.6.96	(PDO)
Bleu d'Auvergne	France	21.6.96	(PDO)
Emmental de Savoi	France	21.6.96	(PGI)
Mozzarella di Bufala Campana	Italy	21.6.96	PDO
Single Gloucester	United Kingdom	21.6.96	(PDO)
Dorset Blue Cheese	United Kingdom	23.12.98	(PGI)

CONCLUSION

Protection of authentic products shows more importance due to the increasing demand in markets. Cheeses are more important in this perspective. The explained protocol mentioned throughout the article is easy to apply and sustainable for future extensions.

Authentication of cheeses will help producer to sustain their authenticity and fulfill the demand. Even there exists an ethical question about some PGI products the authentication process must be applied by all countries.

REFERENCES

Anonymous, 2004, Protection of geographical indications, designations of origin and certificates of specific character for agricultural products and foodstuffs, Working document of commission services, Guide to community regulations, 2nd Ed., European Commission Directorate General for Agriculture Food Quality Policy in the European Union.

Anonymous, 1992a, Council Regulation (EEC) No 2081/92 of 14 July 1992 on the protection of geographical indications and designations of origin for agricultural products and foodstuffs *OJ L 208 24.07.1992 p.1.*

Anonymous, 1992b, Council Regulation (EEC) No 2082/92 of 14 July 1992 on certificates of specific character for agricultural products and foodstuffs *OJ L 208 24.07.1992 p.9.*

Anonymous, 1993a, Commission Regulation (EEC) No 1848/93 of 9 July 1993 laying down detailed rules for the application of Council Regulation (EEC) No 2082/92 on certificates of specific character for agricultural products and foodstuffs *OJ L 168 10.07.1993 p.35.*

Anonymous, 1993b, Commission Regulation (EEC) No 2037/93 of 27 July 1993 laying down detailed rules of application of Council Regulation (EEC) No 2081/92 on the protection of geographical indications and designations of origin for agricultural products and foodstuffs *OJ L 185 28.07.1993 p.5.*

Anonymous, 1996a, Commission Regulation (EC) No 1107/96 of 12 June 1996 on the registration of geographical indications and designations of origin under the procedure laid down in Article 17 of Council Regulation (EEC) No 2081/92 *OJ L 148 21.06.1996 p.1.*

Anonymous, 1996b, Commission Regulation (EC) No 2400/96 of 17 December 1996 on the entry of certain names in the 'Register of protected designation of origin and protected geographical indications' provided for in Council Regulation (EEC) No 2081/92 on the protection of geographical indications and designations of origin for agricultural products and foodstuffs *OJ L 327 18.12.1996 p.11.*

Anonymous, 1997, Commission Regulation (EC) No 2301/97 of 20 November 1997 on the entry of certain names in the 'Register of certificates of specific character' provided for in Council Regulation (EEC) No 2082/92 on certificates of specific character for agricultural products and foodstuffs *OJ L 319, 21.11.1997 p.8-9.*

Anonymous, 2004, Commission Regulation (EC) No 383/2004 of 1 March 2004 laying down detailed rules for applying Council Regulation (EEC) No 2081/92 as regards the summary of the main points of the product specifications *OJ L 64 02.03.2004 p.16.*

Jordana, 2000, Traditional foods: challenges facing the European food industry, *Food Research International*, 33 (2000) 147-152.

Larson J, 2007, Relevance of geographical indications and designations of origin for the sustainable use of genetic resources. Global Facilitation Unit for Underutilized Species Via dei Tre Denari, 472/a, 00057 Maccarese Rome, Italy

Unlu T., Koluman A., Burkan ZT, Akçelik EN, Calim HD., Ata Z., 2010, Incidence and antimicrobial resistance of generic *E.coli* isolated from cheese. *J Food Safety*, Accepted for publication.

In: Cheese: Types, Nutrition and Consumption
Editor: Richard D. Foster, pp. 89-105

ISBN 978-1-61209-828-9
© 2011 Nova Science Publishers, Inc.

Chapter 4

SPANISH BLUE CHEESES: FUNCTIONAL METABOLITES

Sivia M. Albillos[1], Carlos García-Estrada[1] and Juan-Francisco Martín[1,2]

[1] Instituto de Biotecnología de León (INBIOTEC), Avda. Real n°. 1, Parque Científico de León, 24006 León, Spain

[2] Área de Microbiología, Departamento de Biología Molecular, Universidad de León, Campus de Vegazana s/n; 24071 León, Spain

ABSTRACT

Blue cheeses are produced from cow's milk, sheep's milk, or goat's milk depending on the variety. They always have *Penicillium* cultures added, along with the lactic acid bacteria starter cultures (*Lactococcus lactis* and *Leuconostoc cremoris*), so that the final product is spotted or veined throughout with blue, blue-gray or blue-green mold. The aftertaste is a little salty and sharp and its characteristic smell is often produced by metabolites released by the bacteria *Brevibacterium linens*. *Penicillium roqueforti* utilizes β-ketoacyl-CoA deacylase (thiohydrolase) and β-ketoacid decarboxylase to provide the compounds typical for the aroma of the blue semi-soft cheeses. The production of blue cheeses is basically concentrated on a few countries around the world, such as France, Spain, Italy, England and Denmark. Throughout history, there are vestiges that the Roquefort region produced cheese as long as 3,500 years ago, being often considered a delicatessen and prohibitive because of its costly price and political reasons. Roquefort has been named as the "king of cheeses" or the "cheese of the king" due to the veneration that the emperor Charlemagne and several French kings had for this type of product.

In Spain, several blue-veined cheeses of excellent quality are produced, being the region on the north area of Picos de Europa the one with more varieties (Cabrales, Valdeón, Bejes-Tresviso, Picón, among others that carry a legally Protected Designation of Origin). Our research group has recently studied some of these varieties and characterized the *Penicillium* species present in the blue cheese. Interestingly, we have found that *P. roqueforti*, the main of these species, produces important secondary metabolites with functional properties, such as the antitumor andrastins and mycophenolic acid, together with mycotoxins (roquefortine C and PR toxin). Efforts have been made by our group in order to shed light on the biosynthetic pathways for those secondary metabolites with the aim of engineering *P. roqueforti* strains with an added value for the cheese industry.

1. INTRODUCTION

The denomination of blue cheese includes a broad variety of cheeses such as the French Bleu and Roquefort, the Italian Gorgonzola, the English Stilton, and many others from Spain, Denmark and the United States. The production processes present some minor differences depending on the cheese variety, but all of them bear in common as their main maturation agent, the fungus *Penicillium roqueforti*.

The manufacture process of these cheeses begins with milk batches that contain high levels of fat, due to the relevant role of lipolysis in the development of their characteristic flavor. Roquefort cheese is elaborated with sheep's milk, while Gorgonzola and Stilton are made of cow's milk with some addition of cream if the fat content is low. Raw milk is used frequently allowing the lipolytic contribution of the natural lipase of milk. As fermenting agents, mesophilic lactic acid bacteria: *Streptococcus lactis, Streptococcus lactis* subsp. *diacetylactis* and *Leuconostoc* spp. are used.

The inoculation of *P. roqueforti* is generally done in liquid culture suspensions added either to the milk or the curd. Some blue cheeses are injected with spores before the curds form and others have spores mixed in with the curds after they form. Cheeses are perforated during maturation in order to increase the oxygen access that may facilitate the fungal growth and development of the fungal metabolism.

The curd is usually cut in cubical shapes and introduced in molds, which are frequently turned over in order to favor the elimination of whey and curd consolidation. The process of salting is done on the curd before molding, or by spreading salt on the surface when the cheese is in the mold. A considerable increase in the acidity occurs in a slow and continued way reaching a pH of 4.5 to 4.7 in 24 hours caused by the lactic bacteria.

Maturation takes place at the initial stages in chambers at 10-13°C and relative humidity of 96%. *P. roqueforti* appears after 8-10 days, spreads through the holes or fissures, reaching the maximum of growth at 30-90 days. Then the cheeses are wrapped in aluminum foil and placed in chambers at lower temperatures (3-6°C), until the end of the aging process. Local varieties of blue cheeses are typically aged in caves, as these have temperature and moisture nearly constant environments, as well as favorable conditions for growth of many varieties of mould. The smell of this food is due to the types of bacteria encouraged to grow on the cheese: the bacterium *Brevibacterium linens* is responsible for the aroma of many blue cheeses (Deetae *et. al.*, 2007).

2. SPECIFICITY OF THE SPANISH BLUE CHEESES

Traditional Spanish blue cheeses are produced in the mountain region of "Picos de Europa", in the geographic area between the provinces of Asturias, Santander and León (north of Spain). The most famous are shown in Figure 1.

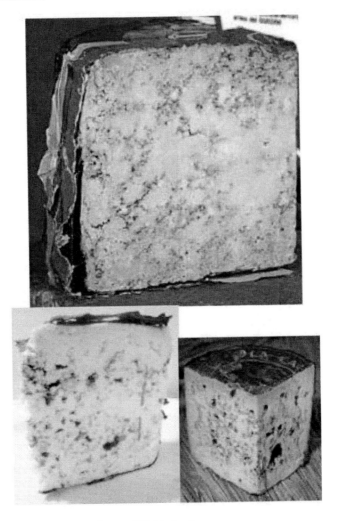

Figure 1. Cabrales, Picón Bejes-Tresviso, and Valdeón cheeses.

The better-known variety of the mould-ripened cheeses is Cabrales, with the major part of the blue cheese production (regulated since 1981 as a Protected Denomination of Origin following the norm EN-45011). The annual production of Cabrales cheese in the year 2009 was ~450,000 kg (298,386 pieces), with an increase of 88.9% since 1974 and shared by 35 certified producers (data published by the Protected Designation of Origin in 2010).

According to an interesting article by Arroyo (2000) on historical data of the Cabrales cheese, the first reference found goes back to the year 962 in a document of May 15th, in the book "Beato de Liébana", indicating that a vineyard was exchanged for a pig, a male goat and seven cheeses. In the X and XI century cheese was a common trade good having monetary value. There is another interesting document of year 980 where a list of cheeses "Nodicia de kesos" is kept by the monk in charge of the pantry in the monastery of Saint Justo and Pastor in La Rozuela (León). This document is one of the first writings in Spanish language following the degeneration of the Latin language (Menéndez Pidal, "Origins of the Spanish language", 27). Cabrales cheese was later cited in the Tratado de Lechería or Dairy Treatise (Fleischmann, 1924), in the Milk Encyclopedia (Agenjo, 1956), in the Larousse des Fromages

(Courtine, 1973) and it is included in the Spanish Cheese Catalog from the Ministry of Agriculture of Spain (since 1974).

The initial studies on the microbiota of the Cabrales cheese were performed by Burgos *et al.* (1971) and focused on the content of lactobacilli during maturation. Results indicated that the maximum level of these bacteria was achieved after 12 days, though counts followed until day 28, with values of $1.2 \times 10^{11} g^{-1}$. One strain was identified as *L. plantarum* and five others as *L. casei* var *casei*. In mature cheese, *P. roqueforti, Penicillium chrysogenum* and *Mucor mucedo* were identified (Sala *et al.*, 1971). Yeasts found were *Kluyveromyces lactis, Candida krusei* and *Trichosporon penicillatum* (Sala and Burgos, 1972).

Arroyo published on 1974 a book (2nd edition 1983) on the industrial improvement of Cabrales cheese, focusing on the analysis of milk, the natural conditions in the caves in the Cabrales area, identifying *P. roqueforti* as the organism responsible for the maturation of this variety of cheese (Fernández-Bodega *et al.*, 2009).

The microbiota evolves throughout the process of elaboration and maturation of the Cabrales cheese (Núñez, 1978); inside the product the main flora are lactic streptococci with a maximum level after 4 days. During the first period of maturation, there is a majority of streptococci and yeasts, while fungi and lactobacilli comprise the dominant flora during the second stage of maturation. On the cheese surface, lactic streptococci are dominant until salting and streptococci, micrococci and leuconostoc are predominant in the second maturation stage. Coliforms present in curd disappear before the first month.

The cheese is produced with raw cow's milk adding small percentages of goat's and ewe's milk. The farmhouse cheeses were elaborated by mixing the milks produced by the cattle. Traditionally, in local cheese-making no lactic bacteria, nor fungi spores, were inoculated. The coagulation of milk was accomplished by adding lamb or kid-goat rennet; this method has been more recently substituted by industrially prepared rennet. Milk is curdled at 28-30°C for 1-2 hours. The cheese curd used to be cut in cubes of 2-4 cm per edge with an instrument with the shape of a spoon two hours after curdling. Soon after, the cut curd is introduced into cylindrical molds kept at 16-18°C for 48 hours. Cheeses are turned over after 24 hours. As no pressure is applied, the final cheeses weight 3-4 kg and have a diameter of 20-22 cm with a height of 8-10 cm. Salting is done covering the cheeses with thick-grain salt during 48 hours at 16-18°C and a turnover after 24 hours. The maturation is performed in two stages: the first one in dry, well-vented rooms, during 10-15 days at 10-12°C, and the second one in natural caves in the mountain for 2-4 months at constant temperatures of 9-10°C and relative humidity of 90-95%, placing the cheeses on their flat sides and turning them over periodically. Sometimes they are perforated to improve air transfer and fungal growth. Once ready, cheeses used to be wrapped in *Acer pseudoplatanus* leaves for their commercialization or storage in refrigerated rooms; actually they are wrapped in aluminum foil.

3. PRODUCTION OF SECONDARY METABOLITES BY *P. ROQUEFORTI*

There is considerable evidence to indicate that most strains of *P. roqueforti* are capable of producing important secondary metabolites (Figure 2) with functional properties, such as the antitumor andrastins and mycophenolic acid (Bentley, 2000; Schneweis *et al.*, 2000; Nielsen *et al.*, 2005; 2006; Fernández-Bodega *et al.*, 2009). In addition, harmful secondary metabolites, such as the PR mycotoxin and its precursors eremofortins A-E, are also produced under certain growth conditions (Teuber and Engel, 1983; López-Díaz et al., 1996). However, these mycotoxins are not found in cheeses, where the related PR-imine and PR-amide are detected instead (Moreau et al., 1980; Chang et al., 1993). Another secondary metabolite that can be found in blue cheeses is roquefortine C (Finoli et al., 2008). This diketopiperazine-alkaloid, which is produced by *P. roqueforti* and other species of the genus *Penicillium*, such as *P. chrysogenum* (Ohmono et al., 1975; Scott et al., 1976; de la Campa et al., 2007), has been described as a mycotoxin (Wagener et al., 1980), although it has been suggested that there is no significant toxicological data to support this premise (Tüller et al., 1998). In fact, the toxicity of roquefortine C is relatively low in comparison with other mycotoxins.

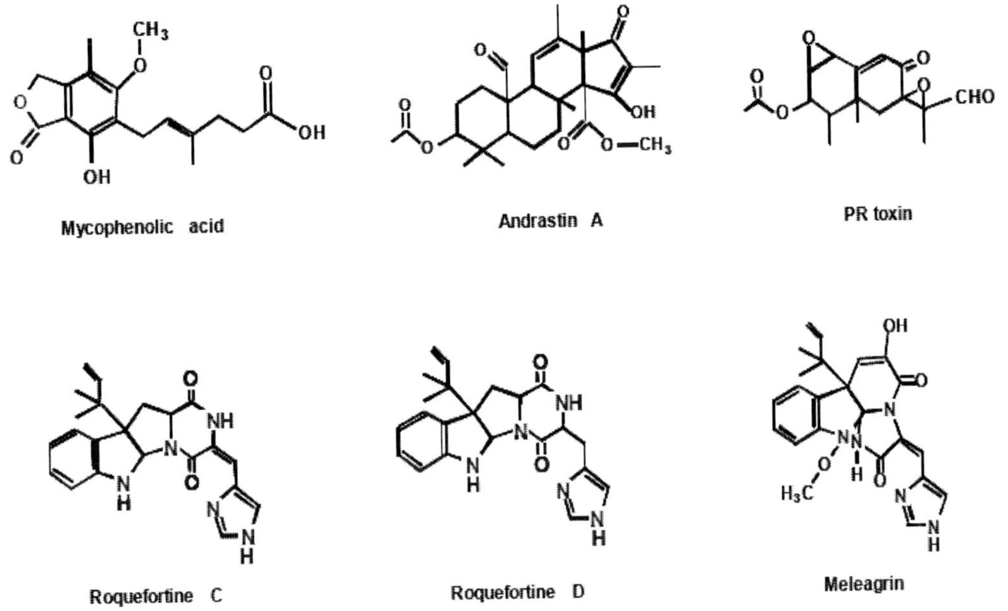

Figure 2. Some secondary metabolites produced by *P. roqueforti*.

3.1. Secondary Metabolites with Potential Beneficial Effects on Human Health: Mycophenolic Acid and Andrastins

3.1.1. Mycophenolic Aacid

Mycophenolic acid ($C_{17}H_{20}O_6$) or 6-(4-hydroxy-6-methoxy-7-methyl-3-oxo-5-phthalanyl)-4-methyl-4-hexenoic acid is a weak organic acid used by the pharmaceutical industry because of its antifungal, antibacterial and antiviral activities (Abraham, 1945; Abrams and Bently, 1959; Cline et al., 1969). This compound is produced by *P. roqueforti* and *Penicillium carneum* (Nielsen et al., 2006) and it naturally occurs in some blue-moulded cheeses and silages (Lafont et al., 1979; Schneweis et al., 2000), but it has never been implicated in livestock health problems due to its apparent low acute toxicity to mammals (Cole and Cox, 1981). Mycophenolic acid is also an immunomodulator, blocking the proliferative response of T and B lymphocytes and inhibiting both antibody formation and the production of cytotoxic T cells (Eugui et al., 1991). This is because mycophenolic acid acts as a noncompetitive inhibitor of eukaryotic inosine monophosphate dehydrogenase (Lee et al., 1985), blocking the *de novo* biosynthesis of purines, which is essential for T and B lymphocytes. Mycophenolic acid and its derivatives have been described as having immunosuppressive and antitumor effects (Ohsugi et. al., 1976, Domhan et. al., 2008) and it is used for the prevention of organ transplant rejection. It has other uses in psoriasis treatment, and produces diarrhea and nausea when the oral dose is too high (Scott, 1981).

The presence of mycophenolic acid in 38% of cheese samples was demonstrated by Lafont et al. (1979), with 0,01-15 ppm and a higher incidence in Roquefort variety (84%). Engel et al. (1982) found after examining 62 strains of *P. roqueforti* that only 7 were able to synthesize mycophenolic acid in YES medium, some of them reaching levels in cheese of up to a maximum of 5 mg kg^{-1}. The production in YES media was of 600 mg ml^{-1}.

3.1.2. Andrastins

Andrastins, which were initially discovered in an antitumor search program at the Kitasato Institute (Tokyo, Japan) (Uchida et al., 1996a; 1996b; Omura et al., 1996), are particularly interesting anticancer drug candidates due to their ability to inhibit the activity of the farnesyltransferases, especially the farnesyltransferase of the RAS proteins. These proteins are subjected to post-translational farnesylation at a cysteine residue, in which a farnesyltransferase is involved. Prenylation of the RAS protein is required for stabilization and binding of the protein to the plasma membrane, which allows the protein to regulate mitogenic signaling pathways and control cell division and the development of cancer (Rho et al., 1998; Uchida et al., 1996a; 1996b; Overy et al., 2005). Andrastins can also inhibit the efflux of antitumor agents and enhance their accumulation in vincristine-resistant cancer cells (Rho et al., 1998). For these reasons, andrastins are potentially important chemotherapeutic compounds.

Four types of andrastins (A, B, C and D) have been described so far (Omura et al., 1996; Nielsen et al., 2005) and all of these types have been detected in different blue cheeses (Nielsen et al., 2005; Fernández-Bodega et al., 2009). Andrastin A appears to be produced in significant amounts by *P. roqueforti* during blue cheese ripening, together with minor amounts of other andrastins (Nielsen et al., 2005). The biosynthetic pathway for andrastins has not yet been elucidated, but it has been suggested that a farnesylpyrophosphate and a tetraketide (the basic molecular structure of the orsellinic acid) are precursor molecules involved in their biosynthesis (Uchida et al., 1996a).

Table 1. Production of andrastins of several mutants of *P. roqueforti* obtained by UV mutagenesis. Percentages of production compared versus the control strain CECT 2905

Strain	Andrastin B µg/ g DM	Andrastin A µg/ g DM	SD Andr. B µg/ g DM	SD Andr. A µg/ g DM	% Andr. B	% Andr. A
CECT 2905	1370.31	15558.61	97.57	743.01	100.00	100.00
Mut 209	1976.18	29557.08	529.27	989.87	144.21	189.97
Mut 231	980.62	11287.96	153.36	746.41	71.56	72.55
Mut 245	541.03	5666.14	40.18	544.80	39.48	36.42
Mut 264	1061.95	12384.49	30.43	890.08	77.50	79.60

SD: Standard Deviation. Mut 209 overproducer. DM: Dry Matter.

Since genetic engineering of *P. roqueforti* to modify this biosynthetic pathway is still difficult, we obtained by random UV mutagenesis *P. roqueforti* strains that overproduce andrastins (Table 1). These strains might be of interest for the cheese industry.

3.2. Mycotoxins

Mycotoxins are secondary metabolites produced by fungi that can produce toxic, carcinogenic, teratogenic and mutagenic effects by acting on cell division, depressing immunologic processes, complexing with the DNA or inhibiting protein synthesis. The biosynthesis of toxins is highly dependent on the water activity (humidity), temperature, pH, substrate composition, oxygen concentration and microbial competition (Northolt and Bullerman, 1982). It has been proven that the presence of mycotoxins is usually very low, with small or even null values in numerous moldy food products. The mycotoxin problems in the cheese industry may come from cheese contamination during maturation or storage or from the inherent presence of mycotoxins in mould ripened cheeses, making necessary high precaution in selecting the fungal ferments and the manufacture and storage conditions. Several are the mycotoxins detected from *P. roqueforti* cultures, some isolated from cheese, such as patulin, penicillic acid, citrinin, PR-toxin and alkaloids.

3.2.1. The PR Toxin

The PR toxin ($C_{17}H_{20}O_6$) is a mycotoxin that belongs to the group of sesquiterpenoids. It is one of the fungal secondary metabolites isolated from cultures of different *P. roqueforti* strains grown on a semisynthetic medium (Wei *et al.*, 1973; 1978). They obtained considerable amounts of toxin from extracts of *P. roqueforti* NRRL 849 incubated during 14 days at 25°C in YES liquid medium in stationary conditions. The toxin had DL_{50} values in rats of 11 and 115 mg kg^{-1} intraperitoneally and orally, respectively. The PR-toxin is a very acute toxin inhibiting "in vivo" the hepatic proteins in rats. It has been described to have inhibitory effect on the mitochondrial HCO-3-ATPase of rat brain, liver and heart (Hsieh *et. al.*, 1986).

The chemical structure of this toxin is well-kwown (Wei et al., 1975) and contains several functional groups: an aldehyde, an acetoxy group, an α, 4-unsaturated ketone and two stable epoxides. The aldehyde group, which is located on C12, appears to be responsible of the biological activity (Moulé *et al.*, 1977; Wei *et al.*, 1979), which is due to the inhibition of protein and RNA synthesis (Moulé *et al.*, 1976; 1978). The PR toxin is lethal in rats and mice by either oral administration or intraperitoneal injection (Wei *et al.*, 1973; 1976; Chen *et al.*, 1982).

The PR toxin biosynthesis has been suggested to proceed via an isoprene biosynthetic pathway (Chalmers *et al.*, 1981), where eremofortin C is the direct precursor of the toxin (Moreau *et al.*, 1980). The skeletons of the PR toxin and eremofortin C are similar to each other and differ only by a hydroxyl functional group in eremofortin C and an aldehyde functional group in the PR toxin at the C12 position (Moreau *et al.*, 1977; Wei *et al.*, 1975). Eremofortin C was isolated and characterized in 1977 by Moreau and co-workers and up to four eremofortins have been described so far (A, B, C and D), none of them showing significant toxicity in laboratory animals (Moulé *et al.*, 1977). According to the proposed biosynthetic pathway (Moreau *et al.*, 1980) eremofortin C seems to be formed after C12 hydroxylation of eremofortin A. In addition to direct isolation from *P. roqueforti* culture medium, eremofortin C can also be obtained by biotransformation of PR toxin and eremofortin A in a reaction catalyzed by liver mixed-function oxidases (Cacan *et al.*, 1977; Moreau *et al.*, 1977). In 1985, Chang and co-workers carried out the isolation or characterization of the 40-kDa oxidase responsible for the conversion of eremofortin C into PR toxin. In addition, chemical transformation of eremofortin C into PR toxin was also achieved through chemical oxidation with a chromic anhydride-pyridine complex (Li *et al.*, 1985).

3.2.1.1. Biosynthesis of Aristolochene: The Precursor Molecule of the PR Toxin

It is believed that the (+) enantiomer of aristolochene is the likely parent compound for several sesquiterpenoid toxins, including the PR toxin, produced by filamentous fungi (Wei *et al.*, 1976; Cane *et al.*, 1987; Kenfield *et al.*, 1989). Cyclization of the isoprenoid pathway intermediate trans, trans-farnesyl pyrophosphate (FPP) is the first step in the biosynthesis of the majority of sesquiterpenoids. This reaction is catalyzed by sesquiterpene cyclases, such as the aristolochene synthase Ari1. This protein was isolated from *P. roqueforti* and consists of a 37-kDa monomer, which showed properties similar to sesquiterpene cyclases (Hohn and Plattner, 1989). The crystal structure of Ari1 revealed active site features that participate in the cyclization of the universal sesquiterpene cyclase substrate, farnesyl pyrophosphate, to form the bicyclic hydrocarbon aristolochene (Caruthers *et al.*, 2000).

The *P. roqueforti* gene encoding Ari1 was isolated and characterized by Proctor and Hohn (1993). The 1129-bp *ari1* gene is present as a single copy in the *P. roqueforti* genome and contains two introns. The protein deduced from this nucleotide sequence contains 342 amino acids with a calculated molecular mass of 39.200 kDa, which is coincident with the molecular mass of the Ari1 protein previously isolated from *P. roqueforti* (Hohn and Plattner, 1989). The *ari1* gene is expressed in stationary phase cultures, where the aristolochene synthase activity is higher and the PR toxin is produced, and appears to be transcriptionally regulated (Proctor and Hohn, 1993).

3.2.1.2. Secondary Metabolites Derived From the Degradation of the PR Toxin

It is well known that the PR toxin is unstable in the presence of blue cheese extracts, amino acids or tryptamine (Scott and Kanhere, 1979). It was proposed that the amino groups from aminoacids and other nitrogen molecules may react with the aldehyde group of the PR toxin, degrading this mycotoxin into PR-imine ($C_{17}H_{21}O_5N$) and PR-amide ($C_{17}H_{21}O_6N$) derivatives in the culture medium of *P. roqueforti* (Chang *et al.*, 1993). Unlike the PR toxin and eremofortins, the PR-imine and PR-amide derivatives can be found in blue cheeses (Moreau *et al.*, 1980; Chang *et al.*, 1993). Unlike the PR-imine, the PR-amide is a stable molecule. The PR-imine was detected when the PR toxin was degraded in the culture medium and it was concluded that the PR-imine was the final product resultant from the degradation of the PR toxin.

Another secondary metabolite derived from the degradation of the PR toxin in the culture medium of *P. roqueforti* is the PR-acid (Chang *et al.*, 1996). The structures of PR-acid ($C_{17}H_{20}O_7$) and PR toxin ($C_{17}H_{20}O_6$) are closely related. The enzyme catalyzing this reaction is the PR oxidase, a monomeric extracellular enzyme (88 kDa) that was purified from the culture broth of *P. roqueforti*. This enzyme is specific for PR toxin and cannot use eremofortin C as substrate (Chang *et al.*, 1998). The characterization of the PR-amide synthetase has provided more information about the PR toxin degradation pathway. This enzyme, which is a 66-kDa monomer, is involved in the conversion of PR-acid into PR-amide and was purified from the culture of *P. roqueforti* (Chang *et al.*, 2004). The PR-amide may simply be formed by the action of a transaminase or an aminotransferase, using glutamine or glutamic acid as aminodonors.

3.2.2 Patulin, Penicillic Acid and Citrinin

Engel and Prokopek (1980) observed an optimal growth of three strains of *P. roqueforti* in blue cheese at 8°C and 15°C without any production of patulin, penicillic acid or citrinin during a maturation period of 80 days. Nevertheless, in YES liquid medium, levels of 340 mg ml^{-1} of patulin at 8°C and 600 mg ml^{-1} of penicillic acid at 15°C were produced.

Patulin does not seem to be synthesized in cheese and penicillic acid does very seldom, according to data from samples of blue cheese (Siriwardana and Lafont, 1979; Erdogan and Sert, 2004). Moreover, the instability of these toxins in the final product (Lieu and Bullerman, 1977) suggests that blue cheese consumption does not pose any risk relating to these mycotoxins.

On the other hand citrinin has been detected in wild type strains of *P. roqueforti*, but not in commercial strains or strains isolated from blue cheese (Scott, 1981).

3.2.3. Roquefortin C and Other Alkaloids

The first article describing the production by *P. roqueforti* of the three alkaloids roquefortin C, roquefortin A and festuclavine, was published in 1975 by Ohmomo *et. al.* The structures of roquefortine and isofumigaclavine A were determined by Scott and Kennedy (1976). The isofumigaclavines A and B correspond to the roquefortines A and B described by Ohmomo and co-workers (1975). The levels of roquefortine A (isofumigaclavin A) found in five cheeses were 0.2-3.6 mg kg^{-1} with traces of festuclavine, roquefortine C and B (Ohmomo *et al.*, 1975). In another study of 12 samples of blue cheese, the levels found were in the average of 424 ng g^{-1} of roquefortine (Ware *et. al.*, 1980).

Roquefortine C is a diketopiperazine-alkaloid mycotoxin that is consistently produced in blue cheeses (Finoli *et al.*, 2001). This alkaloid was isolated from the mycelium of *P. roqueforti* in the 70's (Ohmomo *et al.*, 1975; Scott and Kennedy, 1976) and later from cultures of other *Penicillium* species growing on contaminated feed grain (Häggblom, 1990), onions (Overy *et al.*, 2005), beer (Cole *et al.*, 1983) and wine (Möller *et al.*, 1997). Roquefortine C contamination of food and feedstuff is of great interest because this alkaloid possesses neurotoxic properties in mice (Polonsky *et al.*, 1977) and chicks (Wagener *et al.*, 1980). In addition to the neurotoxic properties, roquefortine C also has antibiotic activity against Gram-positive microorganisms that contain hemins, while the *Clostridium* species, lactic acid bacteria and Gram-negative are not affected by this alkaloid (Kopp-Holtwiesche and Rehm, 1990). It is proved roquefortine's interaction with the cytochrome p450 from rat and human liver (Aninat *et. al.*, 2001). Another aspect of roquefortine is that it inhibits bacterial protein, RNA and DNA synthesis, according to studies by Kopp-Holtwiesche and Rehm (1981) on *Corynebacterium flaccumfaciens*, affecting essentially the RNA synthesis.

The status of roquefortine C as a mycotoxin remains unclear. No toxicity has been detected in feeding experiments despite the wide absorption and distribution of this compound through the tissues examined (Tüller *et al.*, 1998). However, a more recent study showed that roquefortine C is highly toxic when inhaled (Rand *et al.*, 2005), supporting the initial observations on the toxicity of roquefortine C (Ohmomo, 1982).

3.2.3.1. Precursors of the Roquefortine C Biosynthesis

Precursor feeding experiments revealed that tryptophan, histidine and mevalonate are involved in the biosynthesis of roquefortine C (Barrow *et al.*, 1979; Gorst-Allman *et al.*, 1982). In addition to roquefortine C, roquefortine D was also isolated from cultures of *P. roqueforti* (Ohmomo *et al.*, 1978). In parallel, Kozlovskii and co-workers (1980) also identified an alkaloid related to roquefortine C from *P. roqueforti*. This compound was named 3,12-dihydroroquefortine (or isoroquefortine C) and its chemical structure corresponded to that of the roquefortine D. The latter compound has been directly involved in the biosynthetic pathway of roquefortine C, which would be synthesized after dehydrogenation of isoroquefortine C (Richard *et al.*, 2004).

The diketopiperazine precursor of the roquefortine family may originate from tryptophan (or from dimethylallyltryptophan) and histidine activated by a two-module nonribosomal peptide synthetase. Recent evidences from other diketopiperazine alkaloids suggest that the diketopiperazine intermediate is then modified by isoprenylation at C3, ring closure between C2 and N11 to roquefortine D and dehydrogenation to roquefortine C.

Prenylated indole alkaloids are widely distributed in nature, particularly in filamentous fungi (Stocking *et al.*, 2000; Williams *et al.*, 2000; Li, 2009). Interestingly, prenylated indole alkaloids have diverse chemical structures. The isopentenyl group is present in different prenylated trytophan derivatives in almost every position of the indole or indoline ring (Li, 2009). In some of the compounds, the prenyl (isopentenyl) moiety is attached to the indole ring in a 'reverse' mode, i.e. by a connection via its C3' carbon atom. A series of natural products carrying reverse prenyl moieties at position C3 of the indoline rings and an additional ring between the indoline and the diketopiperazine moieties (or their analogues) were identified in different ascomycetes, e.g. roquefortine C from *Penicillium* strains (Finoli *et al.*, 2001; Rundberget *et al.*, 2004) and acetylaszonalenin from *Aspergillus* and *Neosartorya* strains (Kimura *et al.*, 1982; Capon *et al.*, 2003; Wakana *et al.*, 2006; Yin *et al.*, 2009). Recently, it has been reported that formation of the additional ring between the indoline and the diketopiperazine moieties involves a P450 monooxygenase followed by dehydration (Kato *et al.*, 2009).

3.2.3.2. Genes for the Biosynthesis of Roquefortine C and Meleagrin

Although roquefortine C production is best characterized in *P. roqueforti*, there is no information on the genes or enzymes involved in the biosynthesis of this compound. Only the partial sequence of the *dmaW* gene, which encodes a putative dimethylallyl-tryptophan synthase (the first enzyme in the pathway catalysing the prenylation of tryptophan), has been reported. However, data obtained in our laboratory indicate that the protein encoded by this gene might not be involved in the biosynthesis of roquefortine C. Work is now in progress in our laboratory to characterize the roquefortine gene cluster.

CONCLUSION

The present chapter describes relevant characteristics of the elaboration process of the main Spanish blue cheese (Cabrales variety) and explains thoroughly the biochemistry of the most important secondary metabolites produced by *P. roqueforti*, present in this type of cheese. The potential functional properties of the andrastins and mycofenolic acid are described, along with the interest in reducing the excretion by *P. roqueforti* strains of harmful mycotoxins. The chapter has shown the importance and potential of biotechnology in tailoring fungal strains lacking the enzymes involved in the production of toxins while improving the content of beneficial fungal secondary metabolites (Fernández-Bodega *et al.*, 2009). This is extremely relevant for a food market more and more interested in the elaboration of functionalized foods.

REFERENCES

Abraham, E.P. (1945). "The effect of mycophenolic acid on the growth of *Staphylococcus aureus* in heart broth". *Biochem. J.* 39: 398–404.

Abrams, R., and Bently, M. (1959). "Biosynthesis of nucleic acid purines". *Biochim. Biophys. Acta.* 79: 91–97.

Agenjo, C. (1956). Enciclopedia de la leche. Ed. Espasa Calpe, Madrid.

Aninat, C., Hayashi, Y., André, F. and Delaforge, M. (2001). "Molecular requirements for inhibition of cytochrome p450 activities by roquefortine". *Chem. Res. Toxicol.* 14, 1259-1265.

Arroyo M. (2000). Revista Cabrales. Reference from "Beato de Liébana". Cartulario, folio 45, número 162.

Arroyo, M. (1974). Fabricación y estudio del queso de Cabrales. ISBN 84-400-0749-3. Santander.

Barrow, K.D., Colley, P.W., and Tribe, D.E. (1979). "Biosynthesis of the neurotoxin alkaloid roquefortine". *J. Chem. Soc., Chem. Commun.* 225 – 226.

Bentley, R. (2000). "Mycophenolic acid: a one hundred year odyssey from antibiotic to immunosuppressant". *Chem. Rev.* 100: 3801-3826.

Burgos, J.; López, A. and Sala, F.J. (1971). Maduración del queso "Cabrales". Microflora I. Lactobacilos. *An. Fac. Vet. León, 17,* 109.

Cacan, M., Moreau, S., and Tailliez, R. (1977). "In vitro metabolism of *Penicillium roqueforti* toxin (PRT) and a structurally related compound, eremofortin A, by rat liver". *Toxicology* 8: 205-212.

Cane, D.E., Rawlings, B.J., and Yang, C.C. (1987). "Isolation of (-)-gamma-cadinene and aristolochene from *Aspergillus terreus*". J. Antibiot. 40: 1331-1334.

Capon, R.J., Skene, C., Stewart, M., Ford, J., O′Hair, R.A.J., Williams, L., Lacey, E., Gill, J.H., Heiland, K., Friedel, T. (2003). Aspergillicins A–E: five novel depsipeptides from the marine-derived fungus *Aspergillus carneus*. *Org. Biomol. Chem.* 1: 1856–1862.

Caruthers, J.M., Kang, I., Rynkiewicz, M.J., Cane, D.E., Christianson, D.W. (2000). "Crystal structure determination of aristolochene synthase from the blue cheese mold, *Penicillium roqueforti*". *J. Biol. Chem.* 275: 25533-25539.

Chalmers, A.A., de Jesus, A.E., Gorst-Allman, C.P., Steyn, P.S. (1981). Biosynthesis of PR toxin by *Penicillium roqueforti*". *J. Chem. Soc. Perkin Trans.* 1: 2899-2903.

Chang, S.C., Wei, Y.H., Liu, M.L., Wei, R.D. (1985). "Isolation and Some Properties of the Enzyme That Transforms Eremofortin C to PR Toxin". *Appl. Environ. Microbiol.* 49: 1455-1460.

Chang, S., Lu, K., Yeh, S. (1993). "Secondary metabolites resulting from degradation of PR-toxin by *Peniciffium rogueforti*". *Appl. Environ. Microbiol.* 59: 981-986.

Chang, S.C., Yeh, S.F., Li, S.Y., Lei, W.Y., Chen, M.Y. (1996). "A novel secondary metabolite relative to the degradation of PR toxin by *Penicillium roqueforti*". *Curr Microbiol.* 32: 141-146.

Chang, S.C., Lei, W.Y., Tsai, Y.C., Wei, Y.H. (1998). "Isolation, purification, and characterization of the PR oxidase from *Penicillium roqueforti*". *Appl. Environ. Microbiol.* 64: 5012-5015.

Chang, S.C., Ho, C.P., and Cheng, M.K. (2004). "Isolation, purification, and characterization of the PR-amide synthetase from *Penicillium roqueforti*". *Fung. Sci.* 19: 117–123.

Chen, F.C., Chen, C.F., and Wei, R.D. (1982). "Acute toxicity of PR toxin, a mycotoxin from *Penicillium roqueforti*". *Toxicon* 20: 433-441.

Cline, J.C, Nelson, J.D., Gerzon, K., Williams, R.H., Delong, D.C. (1969). "In vitro antiviral activity of mycophenolic acid and its reversal by guanine compounds". *Appl. Microbiol.* 18: 14–20.

Cole, R.J., and Cox, R.H. (1981) Handbook of toxic fungal metabolites. Academic Press, New York.

Cole, R.J., Dorner, J.W., Cox, R.H., Raymond, L.W. (1983). "Two classes of alkaloid mycotoxins produced by *Penicillium crustosum* Thom isolated from contaminated beer". *J. Agric. Food Chem.* 31: 655-657.

Courtine, R. (1973). Larousse des Fromages. Ed. Librarie Larousse, Paris.

de la Campa, R., Seifert, K., Miller, J.D. (2007). "Toxins from strains of *Penicillium chrysogenum* isolated from buildings and other sources". *Mycopathologia.* 163(3): 161-168.

Deetae P, Bonnarme P, Spinnler HE, Helinck S (October 2007). "Production of volatile aroma compounds by bacterial strains isolated from different surface-ripened French cheeses". *Appl. Microbiol. Biotechnol.* 76 (5): 1161–71.

Domhan, S., Muschal, S., Schwager, C., Morath, C., Wirkner, U., Ansorge, W., Maercker, C., Zeier, M., Huber, P.E. and Abdollahi, A. (2008). "Molecular mechanisms of the antiangiogenic and antitumor effects of mycophenolic acid". *Mol. Cancer Ther.*, 6, 1656-68.

Engel, G. and Prokopek, D. (1980). "Kein nachweis von patulin und penicillinsäure in mit patulin und penicillinsäure-bildenden *P. roqueforti* stämmen hergestellten käse". *Milchwissenschaft, 35,* 218-220.

Engel, G., Milczewski, K.E. von, Prokopek, D. and Teuber, M. (1982). "Strain-specific synthesis of mycophenolic acid by *Penicillium roqueforti* blue-veined cheese". *Appl. Environ. Microbiol., 42,* 1034-1040.

Erdogan, A., Sert, S. (2004). "Mycotoxin-forming ability of two *Penicillium roqueforti* strains in blue mouldy tulum cheese ripened at various temperatures". *J. Food Prot., 67,* 533-555.

Eugui, A.M., Almquist, S., Muller, C.D., Allison, A.C. (1991). "Lymphocyte-selective cytostatic and immunosuppressive effects of mycophenolic acid in vitro: role of deoxyguanoside nucleotide depletion". *Scand. J. Immunol.* 33: 161–173.

Fernández-Bodega, M.A., Mauriz, E., Gómez, A., Martín, J.F. (2009). "Proteolytic activity, mycotoxins and andrastin A in *Penicillium roqueforti* strains isolated from Cabrales, Valdeón and Bejes-Tresviso local varieties of blue-veined cheeses". *Int. J. Food Microbiol.* 136: 18-25.

Finoli, C., Vecchio, A., Galli, A., Dragoni, I. (2001). "Roquefortine C occurrence in blue cheese". *J. Food. Prot.* 64 (2): 246–51.

Fleischmann, W. (1924). Tratado de lechería. Ed. G. Gili, Barcelona.

García-Rico, R.O., Fierro, F., Mauriz, E., Gómez, A., Fernández-Bodega, M.A., Martín, J. F. (2008). "The heterotrimeric Gα protein Pga1 regulates biosynthesis of penicillin, chrysogenin and roquefortine in *Penicillium chrysogenum*". *Microbiology.* 154: 3567-3578.

Gorst-Allman, C.P., Steyn, P.S., and Vleggaar, R. (1982). "The biosynthesis of roquefortine. An investigation of acetate and mevalonate incorporation using high field n.m.r. spectroscopy". *J. Chem. Soc., Chem. Commun.* 652 – 653.

Häggblom, P. (1990). "Isolation of roquefortine C from feed grain". *Appl. Environ. Microbiol.* 56: 2924-2926.

Hohn, T.M., and Plattner, R.D. (1989). "Purification and characterization of the sesquiterpene cyclase aristolochene synthase from *Penicillium roqueforti*". *Arch. Biochem. Biophys.* 272: 137-143.

Hsieh, K.P., Yu, S., Wei, Y.H., Chen, C.F. and Wei, R.D. (1986). "Inhibitory effect *in vitro* of PR toxin, a mycotoxin from Penicillium roqueforti, on the mitochondrial HCO-3-ATPase of the rat brain, heart and kidney". *Toxicon., 24,* 153-160.

Kato, N., Suzuki, H., Takagi, H., Asami, Y., Kakeya, H., Uramoto, M., Usui, T., Takahashi, S., Sugimoto, Y., Osada, H. (2009). "Identification of cytochrome P450s required for fumitremorgin biosynthesis in *Aspergillus fumigatus*". *Chembiochem.* 10: 920-928.

Kenfield, D., Bunkers, G., Strobel, G., and Sugawara, F., in Phytotoxins and Plant Pathogenesis, Graniti, A., Durbin, R.D., and Ballio, A., Eds., Berlin: Springer, (1989), pp. 319–335.

Kimura, Y., Hamasaki, T., Nakajima, H., Isogai, A. (1982). "Structure of aszonalenin, a new metabolite of *Aspergillus zonatus*". *Tetrahedron Lett.* 23: 225–228.

Kopp-Holtwiesche, B. and Rehm, H.J. (1981). "Studies in the inhibition of bacterial macromolecule synthesis by roquefortine, a mycotoxin from *Penicillium roqueforti*". *European J. Appl. Microbiol. Technol., 13,* 232-235.

Kopp-Holtwiesche, B., and Rehm, H.J. (1990). "Antimicrobial action of roquefortine". *J. Environ. Pathol. Toxicol. Oncol.* 10: 41-44.

Kozlovsky, A.G., Solovieva, T.F., Reshetilova, T.A., Skryabin, G.K. (1980). "Biosynthesis of roquefortine and 3,12-dihydroroquefortine by the culture *Penicillium farinosum*". *Experientia.* 37: 472-473.

Lafont, P., Siriwardana, M.G., Combemale, I. and Lafont, J. (1979). "Mycophenolic acid in marketed cheeses". *Food Cosmet. Toxicol., 17,* 147-149.

Lee, H.J., Pawlak, K., Nguyen, B.T., Robins, R.K., Sadee, W. (1985). "Biochemical differences among four inosinate dehydrogenase inhibitors, mycophenolic acid, ribavirin, tiazofurin, and selenazofurin, studied in mouse lymphoma cell culture". *Cancer Res.* 45: 5512–5520.

Li, S.Y., Chang, S.C., and Wei, R.D. (1985). Chemical transformation of eremofortin C into PR toxin. *Appl. Environ. Microbiol.* 50: 729-731.

Li, S.M. (2009). "Evolution of aromatic prenyltransferases in the biosynthesis of indole derivatives". *Phytochemistry.* 70: 1746-1757.

Lieu, F.Y. and Bullerman, L.B., (1977). "Production and stability of aflatoxins, penicillic acid and patulin in several substrates". *J. Food Sci., 42,* 1222–1224.

López-Díaz, T.M., Román-Blanco, C., García-Arias, M.T., García-Fernández, M.C., García-López, M.L. (1996). Mycotoxins in two Spanish cheese varieties. *Int. J. Food Microbiol.* 30(3): 391-395.

Möller, T., Akerstrand, K., and Massoud, T. (1997). "Toxin-producing species of *Penicillium* and the development of mycotoxins in must and homemade wine". *Nat. Toxins.* 5: 86-89.

Moreau, S., Cacan, M., and Lablache-Combier, A. (1977). "Eremofortin C. A new metabolite obtained from *Penicillium roqueforti* cultures and from biotransformation of PR toxin". *J. Org. Chem.* 42: 2632-2634.

Moreau, S., Lablache-Combier, A., Biguet, J. (1980). "Production of eremofortins A, B, and C relative to formation of PR toxin by *Penicillium roqueforti*". *Appl. Environ. Microbiol.* 39: 770-776.

Moulé, Y., Jemmali, M., Rousseau, N. (1976). "Mechanism of the inhibition of transcription by PR toxin, a mycotoxin from *Penicillium roqueforti*". *Chem. Biol. Interact.* 14: 207-216.

Moulé, Y., Moreau, S., and Bousquet, J.F. (1977). "Relationship between the chemical structure and the biological properties of some eremophilane compounds related to PR toxin". *Chem. Biol. Interact.* 17: 185-192.

Moulé, Y., Jammali, M., Darracq, N. (1978). "Inhibition of protein synthesis by PR toxin, a mycotoxin from *Penicillium roqueforti*". *FEBS Lett.* 88: 341-344.

Nielsen, K.F., Dalsgaard, P.W., Smedsgaard, J., Larsen, T.O. (2005). Andrastins A-D, *Penicillium roqueforti* metabolites consistently produced in blue-mold-ripened cheese. *J. Agric. Food Chem.*53(8): 2908-2913.

Nielsen, K.F., Sumarah, M.W., Frisvad, J.C., Miller, J.D. (2006). "Production of metabolites from the *Penicillium roqueforti* complex". *J. Agric. Food Chem.* 54(10): 3756-3763.

Northolt, M.D. and Bullerman, L.B. (1982). "Prevention of mold growth and toxin production through control of environmental conditions". *J. Food Prot., 45,* 519-526.

Núñez, M. (1978). "Microflora of Cabrales cheese: changes during maturation". *J. Dairy Res., 45,* 501-508.

Ohmomo, S. (1982). "Indole alkaloids produced by *Penicillium roqueforti*". *J. Antibact. Antifung. Agents* 10: 253-264.

Ohmomo, S., Sato, T., Utagawa, T. and Abe, M. (1975). "Isolation of festuclavine and three new indole alkaloids, roquefortine A, B and C from cultures of *Penicillium roqueforti*". *Agr. Biol. Chem., 39,* 1333-1334.

Ohmomo, S., Oguma, K., Ohashi, T., Abe, M. (1978). "Isolation of a new indole alkaloid roquefortine D, from the cultures of *Penicillium roqueforti*". *Agric. Biol. Chem.* 42: 2387-2389.

Ohsugi, Y., Suzuki, S. and Takagaki, Y. (1976). "Antitumor and Immunosuppressive Effects of Mycophenolic Acid Derivatives". *Cancer Res., 36,* 2923-2927.

Omura, S., Inokoshi, J., Uchida, R., Shiomi, K., Masuma, R., Kawakubo, T., Tanaka, H., Iwai, Y., Kosemura, S., Yamamura, S. (1996). "Andrastins A-C, new protein farnesyltransferase inhibitors produced by Penicillium sp. FO-3929. I. Producing strain, fermentation, isolation, and biological activities". *J. Antibiot.* 49: 414-417.

Overy, D.P., Larsen, T.O., Dalsgaard, P.W., Frydenvang, K., Phipps, R., Munro, M.H., Christophersen, C. (2005). "Andrastin A and barceloneic acid metabolites, protein farnesyl transferase inhibitors from *Penicillium albocoremium*: chemotaxonomic significance and pathological implications". *Mycol. Res.* 109: 1243-1249.

Polonsky, J., Merrien, M.A., and Scott, P.M. (1977). "Roquefortine and isofumigaclavine A, alkaloids from *Penicillium roqueforti*". *Ann. Nutr. Aliment.* 31: 963-968.

Proctor, R.H., and Hohn, T.M. (1993). "Aristolochene synthase. Isolation, characterization, and bacterial expression of a sesquiterpenoid biosynthetic gene (Ari1) from Penicillium roqueforti". *J. Biol. Chem.* 268: 4543-4548.

Protected Denomination of Origin, published data of 2009 production. http://www.quesocabrales.org

Rand, T.G., Giles, S., Flemming, J., Miller, J.D., Puniani, E. (2005). "Inflammatory and cytotoxic responses in mouse lungs exposed to purified toxins from building isolated *Penicillium brevicompactum* Dierckx and *P. chrysogenum*". *Thom. Toxicol. Sci.* 87: 213-222.

Rho, M.C., Toyoshima, M., Hayashi, M., Uchida, R., Shiomi, K., Komiyama, K., Omura, S. (1998). "Enhancement of drug accumulation by andrastin A produced by *Penicillium* sp. FO-3929 in vincristine-resistant KB cells". *J. Antibiot.* 51 :68-72.

Richard, D.J., Schiavi, B., and Joullié, M.M. (2004). "Synthetic studies of roquefortine C: synthesis of isoroquefortine C and a heterocycle". *Proc. Natl. Acad. Sci. U.S.A.* 101: 11971-11976.

Rundberget, T., Skaar, I., and Flaoyen, A. (2004). "The presence of *Penicillium* and *Penicillium* mycotoxins in food wastes". *Int. J. Food Microbiol.* 90: 181–188.

Sala, F.J. and Burgos, J. (1972). Maduración del queso "Cabrales". Microflora III. Levaduras. *An. Bromatol. León, 24,* 83.

Sala, F.J.; Burgos, J. and Ordoñez, J.A. (1971). Maduración del queso "Cabrales". Microflora II. Mohos. *Ann. Fac. Vet. León, 17,* 115.

Schneweis, I., Meyer, K., Hörmansdorfer, S., Bauer, J. (2000). "Mycophenolic acid in silage". *Appl. Environ. Microbiol.* 66(8): 3639-3641.

Scott, P.M. (1981). "Toxins of *Penicillium* species used in cheese manufacture". *J. Food Prot., 44,* 702-710.

Scott, P.M. and Kennedy, B.P.C. (1976). "Analysis of blue cheese for roquefortine and other alkaloids from *Penicillium roqueforti*". *J. Agric. Food Chem., 24,* 865-868.

Scott, P.M., Kanhere, S.R. (1979). "Instability of PR toxin in blue cheese". *J. Assoc. Off Anal. Chem.* 62: 141-147.

Siriwardana, M.G. and Lafont, P.(1979). "Determination of mycophenolic acid, penicillic acid, patulin, sterigmatocystin, and aflatoxins in cheese". *J Dairy Sci., 62,* 1145-1148.

Stocking, E.M., Williams, R.M., Sanz-Cervera, J.F. (2000). "Reverse prenyl transferases exhibit poor facial discrimination in the biosynthesis of paraherquamide A, brevianamide A, andaustamide". *J. Am. Chem. Soc.* 122: 9089-9098.

Teuber, M., and Engel, G. (1983). "Low risk of mycotoxin production in cheese". *Microbiol. Aliment. Nutr.* 1: 193-197.

Tüller, G., Armbruster, G., Wiedenmann, S., Hnichen, T., Schams, D., Bauer, J. (1998). "Occurrence of roquefortine in silage. Toxicological relevance to sheep". *J. Anim. Physiol. Anim. Nutr.* 80: 246–249.

Uchida, R., Shiomi, K., Inokoshi, J., Sunazuka, T., Tanaka, H., Iwai, Y., Takayanagi, H., Omura, S. (1996a). "Andrastins A–C, new protein farnesyltransferase inhibitors produced by *Penicillium* sp. FO-3929. II. Structure and biosynthesis". *J. Antibiot.* 49: 418–424.

Uchida, R., Shiomi, K., Inokoshi, J., Tanaka, H., Iwai Y., Omura, S.A. (1996b). "Andrastin D, novel protein farnesyltransferase inhibitor produced by *Penicillium* sp. FO-3929". *J. Antibiot.* 49: 1278-1280.

van den Berg, M.A., Albang, R., Albermann, K., Badger, J.H., Daran, J.M., Driessen, A.J., Garcia-Estrada, C., Fedorova, N.D., Harris, D.M., Heijne, W.H., Joardar, V., Kiel, J.A., Kovalchuk, A., Martín, J.F., Nierman, W.C., Nijland, J.G., Pronk, J.T., Roubos, J.A., van der Klei, I.J., van Peij, N.N., Veenhuis, M., von Döhren, H., Wagner, C., Wortman, J., Bovenberg, R.A. (2008). "Genome sequencing and analysis of the filamentous fungus *Penicillium chrysogenum*". *Nat. Biotechnol.* 26: 1161-1168.

Wagener, R.E., Davis, N.D., Diener, U.L. (1980). "Penitrem A and Roquefortine Production by *Penicillium commune*". *Appl. Environ. Microbiol.* 39(4): 882-887.

Wakana, D., Hosoe, T., Itabashi, T., Nozawa, K., Okada, K., Takaki, G.M., D.C., Yaguchi, T., Fukushima, K., Kawai, K.I. (2006). "Isolation of isoterrein from *Neosartorya fischeri*". *Mycotoxins.* 56: 3–6.

Ware, G.M., Thorpe, C.W. and Pohland, A.E. (1980). "Determination of roquefortine in Blue cheese and Blue cheese dressing by high pressure liquid chromatography with ultraviolet and electrochemical detectors". *J. Assoc. of Anal. Chem.*, 63, 637-641.

Wei, R.D., Still, P.E., Smalley, E.B., Schnoes, H.K. and Strong, F.M. (1973). "Isolation and partial characterization of a mycotoxin from *Penicillium roqueforti*". *Appl. Microbiol.*, 25, 111-114.

Wei, R.D., Schnoes, H.K., Hart, P.A. and Strong, F.M. (1975). "The structure of PR-toxin, a mycotoxin from *Penicillium roqueforti*". Tetrahedron, 31, 109-114.

Wei, R.D., Schnoes, H.K., Smalley, E.B., Lee, S.S., Chang, Y.N., Strong, F.M. (1976). Production, isolation, chemistry, and biological properties of *Penicillium roqueforti* toxin, p.137-144. In A. Ohsaka, K. Hayashi, and Y. Sawai (ed.), Animal, plant, and microbial toxins, vol. 2. Plenum Publishing Corp., New York.

Wei, R.D., and Liu, G.X. (1978). "PR toxin production in different *Penicillium roqueforti* strains". *Appl. Environ. Microbiol.* 35: 797-799.

Wei, R.D., Ong, T.M., Whong, W.Z., Frezza, D., Bronzetti, G., Zeiger, E. (1979). "Genetic effects of PR toxin in eukaryotic microorganisms". *Environ. Mutagen.* 1: 45-53.

Williams, R.M., Stocking, E.M., and Sanz-Cervera, J.F. (2000). "Biosynthesis of prenylated alkaloids derived from tryptophan". *Topics Curr. Chem.* 209: 97–173.

Yin, W.-B., Grundmann, A., Cheng, J., Li, S.M. (2009). "Acetylaszonalenin biosynthesis in Neosartorya fischeri: identification of the biosynthetic gene cluster by genomic mining and functional proof of the genes by biochemical investigation". *J. Biol. Chem.* 284: 100–109.

In: Cheese: Types, Nutrition and Consumption
Editor: Richard D. Foster, pp. 105-118

ISBN 978-1-61209-828-9
© 2011 Nova Science Publishers, Inc.

Chapter 5

SODIUM IN DIFFERENT CHEESE TYPES: ROLE AND STRATEGIES OF REDUCTION

Mamdouh El-Bakry[1,2]

[1]UCD School of Agriculture, Food Science and Veterinary Medicine, Dublin, Ireland
[2]Department of Dairy Science and Technology, Faculty of Agriculture, Cairo University, Giza, Egypt

ABSTRACT

Cheese is a versatile, nutrient-dense dairy food, i.e. a good source of protein, vitamins and minerals particularly calcium and phosphorus, which is an important component in highly consumed convenience foods (O'Brien and O'Connor, 2004). However, cheese is perceived as being high in saturated fat, which might contribute to risks of atherosclerosis, and sodium (Johnson et al., 2009). There is considerable evidence that high sodium intake, which is the case in Western countries, is associated with hypertension and strokes, hence, dietary guidelines recommend that sodium intake be reduced.

This chapter covers the scientific and technological aspects of the role of sodium in cheese manufacture and functional properties and highlights various strategies for reducing the sodium. The focus is on natural cheese, made from milk by acid and/or rennet-coagulation, and process cheese. This cheese differs from natural cheese in that it is made from natural cheese or casein, which is blended with the necessary emulsifying salts and in the presence of heat, leading to the formation of a homogeneous product with extended shelf-life (Zehren and Nusbaum, 2000). Process cheese has numerous end-use applications in processed foods, which counts for ~75% of the dietary sodium in industrialized diets (Doyle and Glass, 2010).

The source of sodium in cheese is mainly the added salt (sodium chloride). Salt acts primarily as food preservative and flavor enhancer and also interacts with major components in the cheese and thereby affecting the functionality, e.g. salt increases the protein hydration during manufacture which affects the stability and textural properties (Johnson et al., 2009). Process cheese contains much higher sodium content, compared to natural cheese, due to the necessity of using emulsifying salts, such as sodium citrate and phosphate. These salts are crucial for the hydration of the protein, emulsification of fat and the stability of the final product.

Strategies for reducing sodium in cheese are mainly outlined in the reduction of the salt and/or emulsifying salts used and their substitution by the potassium equivalents salts. However, these strategies present many challenges, such as adverse effects on flavor and microbiological stability. In process cheese, a high reduction of emulsifying salts does not allow for the formation of a homogeneous end product. Recent approaches of reducing emulsifying salts used are also discussed, such as utilizing of emulsifiers or protein hydrolyzates in the manufacture of cheese (Zehren and Nusbaum, 2000).

A final section in this chapter is about the future of low sodium cheese manufacture, including suggestions for reducing sodium which has not been systematically investigated in research on various cheese types.

1. INTRODUCTION

Although cheese production is a very ancient and traditional craft, it enjoys a consistent and substantial growth rate, with a healthy and positive image. It could be regarded as the original convenience food which may be consumed as the main component of a meal, as a dessert, as a snack, as a condiment, or as a food ingredient. In addition, new varieties continue to be developed, despite the fact that there are 500 types, e.g., Jarlsberg and Araglin (Fox and McSweeney, 2004).

Cheese is a nutritionally valued dairy product that contains a high concentration of essential nutrients relative to its energy content, i.e. cheese contributes ~9% of the protein, 11% of the phosphorus, and 27% of the calcium in the U.S. food supply (O'Brien and O'Connor, 2004). Regarding the vitamin content of the cheese, most cheeses are good sources of vitamin A, as ~85% of its content in milk is retained in the cheese, riboflavin, vitamin B12, and folate (Holland et al., 1989). Cheese fat generally contains ~66% saturated, 30% monounsaturated and 4% polyunsaturated fatty acids. Thus, cheese represents a significant dietary source of both saturated and unsaturated fatty acids.

However, despite these nutritional benefits, cheese is also perceived as being high in fat and sodium. This might discourages some consumers from including cheese in their diets. Evidence exist that high sodium intake can contribute to hypertension, strokes and cardiovascular diseases, particular in the case of salt-susceptible individuals (Cutler, 1999, Johnson et al., 2009). Adults in Western Societies consume, on average ~5-6g sodium/day, which is much more than the required daily sodium (Taormina, 2010). Salt (sodium chloride), which is mostly the main source of added sodium in cheese, serves several important functions in the cheesemaking process. A wide range of sodium levels are found in cheese due to different amounts of salt added during manufacture.

The objectives of this chapter is to review the scientific and technological aspects of the role of sodium in cheese manufacture and functional properties, highlights the progress made so far of various strategies for reducing the sodium, and to include a review of recent advances in reducing sodium which has not been sufficiently investigated in research on various cheese types.

2. Sources of Sodium in Cheese

In natural cheese, one of the final steps in the manufacture process is the addition of salt (NaCl). In dry salted cheeses like cheddar, the salt is added directly to the curds just before pressing. In pickled cheeses, the salt is added by submersing the cheese in brine containing about 5 to 10% salt for an appropriate storage time. Salt in some cheeses like Ras cheese is rubbed on the outer surface of the cheese. Salt addition is the major source of sodium in natural cheese. The salt content can vary widely, from 0.5% for cheeses like Emmental to 7% for pickeled cheeses like Domiati (Guinee, 2004).

Process cheese, in broad terms, is defined to be a merge of one or more natural cheeses of different ages and types, emulsifying salts, salt, water, and other dairy and nondairy ingredients like whey proteins, starch, preservatives and flavor enhancers (Guinee et al., 2004). This mixture goes through the necessary continuous thermal and mixing energies, i.e. mixing at ~80°C for several minutes, to produce a homogeneous product. The final product is considered to pasteurised and accordingly has an extended shelf life (Zehren and Nusbaum, 2000). A further advantage of this type of cheese is that wide varieties can be produced due to a multitude of ingredients used in the manufacture. In addition, the manufacture of process cheese allows for the upgrading of defective cheese products if the defects could limit the shelf life but the cheese is still edible (Berger et al., 1989). There are three major sources of the sodium in process cheese. These sources include sodium-based emulsifying salts, natural cheese used as ingredient and salt of ~2% of the cheese weight, contributing to approx. 45, 35 and 20% respectively of the total sodium content (Zehren and Nusbaum, 2000).

3. Role of Sodium in Cheese

3.1. Role of Salt (NaCl)

No matter the way or the amount of the salt added to the cheese, it has been an essential component used to for at least a preservative purpose. Controlling growth of pathogens in foods is essential to public health, particularly for high-risk populations including very young children, pregnant women, the elderly, and people whose immune systems are weakened. Salt also maintains the expected flavor, as consumers expect some degree of saltiness in cheese, and body and texture by controlling the activities of enzymes and microorganisms.

3.1.1. Preservative Action of Salt and its Role in Microbial Safety

The classical methods of food preservation, including salting, fermentation, refrigeration and dehydration, are used to preserve cheese. The preservative action of salt is due to its lowering effect on the water activity (a_w) of the medium and therefore prevent microbial growth, as available water is a critical factor affecting microbial growth on and in foods (Betts, 2007). Salt increases the osmotic pressure of the aqueous phase of foods, causing dehydration of bacterial cells and killing them or at least preventing their growth. The amount of salt in the moisture phase (S/M ratio) of the cheese controls the growth of microorganisms, not the total amount of salt in the food (Guinee, 2004). In addition, during manufacture of natural cheeses, salt affects the synersis of the cheese curd formed during manufacture resulting in whey expulsion and thus controlling the final moisture of the cheese, which also influences the growth of microorganisms and enzymes.

Table 1 shows the different a_w values and salt content for various types of cheeses. Cheeses have a high aw of 0.95 to 1 and it has been reported that the water activity of young cheese is determined almost entirely by the concentration of NaCl in the aqueous phase (Christian, 2000). In addition to sodium chloride, proteins decrease a_w like reduced a_w of hard cheeses to 0.90-0.92. It is apparent from Table 1 and 2 that the water activity of most cheese varieties is not low enough to prevent the growth of most bacterial pathogens and spoilage microorganisms, but together with a low pH it is quite effective in controlling the microbial growth. Therefore, by inhibiting or retarding the growth and activity of microorganisms, including pathogenic and food-poisoning microorganisms, the safety of cheeses increases.

Table 1. Salt content and water activity (a_w) of different cheese types

Cheese	Salt (%)	a_w
Cheese Curd, Whey Cheese	0.0	1.00
Cottage, Quarg Cheese	0.5	0.99
Muenster, Process Cheese	1.0-2.0	0.98
Brie, Camembert	1.0-1.5	0.97
Edam, Havarti	1.5-2.0	0.96
Cheddar, Gorgonzola, Gouda	1.5-2.0	0.95
Mozzarella, Stilton	2.0-2.5	0.94
Danablu, Normana	1.5-2.0	0.93
Parmesan, Zamorano	1.5-2.0	0.92
Provolone, Roquefort	2.5-3.0	0.91
Cabrales, Primost	0-1.0	0.90

Adapted from Zehren and Nusbaum, 2000; Guinee and Fox, 2004.

Table 2. Minimum water (a_w) required for the growth of different pathogenic and spoilage microorganisms

Microorganisms	Minimum a_w
Aeromonas hydrophila	0.97
Bacillus cereus	0.93
E. coli	0.94
Staph aureus	0.86-0.91
Yersinia enterocolitica	0.96
Vibrio parahaemolyticus	0.94
Shigella spp.	0.96
Clostridium botulinum	0.94-0.97
Campylobacter jejuni	0.99
Salmonella spp.	0.94

Adapted from Guinee and Fox, 2004.

The literature on food safety of cheeses has been recently reviewed (Bishop and Smukowski, 2006), which was especially related to the storage and distribution temperature of the product. It was recommended that cheeses with ~50% moisture, produced under good manufacturing procedures, with traditional levels of salt, starter culture, pH, and fat be allowed to be distributed at a temperature not exceeding 30°C, if the cheeses contain the necessary content of salt in addition to low pH, which are the main hurdles inherent in maintaining the food safety of these cheeses. Low-fat cheeses have a higher moisture content resulting in a lower S/M ratio, at the same absolute salt content, which negatively affecting the safety and shelf-life especially in the distribution and serving of cheeses.

3.1.2. Flavor and Texture

Saltiness is one of the basic tastes perceived by humans, where sodium is the only edible cations with a taste that is primarily salty. Potassium and calcium contribute to saltiness but they have undesired flavors, which are mostly described as 'metallic' or 'bitter'. Therefore, sodium chloride (table salt) is considered to be the saltiest edible sodium compound. Salt enhances the flavor of cheeses and appears to have a greater impact in low-fat products, as salt is component of the expected taste of the cheese (Johnson et al., 2009; Metzger and Kapoor, 2007). Salt also suppresses or masks bitter flavors.

Salt affects cheese flavor directly and indirectly via its influence on the growth of the microorganisms or starter cultures used, hence, the activities of lipolytic and proteolytic enzymes that produce important characteristic flavor compounds of the cheese type manufacture during the ripening period (Guinee and O'Kennedy, 2007; Johnson et al., 2009). Salt has an impact on the rate and extent of lactose fermentation and thus the final pH obtained in the cheese during the maturation period, where proteolysis and/or lipolysis takes place (Thomas and Pearce, 1985). Proteolysis is necessary for proper flavor and body development. Excessive or insufficient fermentation or proteolysis can lead to defects of both flavor and body of cheese. As an example, cheddar cheese has an intermediate salt content of ~1.5%, which allows for the proteolysis of 95% of the α-casein and 50% of the β-casein, whereas at higher salt content pf above 2%, only 70% of the α-casein and 20% of the β-casein were hydrolysed (Thomas and Pearce, 1985). The high salt content of Roquefort cheese (above 3% salt) is the main aid in selecting growth of the desired mold, *Penicillium roquefortii*, rather than allowing for the growth of salt-sensitive defect-causing microorganisms. In the case of the Parmesan cheese, which is a low-moisture and low a_w cheese, its high salt content of ~2% is the cause of having an extended shelf life of several years. In addition, much of the characteristic fruity flavor of this cheese is due to the action of the microbial lipase. The role and specificity of the lipase enzyme causes the characteristic flavor only at low moisture and low a_w rather than at high moisture and high a_w values (Wolf et al., 2010).

Sodium chloride interacts with other major components in foods thereby affecting the texture of foods. Salt causes changes in cheese proteins that influence cheese texture, protein solubility, and probably protein conformation. For example, salt increases hydration of proteins, which affects the moisture content, and enhances the binding of proteins to each other and to fat. These effects of the salt determine the rheological and textural parameters of the cheese product. In process cheese, during the cooking, moderate concentrations of salt increase the solubilization of casein or para-casein of the natural cheeses used. This will aid in the in the hydration of proteins, which is similar to the effect of the emulsifying salts used

(Guinee and O'Kennedy, 2007; Johnson et al., 2009). Further details about the roles of the emulsifying salts used in the manufacture of process cheese will be discussed in the following section.

3.2. Role of Emulsifying Salts in Process Cheese

During the manufacturing of process cheese, the so called emulsifying or melting salts, such as sodium phosphates and citrates, are essentially added. Generally, sodium salts are used as they do not lead to the formation of a much of a precipitate, i.e. crystals which are obvious after the post-manufacture cooling. These salts have two main functions under the mixing and heating applied during the manufacture. First, they increase the pH of the mixture, which is generally about 5.2 to above 6. Second, these salts lower the calcium ion activity to below 0.2 mM by disrupting the calcium–phosphate protein network (Gupta et al., 1984; Caric et al., 1985; Berger et al., 1989). Under these conditions, the protein becomes soluble, i.e. hydration of the protein, and it is able to act as an emulsifier to emulsify and incorporate the fat that could have been added in its free form, e.g. anhydrous milk fat or vegetable oil, due to the exposure of the hydrophilic and hydrophobic sections of the proteins respectively (Ennis et al., 1998; Lee et al., 2003). It was reported that heating and stirring of cheese in the absence of emulsifying salts does not allow for the sufficient protein hydration and also causes considerable coalescence of the fat globules. The quantity of the emulsifying salt required is approximately 10% of the quantity of protein used, which corresponds to a level of 2% to 3% in the final cheese product.

Post-manufacture, the type and concentration of the emulsifying salts used affect various functional properties such as texture and melting properties (Templeton and Sommer, 1936; Meyer, 1973; Gupta et al., 1984; Berger et al., 1989; Zehren and Nusbaum, 2000). Cavalier-Salou and Cheftel (1991) reported increased melting of process cheese with increased citrate ES content (from 0.25 to 3.0%), in comparison to cheese containing phosphate ES at similar concentrations, which could be due to the higher pH (pH = ~6.5) of the former cheese that increased the degree of casein dissociation or solubilization. This casein dissociation in the high pH cheese may have helped in increasing the cheese melting (Savello et al., 1989). In contrast, pyrophosphates and polyphosphates give harder cheese, showing a poor flow on melting (Swenson et al., 2000). From sensory analyses on process cheese, it is generally recognized that sodium citrates impart a 'clean' flavor with no defects such as bitter or acid tastes, while phosphates, especially orthophosphates, may impart off-flavors described as soapy, chemical or salty (Meyer, 1973; Gupta et al., 1984; Caric and Kalab, 1987). In addition, monosodium orthophosphates and pyrophosphates, if used alone as ES, may cause an overacid flavor and bitterness, respectively, if added at a level of 2% or greater (Fox et al., 1996; Zehren and Nusbaum, 2000). Phopshate emulsifying salts are also used as anti-microbial agents providing food safety and extended shelf-life of process cheese (Chambre and Daurelles, 2000; Tanaka et al., 1986). The general anti-bacterial activity is principally due to the interaction of the phosphates with bacterial proteins and sequestration of calcium, which generally serves as an important cellular cation and cofactor for some microbial enzymes (Stanier et al., 1981). In general microbiology studies, phosphates at concentrations of > 1% showed an anti-microbiological activity against the growth of various *Salmonella* species and many Gram-positive bacteria, including *Staphylococcus aureus, Bacillus subtilis* and *Clostridium* species (Tanaka et al., 1979, 1986; Wagner, 1986; Loessner et al., 1997).

4. STRATEGIES OF SODIUM REDUCTION

There are mainly two general approaches to control the amount of sodium chloride (NaCl) in natural cheese. One is simply to restrict the addition of NaCl. The other means is to replace NaCl by its potassium salt (KCl).

4.1. Reducing Sodium Chloride used in Manufacture

Reducing NaCl content of cheese faces various challenges and complications to cheese manufacturers since salt plays many important roles in cheese, as previously outlined. It is an integral component in cheese, used to maintain shelf-life and contributing to flavor and texture of the final product. Nowadays, many consumers are requesting low-sodium cheeses, as the Western diet has already high sodium content (Taormina, 2010). However, it was reported that that a salt reduction of as little as 25% from typical salt content of cheeses, usually from 1.8% to 1.4% salt, is noticed by consumers and may adversely affect the product acceptability.

As an example of reducing NaCl in natural cheeses, the focus will be on cheddar cheese, which was extensively studied in literature in respect to the salt reduction. In cheddar cheese, Schroeder et al. (1988) investigated the effect of the reduction of sodium chloride, during manufacture and maturation, from 1.44% up to 0.07%. Analysis showed that saltiness was the most important attribute affecting the rating of the overall desirability. The high salt cheeses showed the highest desirability due to the high cheddar intensity flavor and the lack of the unpleasant aftertaste. Similarly, Banks et al. (1993) reported that reduced-fat cheddar cheese at low NaCl content of 1.25% produced a bitter cheese with less cheddar flavor than the one with a higher NaCl content of 1.8% salt. However, the higher salt content produced a firmer cheese. Similar observations were reported by Mistry and Kasperson (1998), who noted a higher firmness when the salt content was increased to 2%. In another study by Rutikowska et al. (2008), cheddar cheeses were manufactured with salt levels ranging from 0.5% to 3.0%. The bacteria of the starter culture and the non-starter lactic acid bacteria substantially survived longer in the case of low salt than in the high salt cheeses with a salt level of above 1.80%. The low-salt cheeses of 0.5% salt had the lowest proteolytic activity resulting in a lower rate of flavor formation and a higher undesired bitterness flavor, which might have been related to the high activity of the non-starter bacteria.

4.2. Replacing Sodium Chloride by Potassium Chloride

Potassium chloride (KCl) is the most chemically similar compound to sodium chloride and accordingly is the most obvious choice for NaCl replacements in cheese products. Potassium chloride is by far the most popular material used to replace sodium chloride in cheeses. From the nutritional viewpoint, the substitution of NaCl by KCl will give an additional benefit since processed foods, in which cheese is used as an ingredient, is already low in potassium which is known to have a significant effect of reducing the blood pressure and, hence, reducing the risk of cardiovascular diseases (Green et al., 2002). Depending on the usefulness and applications of the cheese, the level of substitution is limited by the bitter undesired taste that might be produced by KCl. At levels up to 50% of sodium substitution the bitterness is well masked by the remaining NaCl (Breslin and Beauchamp, 1997). This replacement of the added sodium chloride with potassium chloride might give the perception of saltiness, without undesired flavors, in mild flavored cheeses. However, this approach may not provide a control of the growth and activity of both desired and undesired microorganisms and thus will make it difficult to achieve the desired characteristic flavors of the different cheese types. In addition, as it was shown by Lindsay et al. (1982), most of the panelists under the study preferred high NaCl cheeses over cheeses with partial substitution of KCl with a ratio of 1:1. In another study by Fitzgerald and Buckley (1985) who evaluated the impact of cheddar cheese produced with different salt substitutes at equivalent concentrations of sodium chloride level of 1.5%. The use potassium chloride produced an unacceptable cheese bitter taste and crumbly texture. However, a mixture of 1:1 ratio of sodium chloride and potassium chloride resulted in a cheese comparable to the cheese containing sodium chloride only.

There are several monovalent salts of chloride investigated as a replacement of sodium chloride, including lithium, ammonium, and choline chloride (Fielding and Locke, 1993). The closest salt to NaCl in its taste is the lithium chloride which does not have any bitterness observed. This salt, however, is considered as toxic as even small amounts are causing nausea as an option for salt replacement. Therefore, potassium chloride remains the best option as a replacement for sodium chloride, the typical table salt, if low sodium cheese manufacture is the main aim.

4.3. Process Cheese

Sodium reduction in process cheese involves the modification and/or reduction of one or all the three ingredients, which were previously mentioned as sodium sources, during process cheese formulations and manufacture. Numerous research efforts have been aimed towards the development of low-sodium natural cheese, which is normally used as an ingredient for process cheese manufacture (Karahadian and Lindsay, 1984; Metzger and Kapoor, 2007). In addition to these efforts, attempts have also been directed towards the development of novel formulations in respect to the utilization of potassium-based emulsifying salts (Gupta et al., 1984; Karahadian and Lindsay, 1984; Henson, 1997; Zehren and Nusbaum, 2000; Metzger and Kapoor, 2007), and flavor enhancers (Karahadian and Lindsay, 1984; Metzger and Kapoor, 2007) without causing an adverse effect on the functional properties of the final process cheese product. Recently, in process imitation cheese, it was possible to lower the sodium content by ~ 20% by just changing the emulsifying salts used in the manufacture (El-Bakry et al., 2011). The manufacture of this type of cheese was also successful at reduced levels of salt (NaCl), which usually represents approximately 65% of the total sodium content, up to 0% NaCl without adversely affecting the functionalities of the cheese (El-Bakry et al., 2010). However, the reduction of sodium in process cheese is still facing a lot of difficulties. First of all, there is lack of information regarding clear systematic strategies for low sodium cheese manufacture, as most research studies were performed at different conditions and with various formulations. Accordingly, despite of these research efforts to develop reduced or low sodium process cheese, there are presently no low-sodium process cheeses that are sold in the marketplace throughout most developed countries (GNPD 2008). Second, the area of food safety and maintaining the microbiological stability, which are important aspects that need to be taken into account when trying to reduce the sodium content in the final product, were not completely solved. There are formulation limitations, i.e. the presence of NaCl and sodium phosphate is necessary for a shelf-stable product (Tanaka et al., 1979, 1986), which did not support any changes towards the production of low sodium cheese. There are no food safety-related challenge studies available to quantify the effectiveness of the replacement of the sodium salts by their potassium one in process cheese (Karahadian and Lindsay, 1984, Zehren and Nusbaum, 2000). Third, there are adverse effects of potassium emulsifying salts on the sensory properties of the cheese, when these salts are substituting the traditionally used sodium-based emulsifying salts. In low sodium process cheese, where the potassium equivalent emulsifying salts were used, an unnatural bitter taste, which becomes more pronounced with storage, and an unpleasant aroma were observed (Karahadian and Lindsay 1984; Zehren and Nusbaum, 2000). These adverse organoleptic properties were more pronounced when citrate emulsifying salts, rather than phosphate emulsifying salts, were replaced by their equivalent potassium equivalents.

5. RECENT APPROACHES TO SODIUM REDUCTION IN CHEESE

The most potential sodium reduction strategy is to adapt the preference of consumers for saltiness by reducing sodium in the food products in small steps. However, this is a time-consuming and unfeasible approach that needs to be widely applied to the industry in order to be effective. Therefore, solutions to reduce the sodium in the food stuff are always investigated with the aim of maintaining the same perceived salt taste intensity at lower sodium levels (Doetsch et al., 2009). Currently applied approaches are resulting in sodium reductions between 20–30%. Further reduction will require new technologies and also research into the physiology of salt taste perception and receptors. For instance, Phan et al. (2008) concluded that sodium release during mastication is mainly influenced by the food moisture content, while saltiness perception is limited by the presence of fat. Therefore, a way to reduce salt in cheese without a negative impact on flavor would be to increase the moisture and decrease the fat. Despite these findings, a balance has to be achieved between the composition and structure to produce cheeses that meet the acceptability of the consumers in terms of salty perception, as well as nutritional recommendations. In this section, a brief overview of the approaches used for high sodium reduction, which are still not widely applied in the cheese industry, is presented.

The use of alternatives to sodium chloride has been reviewed in literature, however these alternatives were not applied, to the authors knowledge, in low sodium cheese manufacture. Arginine amino acid has been most often mentioned as contributing to the salty taste. In some studies very large effects are reported, e.g. more than doubling the saltiness of 4.5 g/l NaCl (Breslin, 2004). In addition, combinations of arginine with aspartame amino acids have been shown a higher salty 'sodium chloride' taste (Angus et al., 2005). Sourness is also known to enhance perceived saltiness (Keast and Breslin, 2003; Hellemann, 1992), as it has been reported that specific acids might give an extra salty flavor. Malate and lactate, usually added as potassium salt, was reported to significantly enhance saltiness at low amounts (Angus et al., 2005; Labruni et al., 2003). However, a limitation for replacing salt with "artificial" salt replacers could be the increasing consumer interest in "natural food" (Searby, 2006). Another important disadvantage for using salt replacers is the costs involved in comparison to salt (NaCl), which is one of the cheapest food ingredients available, e.g. a sodium chloride reduction of ~25% increases costs by up to 30%, depending on the product manufactured.

Process cheeses contain much higher levels of Na than natural cheeses owing to the addition of sodium-based emulsifying salts, as previously discussed. In addition, in general, the salt content of process cheese tends to be more than that of many natural cheeses (Meyer, 1973; Zehren and Nusbaum, 2000). Therefore, there might be greater opportunities and more interest to reduce the total sodium content in these cheese products than in natural cheeses. Attempts have been mainly performed to reduce sodium through the lowering of the sodium emulsifying salts used in the manufacture. Recently, the use of casein hydrolysates has been found to reduce the concentrations of sodium emulsifying salts used for the emulsification and formation of a homogeneous stable product (Kwak et al., 2002). However, the use of such hydrolyzates caused an excessive oiling-off when the cheese product was heated. Another approach may involve the use of traditional emulsifiers such as mono- and diglycerides at various levels, where the cheese functionality was not adversely affected (Lucey 2008; Paulus 2008). In a type of process cheese manufactured in Germany called Kochkäse, its manufacture starts with low-fat ripened quarg cheese, which has a pH of about 4.5 (Walstra et al., 2006). This is followed by yeasts growth and the fermentation of lactic acid, raising the pH to about 5.8. Finally, ~1.5% salt, water or milk and butter are mixed for approximately 10min at 90°C. This product has the ability to form a homogeneous mass and melt without the addition of emulsifying salts, due to the low content of calcium present in the quarg cheese used. This process cheese is consumed as a smooth process cheese spreads, which is considered as a light product

CONCLUSION

High sodium intake has been related to diseases like strokes and hypertension (Cutler, 1999; Johnson et al., 2009; Doyle and Glass, 2010). Processed foods, in which cheese is used as an ingredient, contributes to ~75% of the sodium intake in Western diet. Therefore, it is worthwhile from a nutritional and health perspective to review the strategies and recent advances towards the goal of reducing sodium in the cheese products. Current strategies might only allow for a sodium reduction of ~25%. These strategies include mainly a reduction in the salt (sodium chloride) used or replacing it with its potassium salt in some mild taste cheeses up to a maximum of 50% level of substitution. Therefore, it would be beneficial to consider the recent technologies, outlined above, which were shown in few research work done on cheese as well as sensory tests in order to reduce the salt and other sodium ingredients used in the manufacture of cheese products.

REFERENCES

Angus, F., Phelps, T., Clegg, S., Narein, C., Ridder den, C. and Kilcast, D. (2005). Salt in processed foods. Leatherhead Food International (No. 00193).

Banks, J.M., Hunter, E.A. and Muir D.D. (1993). Sensory properties of low-fat Cheddar cheese: effect of salt content and adjunct culture. *Journal of the Society of Dairy Technology,* 46, 119–123.

Berger, W., Klostermeyer, H., Merkenich, K. and Uhlmann, G. (1989). *Processed Cheese Manufacture, A JOHA Guide.* BK Ladenburg GmbH., Wurzburg, Germany.

Bishop, J.R. and Smukowski. M. (2006). Storage temperatures necessary to maintain cheese safety. *Food Production Trends*, 26, 714–24.

Breslin, P. A. and Beauchamp, G. K. (1997). Salt enhances flavor by suppressing bitterness. *Nature*, 387-563.

Breslin, P. A. (2004). Chemosensory Challenges for Industry. Philadelphia, US: Monell Chemical Senses Center,

Caric, M., Gantar, M. and Kalab, M. (1985). Effect of emulsifying agents on the microstructure and other characteristics of process cheese – a review. *Food Microstructure*, 4, 297–312.

Caric, M. and Kaláb, M. (1987). Processed cheese products. In: P. F. Fox (Ed), *Cheese: chemistry, physics and microbiology. Vol. 2: Major cheese groups.* London: Elsevier Applied Science.

Cavalier-Salou, C. and Cheftel, J.C. (1991). Emulsifying salts influence on characteristics of cheese analogs from calcium caseinate. *Journal of Food Science,* 56, 1542-1547, 1551.

Chambre, M. and Daurelles, J. (2000). Processed cheese. In Eck . A. and Gillis,J. (Eds), *Cheesemaking from Science to Quality Assurance,* 2nd edition. Lavoisier Publishers, Paris (pp. 641-657).

Christian, J.H. (2000). Drying and reduction of water activity. In The Microbiological Safety and Quality of Food, Lung, B.M. et al (eds). Gaithersburg, Maryland, USA: Aspen Publishers Inc.

Cutler, J. A. (1999). The effects of reducing sodium and increasing potassium intake for control of hypertension and improving health. *Clinical Experimental Hypertension*, 21, 769-783.

Doetsch, M., Busch, J., Batenburg, M., Liem, G., Tareilus, E., Mueller, R. and Meijer, G. (2009). Strategies to Reduce Sodium Consumption: A Food Industry Perspective. *Critical Reviews in Food Science and Nutrition*, 49: 10, 841 – 851.

Doyle, M.E. and Glass, K.A. (2010). Sodium Reduction and Its Effect on Food Safety, Food Quality, and Human Health. *Comprehensive Reviews in Food Science and Food Safety*, 9, 44-56.

El-Bakry, M., Duggan, E., O'Riordan, E.D. and O'Sullivan, M. (2011). Effect of Chelating Salt Type on Casein Hydration and Fat Emulsification during Manufacture and Functionality of Imitation Cheese. *Journal of Food Engineering*, 102, 145-153.

El-Bakry, M., Beninati, F., Duggan, E., O'Riordan, E.D. and O'Sullivan, M. (2010). Reducing Salt in Imitation Cheese: Effects on Manufacture and Functional Properties. *Food Research International*, doi: 10.1016/j.foodres.2010.12.013.

Ennis, M.P., O'Sullivan, M.M. and Mulvihill, D.M. (1998). The hydration behaviour of rennet caseins in calcium. *Food Hydrocolloids*, 12, 451-457.

Fielding, S. and Locke, K. W. (1993). Choline-containing compositions as salt substitutes and enhancers and a method of preparation. *Interneuron Pharmaceuticals,* 520-604.

Fitzgerald E. and Buckley J. (1985). Effect of total and partial substitution of sodium chloride on the quality of cheddar cheese. *Journal of Dairy Science*, 68, 3127–3134.

Fox, P.F., O'Connor, T.P., McSweeney, P.L.H., Guinee, T.P., and O'Brien, N.M. (1996). Cheese: Physical, biochemical and nutritional aspects. In Taylor, S.L. (Ed), *Advances in Food and Nutrition Research*, 39, 163-328. London, UK: Academic Press.

Guinee, T.P. (2004). Salting and the role of salt in cheese. *International Journal of Dairy Technology,* 57, 2, 99- 109.

Hellemann, U. (1992). Perceived taste of NaCl and acid mixtures in water and bread. *International Journal of Food Science and Technology*, 27, 201–211.

Fox, P.F. and McSweeney, P. (2004). Cheese: An Overview. In Fox, P.F. et al. (Eds.), *Cheese - Chemistry, Physics and Microbiology Vol. 1* (pp. 1-25). Amsterdam, Netherlands: Academic Press.

GNPD. (2008). Global new product database. Chicago, IL: Mintel Group.

Green D.M., Ropper A.H., Kronmal R.A., Psaty B.M., Burke G.L. (2002). Serum potassium level and dietary potassium intake as risk factors for stroke. *Neurology*, 59, 314-320.

Guinee, T.P. and Fox, P.F. (2004). Salt in Cheese: Physical, Chemical and Biological Aspects. In Fox, P.F. et al. (Eds.), *Cheese - Chemistry, Physics and Microbiology Vol. 1* (pp. 207-259). Amsterdam, Netherlands: Academic Press.

Guinee T.P, Carić M. and Kaláb M. (2004). Pasteurized processed cheese and substitute/imitation cheese products. In: Cheese: Chemistry, Physics and Microbiology, Volume 2. Major cheese groups. London, New York: Elsevier Applied Science.

Gupta S.K., Karahdian C. and Lindsay R.C. (1984). Effect of emulsifier salts on textural and flavor properties of processed cheeses. *Journal of Dairy Science*, 67, 764–78.

Holland, B., Unwin, I.D. andBuss, D.H. (1989). Milk products and eggs. In The Fourth Supplement to McCance and Widdowson's The Composition of Foods, 4th edition. Cambridge, UK: Royal Society of Chemistry/Ministry of Agriculture, Fisheries and Food.

Johnson, M.E., Kapoor, R., McMahon, D.J., McCoy, D.R. and Narasimmon, R.G. (2009). Reduction of Sodium and Fat Levels in Natural and Processed Cheeses: Scientific and Technological Aspects. *Comprehensive Reviews in Food Science and Food Safety*, 8, 252-268.

Henson, L.S. (1997). Reduced sodium content process cheese and method for making it. U.S. patent 5871797A1.

Keast, R.S. and Breslin, P.A. (2003). An overview of taste-taste interactions. *Food Quaityl Preference*, 14, 111–124.

Karahadian, C. and Lindsay, R.C. (1984). Flavor and textural properties of reduced sodium process American cheeses. *Journal of Dairy Science*, 61, 1892-1904.

Kwak, H.S., Choi, S.S., Ahn, J. and Lee, S.W. (2002). Casein hydrolysate fractions act as emulsifiers in process cheese. *Journal of Food Science*, 67, 821-825.

Labruni, T., Henry, S., Affolter, M. and Schlichterle-Cerny, H. (2003). Seasoning compositions (EP 1344459).

Lee, S.K., Buwalda, R.J., Euston, S.R., Foegeding, E.A. and McKenna, B. (2003). Changes in the rheology and microstructure of processed cheese during cooking. *LWT-Food Sciend and Technology*, 36, 339–345.

Lindsay R.C., Hargett S.M. and Bush C.S. (1982). Effect of sodium/potassium (1:1) chloride and low sodium chloride concentrations on quality of cheddar cheese. Journal of Dairy Science, 65, 360–370.

Loessner, M.J., Maier, S.K., Schiwek, P. and Scherer, S. (1997). Long-chain polyphosphates inhibit growth of *Clostridium tyrobutyricum* in processed cheese spreads. *Journal of Food Protection*, 60, 493-498.

Lucey, J.A. (2008). Advances in nonfat/lowfat process cheese for melting and ingredient use. *Journal of Dairy Science*, 91, E-Suppl. 1, 153-154.

Metzger, L.E. and Kapoor R. (2007). Novel approach for producing with reduced-fat and reduced sodium content. Journal of Dairy Science, 86(Supplement 1), 198.

Meyer, A. (1973). *Processed Cheese Manufacture*. London, UK: Food Trade Press Ltd.

Mistry, V.V. and Kasperson, K.M. (1998). Influence of salt on the quality of reduced fat Cheddar cheese. *Journal of Dairy Science* 81, 1214–1221.

O'Brien, N.M. and O'Connor, T.P. (2004). Nutritional aspects of cheese. . In Fox, P.F. et al. (Eds.), *Cheese - Chemistry, Physics and Microbiology Vol. 1* (pp. 572-583). Amsterdam, Netherlands: Academic Press.

Paulus, K. (2008). New mozzarella breaks low fat impasse. Wisconsin Center for Dairy Research. *Dairy Pipeline*, 2, 1-6.

Phan VA, Yven C, Lawrence G, Chabanet C, Reparet JM and Salles, C. (2008). In vivo sodium release related to salty perception during eating model cheeses of different textures. *International Dairy Journal*, 18, 956-963.

Rutikowska A, Kilcawley K.N., Doolan I., Alonso-Gomez M., Beresford T.P. and Wilkinson M.G. (2008). Influence of sodium chloride on the quality of cheddar cheese. IDF symposium: 5th IDF symposium on cheese ripening, March 9-13, 2008, Berne, Switzerland.

Savello, P.A., Ernstrom, C.A. and Kalab, M. (1989). Microstructure and meltability of model process cheese made with rennet and acid casein. *Journal of Dairy Science*, 72, 1-11.

Schroeder, C.L., Bodyfeh, E.W., Wyatt, C.J. and McDaniel, M.R. (1988). Reduction of sodium chloride in cheddar cheese: effect on sensory, microbiological, and chemical properties. *Journal of Dairy Science*, 71, 2010-2020.

Searby, L. (2006). Pass the salt. *International Food Ingredients*, 2-3.

Stanier, R.Y., Adelberg, E.A. and Ingraham, J.L. (1981). General Microbiology, 4th edition, The Macmillan Press Ltd, London

Swenson, B.J., Wendorff, W.L. and Lindsay, R.C. (2000). Effects of ingredients on the functionality of fat-free process cheese spreads. *Journal of Food Science*, 65, 822-825.

Taormina, P.J.(2010). Implications of Salt and Sodium Reduction on Microbial Food Safety. *Critical Reviews in Food Science and Nutrition*, 50 (3), 209-227.

Tanaka, N., Goepfert, J.M., Traisman, E. and Hoffbeck, W.M. (1979). A challenge of pasteurized process cheese spread with Clostridium botulinum spores. *Journal of Food Protection*, 42, 787-789.

Tanaka, N., Traisman, E., Plantinga, P., Finn, L., Flom, W., Meske, L. and Guggisberg, J. (1986). Evaluation of factors involved in antibotulinal properties of pasteurized process cheese spread. *Journal of Food Protection,* 49, 526-531.

Templeton, H.L. and Sommer, H.H. (1936). Studies on the emulsifying salts used in processed cheese. Journal of Dairy Science, 19, 561-572.

Thomas, T.D. and Pearce, K.N. (1985). Influence of salt on lactose fermentation and proteolysis in Cheddar cheese. *New Zealand Journal of Dairy Technology*, 16, 253-259.

Wagner, M.K. (1986). Phosphates as antibotulinal agents in cured meats, a review. *Journal of Food Protection*. 49, 482-487.

Walstra, P., Wouters, J. and Geurts, T. (2006). Dairy Science and technology, 2nd edition (pp. 739). New York: Francis and Taylor.

Wolf, I.V, Perotti, M.C., Bernal, S.M. and Zalazar, C.A. (2010). Study of the chemical composition, proteolysis, lipolysis and volatile compounds profile of commercial Reggianito Argentino cheese: Characterization of Reggianito Argentino cheese. *Food Research International*, 43, 1204-1211.

Zehren, V.L. and Nusbaum, D.D. (2000). *Process Cheese*. Madison, Wisconsin, USA: Cheese Reporter Publishing, Co, Inc.

In: Cheese: Types, Nutrition and Consumption
Editor: Richard D. Foster, pp. 119-142

ISBN 978-1-61209-828-9
© 2011 Nova Science Publishers, Inc.

Chapter 6

INVESTIGATION ON A TYPICAL DAIRY PRODUCT OF THE APULIA REGION (ITALY), THE GARGANICO CACIORICOTTA CHEESE, BY MEANS OF TRADITIONAL AND INNOVATIVE PHYSICO-CHEMICAL ANALYSES

A. Sacco, [*] *D. Sacco, G. Casiello, A. Ventrella, and F. Longobardi*

Dipartimento di Chimica, Università di Bari "A. Moro", Via Orabona 4,
70126 Bari (Italy)

ABSTRACT

This work deals with the characterization of a typical goat cheese, cacioricotta, produced in a restricted area (Promontory of Gargano) of the Apulia Region in Southern Italy. For this purpose, conventional (fat, protein, casein, urea, cryoscopy, metals content, fatty acid composition, solid content, moisture, ashes, pH) and innovative physico-chemical analyses, such as Nuclear Magnetic Resonance (NMR) Spectroscopy and Isotope Ratio Mass Spectroscopy (IRMS), have been carried out. The determinations have been done both on the starting goat milk and on the obtained cheese after 20 and 60 days of ripening. The conventional analysis has allowed to follow compositional changes of some elements occurred during the ripening of cacioricotta cheese. The NMR spectra were recorded using two different procedures. In the former, the sample was prepared by means of an aqueous extraction of the cacioricotta, while in the latter, the analysis was performed directly on the cacioricotta sample by using the ^{1}H HR-MAS NMR technique. All spectroscopic results have allowed the identification of the metabolic profile of cacioricotta cheese. Finally, for the first time, the IRMS has been applied on goat milk and cheese. The obtained isotopic results were not easy to understand and required further investigations on a higher number of samples. Moreover, a comparison of results

---

[*] Corrispondent author: Prof. Antonio Sacco, Dipartimento di Chimica, Via Orabona 4, 70126 Bari (Italy). e-mail: antonio.sacco@chimica.uniba.it.

of cacioricotta samples coming from different areas of production could be very interesting.

Keywords: Cacioricotta Cheese, Routine Analyses, NMR, IRMS, Metabolic Profile.

1. INTRODUCTION

The cacioricotta, a seasonal crude and soft cheese, is produced from the milk of goats reared at pasture in the rocky promontory of Gargano, located in the north-eastern Apulia Region in Italy (Figure 1).

Its name derives from the particular coagulation of the milk, that is partly rennet, characteristic of the cheese (*cacio*), and partly thermal, characteristic of ricotta cheese (*ricotta*).

The cacioricotta, with tangy and slightly spicy flavor-ur, is used both as a table product and as cheese for graters.

As a function of aging time, there are two product types: the first is the so called fresh cacioricotta, Figure 2 (a), that undergoes a short ripening up to 20 days; the other is the ripened cacioricotta, Figure 2 (b), left to dry (2-3 months) on wooden supports placed in cool and ventilated locations, that are often covered with a fine mesh to avoid that contact with insects or other animals which makes the product quality poor.

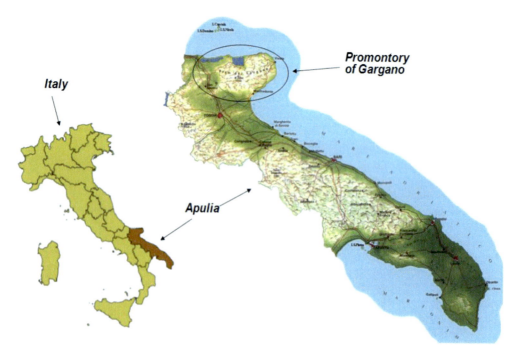

Figure 1. Map of Apulia Region showing the Promontory of Gargano.

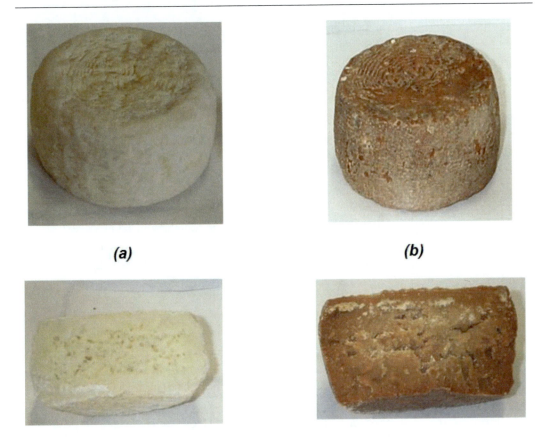

Figure 2. Cacioricotta after 20 (a) and 60 (b) days of ripening.

The fresh cacioricotta is a soft cheese, uniform and white. The fresh product generally loses 30-40% of its original weight after only 15 days from production. Going into the ripening, cacioricotta becomes a semi-hard cheese, slightly riddled and pale yellow in color.

Traditional, Gas Chromatography (GC), Inductively Coupled Plasma Emission Spectroscopy (ICP-AES) and Isotope Ratio Mass Spectrometry (IRMS) analyses on samples of goat milk are reported in this paper. In addition to traditional, GC, ICP-AES and IRMS analyses, investigations based on Nuclear Magnetic Resonance (NMR) spectroscopy were carried out on fresh and aged cacioricotta samples.

In the food chemistry field, there is a growing application of innovative physico-chemical techniques, such as IRMS and NMR, to obtain detailed information on the metabolites of the analyzed matrices and to characterize the geographical origin of products.

NMR is a fast technique that allows to determine a great number of metabolites and is, for this reason, increasingly used in food and dairy research [1-14]. The enormous improvement of the NMR hardware has made this technique rather sensible and applicable on both liquid and solid samples. Another advantage of NMR is that of minimum physico-chemical manipulation necessary to prepare the sample. Since NMR provides exhaustive chemical profiles in a single experiment, we applied this technique to determine the metabolic profile of the cacioricotta cheese. Moreover, in the case of the NMR spectra, we used two different methods of analysis on cacioricotta.

The first consisted in the recording of a spectra of aqueous extracts of cacioricotta, while in the second, we used the technique of ^{1}H HR-MAS NMR which allows to obtain the spectrum directly on the solid sample of cacioricotta.

Indeed, the use of IRMS to characterize origin and animal feeding has been widely investigated [15-17]. The ratio of carbon isotopes (δ^{13}C) in plants is influenced mainly by the pathway of CO_2 fixation used by the plant species, be it the C_3 Calvin cycle, as for wheat, or the C_4 Hatch-Slack cycle, as for corn and maize.

The ratio of oxygen isotopes (δ^{18}O) in milk water reflects the isotope composition of the ground water drunk by animals, which, in turn, is influenced by geographical factors such as altitude, latitude, and distance from the sea [18]. Seasonal effects are also of great importance: in summer, milk water contains higher δ^{18}O content because animals eat fresh plants containing δ^{18}O–enriched water due to evapotranspiration phenomena in leaves.

The ratio of nitrogen isotopes (δ^{15}N) in dairy products reflects, through the plants consumed by animals, the isotope composition of the original soil [19-22] which is influenced by many factors such as agricultural practices (intensive or extensive cultivation) [23], climatic and geographical conditions [24]. The use of massive quantities of organic fertilizers and other factors such as aridity, salinity, and closeness to the sea, tends to increase the ^{15}N/^{14}N isotope ratio in soil, plants and animal products. Moreover, for animal products, the presence of nitrogen-fixing plants in the diet can lead to lower values because these plants use both atmospheric and soil nitrogen as a nitrogen source, which results in lower ^{15}N content than in plants relying only on soil nitrogen (enriched in ^{15}N relative to the atmospheric nitrogen).

All results obtained have provided a complete physico-chemical characterization of cacioricotta, allowing to highlight the quality of the product.

2. MATERIALS AND METHODS

2.1. Methods for Collection of Goat Milk and Cacioricotta Samples

Seven farms in the Promontory of Gargano have provided goat milk samples. The samples divided into two aliquots of 500 ml were numbered from 1 to 7, depending on the origin, and were immediately placed in a refrigerator at 4°C.

The seven farms supplying the milk samples are located at an altitude of 300-400m and have an average consistence of about 150 head of goats, only raised in the wild.

In the same farms, 7 rounds of cacioricotta were collected, after 20 days, obtained from the same previously supplied fresh milk.

The rounds of cacioricotta were also numbered from 1 to 7, in such a way to match the cacioricotta and milk coming from the same supplier.

Finally, after 60 days, in two dairies, which previously had supplied the milk, two rounds of ripened cacioricotta have been taken.

The rounds have been identified with the number 8 and 9 corresponding to the starting milks 5 and 6.

2.2. Milk Samples

2.2.1. Routine Analyses

On the seven samples of goat milk, the following traditional physico-chemical analyses were carried out: fat, protein, lactose, crioscopy, somatic cell count, pH, casein and urea.

Contents of protein, fat, lactose, casein and urea were determined using a Milko Scan FT 120 (Foss Italia, Padova, Italy).

pH was determined by means of a pH-meter Forlab mod. 707.

Cryoscopy measurements were done by Milk Cryoscope AC2 of Advances, Italy.

Somatic cell count (SCC) was determined by a Fossomatic 360 (Foss Electric, Italy) apparatus using the standard procedure [25].

2.2.2. Fatty Acid Composition

The fatty acid composition of goat milk was determined by gas chromatography (GC) as fatty acid methyl esters (FAME). FAME were prepared using saponification/methylation with potassium methylate.

Fresh samples of milk were centrifuged at 15000 rpm for 40 min, so an aliquot of extracted milk fat was saponified for 30 minutes in the water bath at 60–70°C with the methanolic solution of KOH (2 mol/l).

Methyl esters of fatty acids were separated and quantified by using a HR-GC, Carlo Erba gas chromatograph, equipped with a DB Wax-type analytical column, (30 m length x 0.32 mm i.d) coated with 0.5 μm film thickness (100% PEG, polyethylene glycol) (JandW Scientific Inc. Rancho Cordova, CA, USA), and coupled with an FID detector (Varian, Middelburg, The Netherlands). Helium was used as the carrier gas. The injection is performed with a split ratio 1:50 and constant flow operating mode at 50m/sec. The injector temperature and the heated block temperature are both set at 220°C. The injected volume was 1μL. Fatty acids were identified by comparison with retention times of fatty acids in standard samples.

2.2.3. Chromatographic Analyses

Na, K, Mg and Ca contents were measured by means of high performance ion chromatography (HPIC) as described previously [26].

For these determinations, milk ash samples were dissolved in 50 ml of 0.1 N HCl.

2.2.4. Atomic Emission Spectrometric Measurements

The total concentrations of Ni, Se, Cr, Cu, Fe, Al, Mn, Pb, Zn were measured by inductively-coupled plasma atomic emission spectrometry (ICP-AES) on a Varian instrument model Liberty 110 (Varian Inc. Palo Alto, USA) equipped with an ultrasonic nebulizer Cetac model U-5000AT$^+$ (Cetac Tecnologies Inc., Omaha, Nebraska, USA).

Before analysis, the samples were freeze-dried and subjected to a mineralization process: 0.5g of sample was dissolved in 7 ml of 70% HNO_3 Ultrapure Reagent (J.T. Baker, Phillipsburg, USA) and 2 ml of 30% H_2O_2 (J. T. Baker, Phillisburg, USA) and digested in a microwave system Milestone model MLS-1200 MEGA (Milestone, Bergamo, Italy). For each digestion step, a blank sample was prepared with the same amount of reagents.

Normal precautions for trace element analysis were observed throughout. The reaction vessels of microwave ovens were cleaned before each digestion with 5 ml of INSTRA-

Analyzed 70% HNO$_3$ (J.T. Baker, Phillipsburg, USA), heated for fifteen minutes at 600 W and then rinsed with ultra pure water. Glassware was cleaned by soaking overnight in 10% nitric acid solution and then rinsed with ultra pure water obtained from a water deionization system, Millipore model MILLI-Q RG (Millipore, MA, USA).

Calibration was carried out using an external standard solution obtained by diluting a 1000 mg l^{-1} standard solution for inductively-coupled plasma (J.T. Baker, Phillipsburg, USA).

For the freeze-dry process of goat milk, a Heto-Holten A/S LyoLab 3000 instrument was used, connected with a vacuum rotary pump. The freeze-dry process was performed at −55°C.

2.2.5. Stable Isotope Ratio Analyses

The determination of $^{13}C/^{12}C$, $^{15}N/^{14}N$ ratios ($\delta^{13}C$ and $\delta^{15}N$, respectively) of goat milk were carried out on the freeze-dried samples. About 1.5 mg of sample were directly weighed into tin capsules (Santis Analytical Italia, Bareggio, Italy) for these determinations.

The analyses were performed using an isotopic ratio mass spectrometer (IRMS, Finnigan Delta V Advantage, Thermo Fisher Scientific, Bremen, Germany) coupled with an Elemental Analyzer (EA, FlashEA 1112 HT, Thermo Fisher Scientific, Bremen, Germany). The EA was equipped with a combustion reactor for determination of $^{13}C/^{12}C$, $^{15}N/^{14}N$. The EA was connected with an auto-sampler (MAS 200R, Thermo Fisher Scientific, Bremen, Germany) and interfaced with the IRMS through a dilutor (Finningam, Conflo III, Thermo Fisher Scientific, Bremen, Germany) dosing the samples and reference gases. Variations in stable isotope ratios were reported as parts per thousand (‰) deviation from Internationally accepted standards: Pee Dee Belemnite (PDB) for carbon, Atmospheric nitrogen (AIR) for nitrogen. The isotopic values were expressed using the formula:

$$\delta(‰) = [(R_{sample} - R_{standard})/R_{standard}] \times 1000$$

where R is the ratio between the heavy and light isotopes, R_{sample} is the isotopic ratio of the sample and $R_{standard}$ is that of the reference material. Each sample was analyzed twice and values were averaged. The analysis was repeated if the difference between the two values was higher than 0.2‰ for $\delta^{15}N$ and $\delta^{13}C$, respectively. The values were referenced against reference gases (N$_2$, CO$_2$) previously calibrated against International Standards from the International Atomic Energy Agency (IAEA). Moreover, for each run, at least one in-house standard (casein for carbon and nitrogen) was analyzed to check the accuracy of the analysis.

2.3. Cacioricotta Samples

2.3.1. Routine Analyses

On the seven samples of fresh cacioricotta and the two samples of ripened cacioricotta, the following traditional physico-chemical analyses were carried out: solid content, moisture, ashes, fat, pH and NaCl.

Solid content was determined by difference of weighing, leading to dry 10 g of the sample in an oven at 102 °C for 2 hours, then cooling in a desiccator and weighted to constant weight.

Ashes: samples were heated to give dry extracts whose ash content was obtained by heating to 600°C for 6 hours, in muffle.

Moisture and NaCl were determined by standard procedure [27-28].

Fat and pH measurement procedure was reported previously in the milk section.

2.3.2. Chromatographic Analyses and Atomic Emission Spectrometric Measurements

The total concentrations of Na, K, Mg, Ca, Se, Cu, Fe and Zn were measured as previously reported in the case of milk samples.

2.3.3. Stable Isotope Ratio Analyses

The determination of $\delta^{13}C$ and $\delta^{15}N$ of cacioricotta samples were carried out as previously reported in the case of milk samples.

2.3.4. NMR Spectra

2.3.4.1. ^{1}H-NMR Spectra on Aqueous Extract of Cacioricotta

^{1}H NMR spectra were realized on freeze-dried cacioricotta samples. 2 g of sample was dissolved in 7 ml of D_2O containing 0.75% of 3-(trimethylsilyl)propionic-2,2,3,3-d_4 acid, sodium salt (TSP), as reference. The mixture was placed in an ultrasonic bath to ensure solubilization. The aqueous extract obtained was filtered to remove insoluble particles and placed in a 5mm NMR sample tube. Spectra were obtained on a Bruker Avance 500 MHz spectrometer (Bruker Analytik GMBH, Rheinstetten, Germany), using a pre-saturation sequence for water suppression. The following conditions were used: 65000 data points, 200 scans, spectral width of 9.76 ppm, line broadening of 0.3 Hz.

2.3.4.2. ^{1}H HR-MAS NMR Spectra

Spectra were acquired at 300K on an AVANCE 400 MHz (Bruker Analytik GmbH, Rheinstetten, Germany) spectrometer equipped with a high-resolution HR-MAS probe head suitable for 4 mm rotors. The samples were brought to the magic angle respect to the direction of the static magnetic field and they were spun at 4200Hz in order to minimize the chemical shift anisotropy effects. Proton 1D spectra were acquired by using the mono-dimensional version of NOESY sequence, with water signal suppression by pre-saturation. The following experimental conditions were applied: spectral width = 6000 Hz (~15 ppm); time domain = 32K points; acquisition time = 3 sec; number of transients = 160; mixing time = 80 ms. Spectra were processed by applying a 0.3 Hz line broadening factor.

Table 1. Routine analyses of goat milk

Sample	Fat (% p/p)	Protein (% p/p)	Casein (% p/p)	Casein/Protein (%)	Urea (mg/100ml)	Lactose (% p/p)	Crioscopy (°C)	SCC* (Cell/ml)	pH
1	3.0	2.6	2.1	81	36.1	4.6	-0.558	1,079,000	6.43
2	3.6	3.1	2.4	79	51.0	4.4	-0.580	1,015,000	6.24
3	3.9	2.7	2.1	79	51.4	4.3	-0.563	575,000	6.34
4	2.6	2.8	2.2	79	41.8	4.5	-0.558	1,957,000	6.49
5	3.3	2.8	2.2	79	40.8	4.5	-0.557	1,048,000	6.54
6	2.9	2.6	2.1	81	37.6	4.6	-0.563	1,270,000	6.44
7	3.3	3.2	2.6	82	42.5	4.5	-0.566	833,000	6.38
Average	3.2	2.8	2.3	80	43.0	4.5	-0.564	1,111,000	6.41

* Somatic Cell Count.

3. RESULTS AND DISCUSSION

3.1. Goat Milk

3.1.1. Routine Analyses

In Table 1, the results of traditional analyses carried out on the seven samples are reported.

Some comments can be made on the results.

Fat Content

The percentage of fat in Gargano goat milk is relatively low compared to the average values reported in the literature [29]. This unexpected value can be attributed to several causes such as species and breed of animals, animal housing conditions, type of forage and the microclimate in which they live.

Casein

The average value of this parameter is relatively low. This value, coupled with the equally low value for protein, leads to clots generally less consistent than those of cow's milk. In particular, the clot is formed more rapidly but the time of firming is higher. Consequently, the curd has a weak consistency, is more delicate, less resistant to mechanical treatment, and therefore, gives lower yields.

pH

The average value found for goat milk is comparable with that reported in the literature [29].

3.1.2. Fatty Acid Composition.

In Table 2, the composition of fatty acids are shown.

Fatty acids profile is considered essential in the definition of flavors and aroma of typical dairy product called "of niche". Furthermore, fatty acids are able to reflect the narrow link between product and territory since they represent a source of volatile aromatic constituents.

Particularly, the lipid fraction of goat milk is its most distinctive property.

Fat globules of goat milk are smaller in size when compared to that of cow milk. Fatty acids in milk fat are arranged in triglycerides in accordance with a pattern that appears to be universal among ruminants. Although the percent of unsaturated fatty acids (e.g. oleic and linolenic acid) do not differ from the average found for cow milk, a major difference between goat and cow milk is the distribution of specific short chain fatty acids. In fact, goat fatty acids have an appreciably higher proportion of capric, caprylic and caproic acids. These features make goat milk more digestible due to the most specific micellar surface available to lipase attack, and more flavorful. However, heat treatment and hence, pasteurization of milk removes the characteristic smell associated with goat milk and derivates.

Goat milk samples, analyzed in this work, showed higher concentration of fatty acids with short and medium chain, such as caproic, caprylic and capric, as expected.

Table 2. Fatty Acid composition (%) of goat milk

	Fatty Acid	1	2	3	4	5	6	7	Average
C4	Butyric	1.71	1.48	1.19	2.87	2.38	2.34	1.32	1.90
C6	Caproic	1.71	2.15	1.78	3.08	1.32	1.71	1.71	1.92
C8	Caprylic	2.40	3.39	2.15	4.40	3.34	5.85	2.13	3.38
C10	Capric	8.09	10.3	6.95	13.2	8.67	15.5	7.98	10.1
C12	Lauric	3.64	4.23	2.59	4.98	2.31	6.52	2.39	3.81
C14	Myristic	7.04	9.20	5.63	10.4	6.45	13.6	12.9	9.34
C16	Palmitic	17.6	23.0	23.4	28.7	26.0	28.7	19.6	23.9
C18:0	Stearic	7.64	12.7	10.8	14.5	16.2	14.0	15.6	13.1
C18:1c	Oleic	11.8	13.0	26.2	17.6	22.9	10.9	18.3	17.3
C18:2	Linoleic	6.43	3.38	3.24	0	1.42	0	2.17	2.37
C20:0	Arachidic	6.50	4.29	3.37	0	1.51	0	1.23	2.41
C18:3	Linolenic	5.63	3.60	2.67	0	1.17	0	5.67	2.67

3.1.3. Metal Content

In Table 3, the concentrations of metals: Ca, Mg, Na, K, Zn, Cu, Fe, Se, Cr, Al, Ni, Mn, Pb, are reported.

It should be pointed out again that the results in Table 3 were obtained on "freeze-dried" milk samples. Therefore, these values cannot be immediately compared with that reported in the literature for whole goat milk [29]. However, if we consider that the water content in goat milk is on average 86-87%, it is possible to recalculate the data on the basis of water loss due to freeze-drying process. The results obtained are in satisfactory agreement with literature data [29]. For example, if the average value obtained for Na (286 mg/100g) in the lyophilized product is corrected by the average loss of water, a value of 39 mg/100g in the whole milk is obtained, in satisfying agreement with the 40 mg/100g value reported in the literature [29]. The recalculated values of metal concentrations are shown at the bottom of Table 3.

Taking a look at the results, we can draw some considerations.

Goat milk is particularly suitable for children and the elderly due to the high value of Ca, together with a good content of other minerals such as K, Cu, Mn and Fe and the highest digestibility compared to cow milk. Furthermore, the analyzed samples are totally lacking those metals that could be harmful to health. In particular, Cr and Pb concentration, even if calculated in the freeze-dried samples, are always less than the detection limit of the instrument (<0.1 mg/100g). Therefore, we can assert that goat milk, coming from animals fed on pasture, are free from contamination and pollutants.

Table 3. Metals content (mg/100 g) of freeze-dried goat milk

Sample	Ca	Mg	Na	K	Zn	Cu	Fe	Se	Cr	Al	Ni	Mn	Pb
1	1130	96	280	1420	1.10	0.11	0.43	<0.8	<0.1	0.98	<0.6	0.02	<0.1
2	1030	96	250	1260	0.73	0.08	0.22	<0.8	<0.1	0.67	<0.6	0.02	<0.1
3	990	104	310	1630	0.71	0.07	0.30	<0.8	<0.1	0.76	<0.6	0.02	<0.1
4	1140	106	310	1610	0.90	0.11	0.43	<0.8	<0.1	1.35	<0.6	0.03	<0.1
5	1050	95	290	1440	0.84	0.11	0.47	<0.8	<0.1	1.10	<0.6	0.03	<0.1
6	1120	102	270	1410	0.94	0.06	0.24	<0.8	<0.1	0.75	<0.6	0.01	<0.1
7	960	96	290	1520	0.75	0.11	0.48	<0.8	<0.1	1.23	<0.6	0.04	<0.1
Average	1060	99	286	1470	0.85	0.09	0.37			0.98		0.024	

Metals content (mg/100 g) of goat milk [corrected as reported in the text]

	Ca	Mg	Na	K	Zn	Cu	Fe	Se	Cr	Al	Ni	Mn	Pb
Average	146	14	39	201	0.12	0.012	0.05			0.14		0,003	
INRAN*	141	13	40	180	0.31	0.03	0.10			-		-	

* Istituto Nazionale di Ricerca per gli Alimenti e la Nutrizione. Tabelle di composizione degli alimenti, Italy (2009).

3.1.4. IRMS Results

Table 4 shows the values of isotopic ratios $^{13}C/^{12}C$ ($\delta^{13}C$) and $^{15}N/^{14}N$ ($\delta^{15}N$) found in the seven samples of goat milk.

Table 4. $\delta^{13}C$ and $\delta^{15}N$ of goat milk

Sample	$\delta^{13}C$ [‰]	$\delta^{15}N$ [‰]
1	−23.2	5.7
2	−22.1	5.8
3	−22.5	5.2
4	−22.2	5.4
5	−22.4	5.6
6	−22.7	5.3
7	−22.3	5.6
Average	−22.5	5.5

Relative carbon, nitrogen and oxygen stable isotope abundances in milk reflect the isotopic composition of the diet fed to the animals and are also related to the geographical and the climatic factors. Therefore, a statistical treatment on the results of isotopic ratios ($\delta^{13}C$, $\delta^{15}N$ and $\delta^{18}O$) on milk from animals of the same species but from farms located in different geographical areas could be able to distinguish the various products and then characterize their geographical origin. As previously said, the $\delta^{13}C$ value is related to the botanical origin of a plant or its photosynthetic cycle (C3 or C4 plants), while $\delta^{15}N$ and $\delta^{18}O$ are primarily influenced by factors such as climate and geographical conditions. For example, milk from regions dominated by grassland typically shows negative $\delta^{13}C$-values, while in regions dominated by crop cultivation, the $\delta^{13}C$-values are less negative. Furthermore, the $\delta^{13}C$-value in animal products indicates the C3/C4-plant ratio in the feed while the $\delta^{15}N$ and $\delta^{18}O$ values are characteristic of local conditions.

Looking in more detail at the results, it can be observed that the average value of $\delta^{13}C$ found in goat milk does not differ too much from the value obtained for Apulia cow milk [30]. Similar considerations can be made on the average value of $\delta^{15}N$ obtained for goat and cow milk [30]. This fact suggests that this parameter does not depend strongly on the animal species investigated.

However, this study on Gargano goat's milk must be considered a preliminary approach to the problem on the differentiation of goat milk with different geographic origin.

3.2. Cacioricotta Cheese

3.2.1. Routine Analyses

In Tables 5 and 6, the results of traditional analyses on the cacioricotta samples are reported after 20 and 60 days of ripening, respectively.

Table 5. Routine analyses of cacioricotta (20 days ripening)

Sample	Solid content (%)	Moisture (%)	Ashes (%)	Fat (%)	pH	NaCl (g/100g)
1	73	27	10	33.3	5.59	6.9
2	73	27	7	27.9	5.60	3.7
3	75	25	11	29.8	5.45	3.7
4	68	32	8	30.6	5.53	7.3
5	70	30	7	35.2	5.84	6.0
6	73	27	11	30.6	5.52	7.4
7	70	30	9	30.2	5.65	7.2
Average	72	28	9	31.1	5.60	6.0

Table 6. Routine analyses of cacioricotta (60 days ripening)

Sample	Solid Content (%)	Moisture (%)	Ashes (%)	Fat (%)	pH	NaCl (g/100g)
8	82	18	11	33.6	5.31	13.7
9	80	19	11	31.9	5.51	10.9
Average	81	19	11	32.7	5.41	12.3

Looking more in detail at the results obtained, it is possible to make the following considerations.

Solid Content and Moisture

The average values for solid content for fresh and ripened cacioricotta are within the values reported in literature. Similar considerations, since referred to complementary values, could be made for moisture content.

pH

The similar average pH value of fresh and ripened cacioricotta samples shows that this parameter is not linked to the ripening stage but rather to the milk provenance.

Fat

In relation to the fat content (referred to the dry matter), a cheese can be classified as "fat", if containing not less than 42%, "low-fat" if it contains less than 20%, "semi-fat" when fat content ranges between 20 and 42%. Therefore, the Gargano goat cacioricotta may be classified as "semi-fat" cheese.

NaCl

The value of this parameter depends on the salting of the product. The values obtained for the fresh and ripened products are slightly higher than those reported in the literature.

3.2.2. Fatty Acid Composition

In Tables 7 and 8, the results of the composition of fatty acids in the cacioricotta samples are reported after 20 and 60 days of ripening, respectively.

Milk fat is the macro-component more exposed to changes, both quantitative and qualitative, in the process of maturation. The latter is comprised of several fermentation processes involving the release of highly aromatic substances. Goat cheeses are characterized by a more pungent flavor and aroma due to the higher content of specific fatty acids (capronic, caprylic and caprinic), but these features are evident only with ripening, when triglycerides are broken down. Fresh and ripened cacioricotta, herein analyzed, show that saturated fatty acids increase with the ripening, while the oleic acid decreases

Table 7. Fatty Acid composition (%) in cacioricotta (20 days ripening)

Sample	1	2	3	4	5	6	7	Average
C4	2.71	3.24	1.95	3.31	2.57	1.07	2.31	2.45
C6	3.75	3.04	1.47	6.54	7.65	2.85	3.82	4.16
C8	5.10	3.27	2.24	3.31	2.94	1.95	2.78	3.08
C10	17.6	12.7	8.25	12.9	10.2	7.54	11.1	11.5
C12	6.52	5.51	3.97	4.81	3.83	4.06	5.43	4.88
C14	11.7	10.9	9.95	10.7	9.08	11.2	9.92	10.5
C16	28.4	30.3	36.0	27.4	28.8	38.7	30.0	31.4
C18:0	11.3	12.9	15.2	14.5	15.0	9.7	10.5	12.7
C18:1c	13.1	18.1	21.0	16.6	20.0	22.9	24.1	19.4

Table 8. Fatty Acid composition (%) in cacioricotta (60 days ripening)

Sample	8	9	Average
C4	2.38	2.46	2.42
C6	0.57	0.78	0.68
C8	4.53	5.12	4.83
C10	15.9	16.9	16.4
C12	7.60	6.90	7.25
C14	17.1	14.9	16.0
C16	36.6	32.8	34.7
C18:0	7.36	9.33	8.35
C18:1c	8.00	10.9	9.44

3.2.3. Metal Content

In Tables 9 and 10 the concentrations of metals are reported: Ca, Mg, Na, K, Zn, Cu, Fe, Se, obtained on freeze-dried cacioricotta samples after 20 and 60 days of ripening, respectively.

Table 9. Metals content (mg/100 g) of freeze-dried cacioricotta (20 days ripening)

Sample	Ca	Mg	Na	K	Zn	Cu	Fe	Se
1	1220	81	1240	770	1.46	0.20	0.32	<0.8
2	1220	87	1670	760	1.24	0.16	0.49	<0.8
3	1210	81	910	770	1.10	0.16	0.38	<0.8
4	1250	86	1860	730	0.72	0.17	0.48	<0.8
5	950	74	1520	780	0.91	0.29	0.44	<0.8
6	1170	81	1310	940	1.44	0.10	0.59	<0.8
7	1180	82	1420	790	1.62	0.19	0.45	<0.8
Average	1171	82	1419	791	1.21	0.18	0.45	

Metals content (mg/100 g) of cacioricotta (20 days ripening)
[corrected as reported in the text]

	Ca	Mg	Na	K	Zn	Cu	Fe	Se
Average	830	58	1006	561	0.86	0.13	0.32	

Table 10. Metals content (mg/100 g) of freeze-dried cacioricotta (60 days ripening)

Sample	Ca	Mg	Na	K	Zn	Cu	Fe	Se
8	1250	99	3200	120	1.28	0.23	0.75	<0.8
9	1240	94	3010	130	1.54	0.23	0.37	<0.8
Average	1245	97	3105	125	1.41	0.23	0.56	

Metals content (mg/100 g) of cacioricotta (60 days ripening)
[corrected as reported in the text]

	Ca	Mg	Na	K	Zn	Cu	Fe	Se
Average	1012	79	2524	102	1.20	0.18	0.45	

Before making some considerations on the results, it should be remembered that these values are relevant to the lyophilized product. Therefore, as done previously, it is necessary to recalculate the values of metal content taking into account the percentage of water removed during freeze-drying process. The results obtained are reported at the bottom of Tables 9 and 10, respectively.

Calcium

Calcium, like phosphorus, plays a plastic function, because as salt form, it is involved in the formation of bones and teeth. It is found mainly bound to the casein while the soluble fraction (25% of the total) is represented by monocalcium phosphate, monocalcium citrate and calcium ions. Milk calcium has a high bioavailability because, unlike many other vegetable foods, milk does not contain substances that sequester it. In addition, the lactose in milk allows the body to absorb calcium probably through an action on the intestinal mucosa.

Sodium

The significant difference between the average values of sodium in cacioricotta after 20 and 60 days of ripening is clearly due to the salting made during the preparation of the product.

Magnesium

The values of the products with different degrees of ripening are almost comparable.

Potassium

This metal is present in massive amounts in goat milk analyzed samples, while in cacioricotta, both in fresh and ripened, there is a lower quantity.

3.2.4. IRMS

Tables 11 and 12 show the isotopic ratios, $\delta^{13}C$ and $\delta^{15}N$, of cacioricotta for 20 days and for 60 days of ripening, respectively.

Table 11. $\delta^{13}C$ and $\delta^{15}N$ of fresh cacioricotta (20 days ripening)

Sample	$\delta^{13}C$ [‰]	$\delta^{15}N$ [‰]
1	−27.8	3.4
2	−27.7	3.2
3	−27.8	3.4
4	−27.5	3.5
5	−28.2	3.7
6	−27.3	4.2
7	−27.3	4.0
Average	−27.6	3.6

Table 12. $\delta^{13}C$ and $\delta^{15}N$ of cacioricotta (60 days ripening)

Sample	$\delta^{13}C$ [‰]	$\delta^{15}N$ [‰]
8	−26.9	3.8
9	−26.9	3.9
Average	−26.9	3.9

The daily consumption of about 100 grams of cheese is enough to satisfy the requirement of this element.

As expected, the concentration of Ca increases from milk to a more ripened product.

3.2.5. NMR Spectra

3.2.5.1. ¹H-NMR Spectra on Aqueous Extract of Cacioricotta

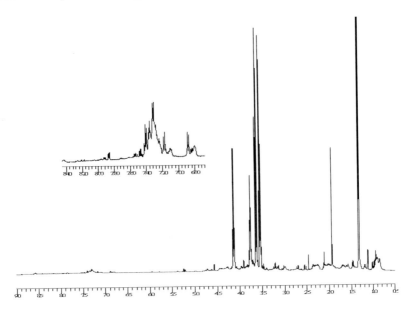

Figure 3. ¹H-NMR spectrum of an aqueous extract of cacioricotta cheese. The insert shows signals due to secondary components.

Table 13. Assignment of resonance in ¹H NMR spectrum of the aqueous extract of cacioricotta cheese

δ^1H (ppm)	Assignment	δ^1H (ppm)	Assignment
0.88	CH₃ butyric acid	3.08	βCH cysteine
0.91	CH₃ isoleucine	3.15	CH tyrosine
0.93	CH₃ leucine	3.27	CH β-glucose
0.95	CH₃ leucine	3.33	Proline
0.97	CH₃ valine	3.39	CH β-glucose
0.99	CH₃ isoleucine	3.40	Proline
1.02	CH₃ valine	3.54	CH₂ glycerol
1.28	CH₂ isoleucine	3.63	CH₂ glycerol
1.32	CH₃ lactic acid	3.75	CH lisine
1.46	CH₃ alanine	3.75	CH glutamate
1.46	CH₂ isoleucine	3.76	CH glycerol
1.54	β CH₂ butyric acid	3.77	CH β-galactose
1.69	CH lisine	3.77	CH alanine
1.72	CH₂ leucine	3.84	CH α-glucose
1.88	CH₂ lisine	3.85	CH β-glucose
1.88	β CH₂ γ-aminobutyric acid	3.89	α CH aspartate

1.92	CH₃ acetic acid	3.91	CH tyrosine
2.01	Proline	3.91	CH β-galactose
2.05	β CH glutamate	3.95	CH α-galactose
2.13	Methionine	3.98	αCH cysteine
2.15	βCH₂ methionine	4.00	αCH asparagine
2.15	α CH₂ butyric acid	4.11	CH lactic acid
2.28	Valine	4.12	Proline
2.28	α CH₂ γ-aminobutyric acid	4.56	CH β-galactose
2.34	Glutamate	4.65	CH β-glucose
2.36	Proline	5.21	CH α-glucose
2.44	CH₂ succinate	5.24	CH α-galactose
2.52	CH₂ citric acid	6.88	C3,C5 tyrosine ring
2.63	γCH₂ methionine	7.18	C2,C6 tyrosine ring
2.68	CH aspartate	7.20	C5 tryptophan ring
2.70	CH₂ citric acid	7.28	C6 tryptophan ring
2.79	CH aspartate	7.54	C7 tryptophan ring
2.87	CH asparagine	7.71	C4 tryptophan ring
2.95	CH asparagine	8.43	CH formic acid
3.00	γ CH₂ γ-aminobutyric acid		
3.02	CH₂ lisine		
3.04	CH tyrosine		

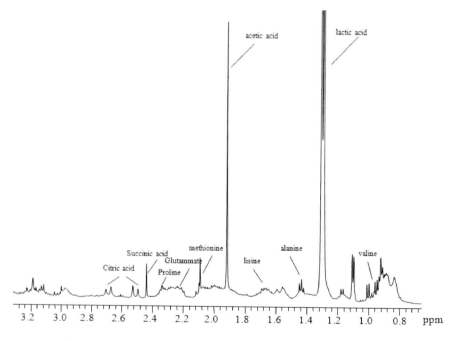

Figure 4. Region of ¹H NMR spectrum of the aqueous extract cacioricotta cheese showing signals of amino acids and organic acids.

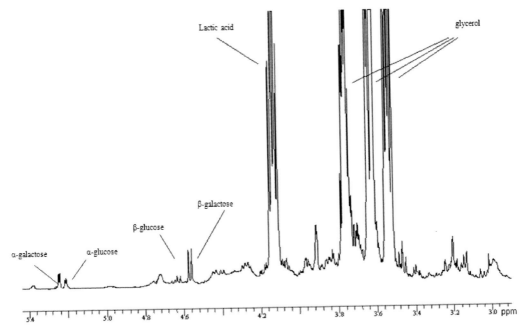

Figure 5. Region of ¹H NMR spectrum of the aqueous extract of cacioricotta cheese showing signal of glycerol and sugars.

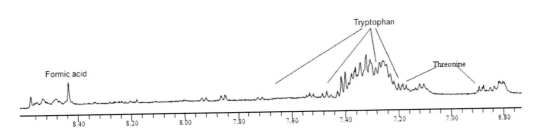

Figure 6. Region of ¹H NMR spectrum of the aqueous extract of cacioricotta cheese showing secondary components.

The ¹H-NMR spectrum is dominated by resonances due to majority components (lactic acid, glycerol), but it can also detect signals due to minority compounds. The assignments of signals in the spectrum, shown in Table 13, were made on the basis of comparison of chemical shifts with those from standard compounds. As it can be seen, the spectrum is very complex, because it contains several signals that are superimposed. For this reason, the complete assignment of signals was possible only through two-dimensional NMR, COSY experiments.

The most interesting region of the spectrum is the high-field one (Figure 4), where different signals due to amino acids (valine, lysine, proline, alanine, glutamate) and organic acids (lactic, acetic, succinic) are recognizable.

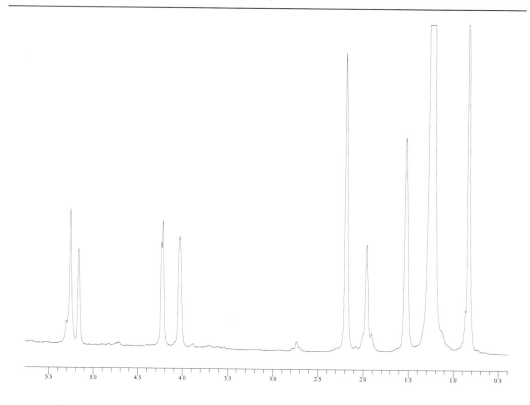

Figure 7. ¹H HR-MAS NMR spectrum of a cacioricotta cheese sample.

Table 14. Assignments of resonances in ¹H HR-MAS NMR spectrum of a fresh cacioricotta sample

δ ¹H (ppm)	Assignment
0.86	CH_3 fatty acids
0.89	CH_3 linolenic and butyric acids
1.25	-$(CH_2)_n$-
1.55	-$\underline{CH_2}$-CH_2-COO-
1.98	-$\underline{CH_2}$-CH=CH-
2.21	-$\underline{CH_2}$-COO-
2.72	-CH=CH-CH_2-CH=CH polyunsaturated acids
4.06	CH_2 glycerol
4.24	CH_2 glycerol
4.64	CH β-glucose
5.18	CH glycerol
5.28	-CH=CH- fatty acids
5.55	-CH=CH- hydroperoxide
5.72	-CH=CH- hydroperoxide

Figure 5 shows the high field region of the spectrum where it is possible to see the resonances due to glycerol and those due to sugars. Glucose and galactose are the most present sugars. Other signals due to minor components such as amino acids and organic acids, are present in this area, but are covered by intense signals due to glycerol and lactic acid.

In the low field area (6.5 to 9.0 ppm) of the spectrum (Figure 6), there are only minority compounds of cacioricotta, like aromatic amino acids, phenolic compounds and formic acid. Due to the low intensity of these signals, it was possible to make only a partial assignment.

3.2.5.2. ^{1}H HR-MAS NMR Spectra

^{1}H HR-MAS NMR spectrum of a cacioricotta sample is shown in Figure 7. As reported previously, this method allows to analyze samples directly in the solid phase without requiring a preliminary extraction process.

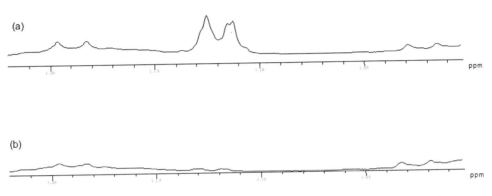

Figure 8. Region of ^{1}H NMR spectrum of an aqueous extract of cacioricotta cheese: (a) Cacioricotta cheese after 20 days of ripening, (b) Cacioricotta cheese after 60 days of ripening.

As it can be seen, the aspect of the spectrum is considerably different from that obtained on aqueous extract, and this is due to the presence of intense signals due to the fat component, which, unlike the other metabolites, is insoluble in water. However, in the spectrum of ^{1}H HR-MAS cacioricotta, it is possible to detect the presence of certain metabolites whose signals are not covered by the signals of fatty acids.

In Table 14, the assignments of signals for the ^{1}H HR-MAS NMR spectrum of a freeze-dried sample of cacioricotta are reported.

^{1}H HR-MAS NMR spectra were acquired for all cacioricotta samples in order to detect any differences between the samples at 20 days and those at 60 days of ripening. The comparison of the areas of the signals, proportional to the amount of fatty acids, were unable to find a significant increase in signal intensity at 5.72 ppm due to the products of oxidation of fat in the sample at 60 days. A reduction in signal intensity due to the protons of the glycerol in the samples at 60 days was also found. This shows the reduction of fat content of cheese, due to hydrolysis of triglycerides and subsequent volatilization of short chain fatty acids. This finding is consistent with the routine determination of total fat content, calculated as a percentage by weight of the dry matter.

However, to generalize the results obtained, we need to extend this search to a larger number of samples, considering a longer period of ripening.

3.3. Comparison between Cacioricotta after 20 and 60 Days of Ripening

The comparison on the spectra carried out on aqueous extracts of fresh and ripened cacioricotta samples does not show significant differences, except for the signal at 1.12 ppm (not assigned). This latest almost disappears in samples at 60 days of ripening (Figure 8).

CONCLUSION

This work was pointed to obtain a physico-chemical detailed description of cacioricotta, since the latter represents an important social and economic issue for the territory of the Gargano Promontory. Unfortunately, although the analyses carried out have demonstrated that cacioricotta is a good dairy product, both from the organoleptic and nutritional points of view, its use and diffusion is very limited. The production of cacioricotta occurs at the final stage of the lactation cycle of the goat, generally between May and September, during which the greater part of the production occurs. Moreover, the marketing of this typical product does not occur evenly throughout the year. In particular, in May, cacioricotta is highly demanded by consumers, as used traditionally for dinner matched with broad beans.

It should be noted, however, that especially in summer months, July and August, due to the flow of tourists and some specific promotion events for the local products, there is an increase in sales.

Typically, the sale of cacioricotta occurs almost exclusively from the same manufacturer that operates the transformation. Although this product, together with caciocavallo, is one of the cheeses that best characterizes the dairy business of the area of Gargano, it is almost unknown in the markets. However, this product seems to have significant potentialities for commercial development, especially if properly advertised in order to make known its peculiar characteristics.

In addition to its excellent organoleptic characteristics, the fresh cacioricotta has nutritional properties of high value. Also, being obtained from boiled milk, it is protected from health risks, such as brucellosis, affecting milk derivatives.

Finally, from the point of view of farmers, it is a reliable product since, thanks to the particular production technique, it incorporates the ricotta cheese, that the companies would not be able to market easily, due to storage and preservation problems, especially in summer.

ACKNOWLEDGMENTS

This work was completely supported by the Gargano Mountain Community (Contract No. 607). We are also grateful to Dr. Antonio Contessa for providing samples of goat milk and cacioricotta cheese.

REFERENCES

[1] Gil, AM; Duarte, IF; Delgadillo, I; Colquhoun, IJ; Casuscelli, F; Humpfer, E; Spraul, M. "Study of the Compositional Changes of Mango during Ripening by Use of Nuclear Magnetic Resonance Spectroscopy". *Journal of Agricultural and Food Chemistry*, 2000, 48, 1524-1536.

[2] Sobolev, AP; Segre, A; Lamanna, R. "Proton high-field NMR study of tomato juice". *Magnetic Resonance in Chemistry*, 2003, 41, 237–245.

[3] Belloque, J; Ramos, M "Application of NMR spectroscopy to milk and dairy products". *Trends in Food Science and Technology*, 1999, 10, 313-320.

[4] Brescia, MA; Monfreda, M; Buccolieri, A; Carrino, C. "Characterisation of the geographical origin of buffalo milk and mozzarella cheese by means of analytical and spectroscopic determinations". *Food Chemistry*, 2005, 89, 139-147.

[5] De Angelis Curtis, S; Curini, R; Delfini, M; Brosio, E; D'Ascenzo, G ; Bocca, B. "Amino acid profile in the ripening of Grana Padano cheese: a NMR study". *Food Chemistry*, 2000, 71, 495-502.

[6] De la Fuente, MA; Juarez, M. "Authenticity assessment of dairy products". *Critical Reviews in Food Science and Nutrition*, 2005, 45, 563-85.

[7] Gianferri, R; Maioli, M; Delfini, M; Brosio E."A low-resolution and high-resolution NMR integrated approach to investigate the physical structure and metabolic profile of Mozzarella di Bufala Campana cheese". *International Dairy Journal*, 2007, 17, 167-176.

[8] Gianferri, R; D'Aiuto, V; Curini, R; Delfini, M; Brosio E. "Proton NMR transverse relaxation measurements to study water dynamic states and age-related changes in Mozzarella di Bufala Campana cheese". *Food Chemistry*, 2007, 105, 720 – 726.

[9] Hu, F; Furuhata, K; Ito-Ishida, M; Kaminogawa, S; Tanokura, M. "Non-destructive Observation of Bovine Milk by NMR Spectroscopy: Analysis of Existing States of Compounds and Detection of New Compounds". *Journal of Agricultural and Food Chemistry*, 2004, 52, 4969–4974.

[10] Kakalis, LT; Kumosinski, TF; Farrell, JHM "The Potential of Solid-State Nuclear Magnetic Resonance in Dairy Research: An Application to Cheese". *Journal of Dairy Science*, 1994, 77, 667-671.

[11] Karoui, R; De Baerdemaeker, J."A review of the analytical methods coupled with chemometric tools for the determination of the quality and identity of dairy products". *Food Chemistry*, 2007, 102, 621-640.

[12] Renou, JP; Depongea, C; Gachonb, P;. Bonnefoyc, JC; Coulonc JB; Gareld, JP; Veritee, R; Ritzf, P."Characterization of animal products according to its geographic origin and feeding diet using Nuclear Magnetic Resonance and Isotope Ratio Mass Spectrometry Part I: Cow milk". *Food Chemistry*, 2004, 85, 63-66.

[13] Shintu, L; Caldarelli, S. "High-Resolution MAS NMR and Chemometrics: Characterization of the Ripening of Parmigiano Reggiano Cheese". *Journal of Agricultural and Food Chemistry*, 2005, 53, 4026-4031.

[14] Shintu, L; Caldarelli, S."Toward the Determination of the Geographical Origin of Emmental(er) Cheese via High Resolution MAS NMR: A Preliminary Investigation". *Journal of Agricultural and Food Chemistry*, 2006, 54, 4148-4154.

[15] Pillonel, L; Badertscher, R; Froidevaux, P; Haberhauer, G; Horn, P; Jacob, A; Pfammatter, E; Piantini, U; Rossmann, A; Tabacchi, R; Bosset, JO. "Stable isotope ratios, major trace and radioactive elements in Emmental cheeses of different origins". *Lebensmittel Wissenschaft und Technologie*, 2003, 36, 615-623.

[16] Brescia, MA; Caldarola, V; Buccolieri, G; Dell'Atti, A; Sacco, A. "Chemometric determination of the geographical origin of cow milk using ICP-OES data and isotopic ratios". *Italian Journal of Food Science*, 2003, 3, 329-336.

[17] Brescia, MA; Monfreda, M; Buccolieri, A; Carrino, C. "Characterization of the geographical origin of buffalo milk and mozzarella cheese by means of analytical and spectroscopic determinations". *Food Chemistry*, 2005, 89, 139-147.

[18] Clark, I; Fritz, P. "Environmental isotopes in Hydrogeology". New York: Lewis Publishers; 1997.

[19] Kornexl, BE; Werner, T; Rossmann, A; Schmidt, HL. "Measurement of stable isotope abundances in milk and milk ingredients - a possible tool for origin assignment and quality control". *Food Research and Technology*, 1997, 205, 19-24.

[20] Rossmann, A; Kornexel, BE; Versini, G; Pichlmayer, F; Lamprecht, G. "Origin assignment of milk from alpine regions by multi-element stable isotope ratio analysis (Sira) ". *La Rivista di Scienza dell'Alimentazione*, 1998, 1, 9-21.

[21] Manca, G; Camin, F; Coloru, G; Del Caro, A; Depentori, D; Franco, MA.; Versini, G. "Characterization of the geographical origin of Pecorino Sardo cheese by casein stable isotope ($^{13}C/^{12}C$ and $^{15}N/^{14}N$) ratios and free amino-acid ratios". *Journal of Agricultural and Food Chemistry*, 2001, 49, 1404-1409.

[22] Chiacchierini, E; Bogoni, P; Franco, MA; Giaccio, M; Versini, G. "Characterization of the regional origin of sheep and cow cheeses by casein stable isotope 13C/12C and 15N/14N ratios". *Journal of Commodity Science*, 2002, 41 (IV), 303-315.

[23] Kreitler, C; Jones, DC. "Natural soil nitrate: the cause of the nitrate contamination of groundwater in Runnels Country, Texas". *Ground Water*, 1975, 13, 53-62.

[24] Heaton, HTE. "The $^{15}N/^{14}N$ ratios of plants in South Africa and Namibia: relationship to climate and coastal/saline environments". *Oceologia* (Berlin), 1987, 74, 236-246.

[25] International Dairy Federation, Brussels, Belgium, Standard n°148A, FIL-IDF (1995).

[26] Brescia, MA; Caldarola, V; De Giglio A; Benedetti, D; Fanizzi, FP; Sacco, A. "Characterization of the geographical origin of Italian red wines based on traditional and nuclear magnetic resonance spectrometric determinations". *Analytica Chimica Acta*, 2002, 458, 177.

[27] International Dairy Federation, Brussels, Belgium, Standard n°58, FIL-IDF (1970).

[28] International Dairy Federation, Brussels, Belgium, Standard n°12B, FIL-IDF (1988).

[29] Istituto Nazionale di Ricerca per gli Alimenti e la Nutrizione (INRAN). Tabelle di composizione degli alimenti, Italy (2009).

[30] Sacco, D; Brescia, M.A.; Sgaramella, A; Casiello, G; Buccolieri, A; Ogrinc N; Sacco A. "Discrimination between Southern Italy and foreign milk samples using spectroscopic and analytical data". *Food Chemistry*, 2009, 114, 1559-1563.

In: Cheese: Types, Nutrition and Consumption
Editor: Richard D. Foster, pp. 143-155

ISBN 978-1-61209-828-9
© 2011 Nova Science Publishers, Inc.

Chapter 7

SLOVAK BRYNDZA CHEESE

Roman Dušinský, Libor Ebringer, Mária Mikulášová, Anna Belicová, and Juraj[*] Krajčovič

Institute of Cell Biology and Biotechnology, Faculty of Natural Sciences, Comenius University, Mlynská dolina, 842 15 Bratislava, Slovakia

ABSTRACT

Slovak Bryndza cheese is a traditional type of cheese closely associated with the history and culture of Slovakia. "Slovenská bryndza" (Slovak Bryndza cheese) has been granted European Protected Geographical Indication (PGI) status. The matured sheep lump cheese alone or mixed with cow cheese is crushed and ground to give rise to soft, spreadable, salty Bryndza cheese. At present, commercially available Bryndza cheese can legally contain up to 49% cow cheese and the traditional technology is influenced by sophisticated milking machines and by thermal processing of the ewes' milk. Characteristic aroma and taste of the traditional Bryndza cheese are the result of the presence of a high amount of natural microorganisms, especially lactic acid bacteria (*Lactobacillus, Enterococcus, Lactococcus*) and partly micromycetes (*Kluyveromyces, Galactomyces, Mucor*) as well. Food safety of the unpasteurized product is ensured by a technological process of fermentation. Keeping sheep on the mountainous meadows makes Bryndza cheese really healthy because of the rich content of unsaturated fatty acids (ALA – alpha linolenic acid, CLA – conjugated linoleic acid), an appropriate amount of minerals and a relatively high content of vitamins and natural positive microflora. Beneficial attributes of the traditional Bryndza cheese in human health and nutrition are being researched. Bryndza cheese is mostly eaten as a topping on small boiled potato dumplings (with pieces of fried bacon) as a Slovak national meal called "Bryndzové halušky" (Bryndza cheese dumplings). It is also often used as a spread on a piece of bread or as a compound of more complex spreads, filling for pasta and pies, or used in a soup. Sheep farming and Bryndza cheese is a part of the unique and specific Slovak folk culture tradition which influenced and boosted tourism, including various annual festivals, e.g. the World Championship of Cooking and Eating Bryndza Cheese Dumplings or "Ovenalie" – Shepherd's Sunday.

---

[*] Corresponding author: E-mail: krajcovic@fns.uniba.sk.

HISTORY

Slovak Bryndza cheese is a traditional type of ewes' milk cheese closely associated with the history and culture of Slovakia. "Slovenská bryndza" (Slovak Bryndza cheese) has been granted European Protected Geographical Indication (PGI) status. There exists several versions about the origin of Bryndza production. Some of them indicate the Wallachian. The Wallachian colonization has brought the use of ewes´ milk in different forms as food – lump cheese, Bryndza cheese and others. In Romania, the term bryndza is used to identify virtually all kinds of cheese but none of those is identical with the Slovak Bryndza. In Russia, bryndza denotes certain salt cheese. Originally, Slovak Bryndza was produced from unpasteurized sheep cheese. The use and form of Bryndza cheese has changed over time until today's soft spreadable form. In the beginning, Bryndza cheese was produced only for the use of sheep owners and shepherds. The primary products of sheep were wool and meat, therefore Bryndza cheese was only a secondary product. In the 16th – 17th century sheep cheese was stored for winter consumption in sheeps' or goats' skin and food stability was improved by salting and smoking. Later procedures involved the sheep cheese being crushed, salted and pressed into clay vessels or wooden barrels. The industrial production of Bryndza began in the second half of the 18th century when Slovakia was a part of Austro-Hungarian empire. Ján Vagač, a merchant and butcher from Stará Turá, started to produce the local variety of Bryndza and in 1787, he founded the first Bryndza factory in Detva. The second factory was founded in Zvolenská Slatina by Peter Molec in 1797. In the 19th century, there was a proliferation of other Bryndza factories. For example, Peter Makovický founded one in Ružomberok (1884) and another one in Tisovec (1897). Since 1921, the Tisovec production has been in hands of the Manica family and produces Bryndza presently. Several small factories started in Liptov, Horehronie (valley along the upper part of the Hron River), Považie (valley along the Váh River).

At the end of the 18th century, Bryndza cheese had gained wide popularity not only in Slovakia but in the whole Habsburg monarchy and later elsewhere. It was an important export article. Firstly, it was transported to Vienna and Budapest on boats or carriages, usually placed in simple fir wood barrels or compressed in a brick shape and mixed with paprika. The version with paprika was popular mainly abroad in Vienna or Munich. J. A. Cronin savored Bryndza in Scotland and positively noticed this product in his roman, The Citadel. Bryndza was known abroad as Liptauerkäse, Liptauer cheese or brinza, brimsen. The export of Bryndza bears testament to its reputation. Before World War I, approximately 3.5 million kilograms of Bryndza were produced, of which more than two-thirds were exported outside the territory of Slovakia, chiefly to Austria and Hungary.

The method of Bryndza production was improved by Teodor Vallo in Zvolen in 1892. He introduced the soft and spreadable Bryndza cheese in the kind known today. He modified the production by using a cylinder mill with different speeds of the cylinders and addition of the salt solution. Famous milk products and socio-intellectual potential of T. Vallo contributed to his election as a Member of the Hungarian Parliament and later as a Member of the Czechoslovak Parliament. He lobbied in both parliaments in favor of Bryndza cheese and other sheep products. Production of Bryndza cheese according to the T. Vallo method expanded throughout Slovakia and this technology principle is presently used in all Slovak factories.

The first important legislative documents for the lawful protection of the Bryndza cheese represent the Regulations of the Czechoslovak government in 1927, 1935 and 1937. These documents describe the procedure of sheep cheese and Bryndza production, quality parameters and ways of market distribution. In 1935, "The Association of Bryndza and cheese industry" was established in Banská Bystrica with aims to enhance the sale of the products, to ensure the standard product quality and solving conflicts among producers. In the same year, on the basis of the government regulation No. 160, "Bryndza syndicate" was established in Turčiansky Svätý Martin and it associated farmers and producers of sheeps' milk products. Since 1955, a professional association, "Guild of Bryndza cheese producers", has been advocating the priorities of producers.

CHEESE MANUFACTURE

Today, the production of Bryndza is manufactured mostly in Bryndza factories which buy the cheese. The farmstead artisan cheese made from raw ewes' milk is placed on a wooden or stainless-steel shelf to ferment. During fermentation for two to three days, the lump of cheese is turned over regularly and its temperature may not be lower than 18 to 20 °C. The cheese reaches maturity in the factory at a temperature around 15°C over a period of three to six days. The matured lump cheese is carefully cleaned by scraping away the dried layer and placed in a pressing vat for two days. Then the sheep cheese alone or mixed with cow cheese is crushed, ground and salted to give rise to soft, spreadable Bryndza cheese. The salt content is up to 2.5% (in the winter season, up to 3%). Traditionally, the Bryndza cheese has been made only from ewes' milk. At present, commercially available Bryndza cheese can legally contain up to 49% cow cheese. The traditional manufacturing is influenced by sophisticated machines of milking and by thermal processing of the ewes' milk.

Bryndza cheese is packaged either in small 1 to 5 kg buckets made of wood or non-toxic plastic material, or in small 0.125 to 1 kg packages overlaid with several layers of aluminium foil, or in the form of a small roll with a wooden case, or a tube in plastic packet.

Slovak Bryndza is characterized as a natural, white, spreadable cheese manufactured according to the traditional method. It has a delicate odor and taste and has a pleasantly sour sheep cheese taste that is slightly spicy and salty. In winter, the only way of producing Bryndza was using surplus summer reserves of sheep cheese. A special preservation method was introduced where a cheese was thoroughly salted (5–6% of salt) and stored in wooden barrels in cellars for several months. Sheep cheese preserved this way (barrel cheese) is ground and mixed with cow cheese and processed to produce so called "winter" Bryndza.

The specific attribute of the production of Slovak Bryndza is the crushing and milling of matured lump cheese in a cutting machine and then in a cylinder mill with different speeds of the cylinders. The cheese is then mixed with salt or a saturated salt solution to process the ingredients into a delicate spreadable cheese. This specific procedure diversifies Slovak Bryndza from other sheep cheese products made in other countries. Characteristic sensory properties originate from the natural microflora present in the lump cheese, which is produced from raw ewes' milk using a specific technique.

MICROORGANISMS AND THEIR ROLE

During the first stage of cheese production – the fermentation, microorganisms ferment mainly milk sugar, whereby lactic acid, as well as other organic acids in small amounts, are formed. These acids and inhibitory compounds (bacteriocins, H_2O_2) destroy many potential food pathogens mainly *Salmonella, Shigella, Listeria*, and *Escherichia*. In the second stage of cheese production – the maturation, further microbiological and biochemical processes, especially proteolytic and lipolytic, take place.

The specific microflora of Bryndza and its connection to the quality of the product were already noted in the Codex Alimentarius Austriacus, Volume III, Vienna 1917. The old name "Karpathenkokkus" was used by Professor Otakar Laxa in 1924 for the natural mixture of lactic acid bacteria. He also used the name "Oidium Lactis" for a noble mold known as *Galactomyces geotrichum* in the current classification (EU Official Journal C 232, 04/10/2007). Slovak Bryndza cheese contains a broad range of naturally occurring microorganisms, predominantly lactic acid bacteria and microscopic fungi. Our group published several scientific papers on Bryndza cheese enterococci and their properties (Jurkovič et al, 2006a, b; Jurkovič et al. 2007; Belicová et al. 2007; Dušinský et al. 2010; Belicová et al. 2011). We have found a high number of enterococci in Bryndza cheese. An average number of enterococci ranged from 10^7 to 10^8 CFU g^{-1} (colony forming units). Species *Enterococcus faecium, E. durans, E. faecalis, E. italicus, E. gallinarum, E. casseliflavus* and *E. hirae* were identified (Jurkovič et al. 2006a, b). The enterococcal composition of Bryndza cheese corresponds with those of other European artisanal cheeses, where *E. faecium* and *E. faecalis* represent the dominant enterococcal microflora (Giraffa et al. 1997; Franz et al. 1999), although there are exceptions. Using molecular DNA techniques, we have shown that there is a considerable genetic variability among enterococci isolates among various Bryndza distributors, but also at one distributor at different intervals during one year.

The genus *Enterococcus* is the most controversial group of lactic acid bacteria. Unlike most lactic acid bacteria, enterococci are not considered GRAS (generally recognized as safe). They are potentially dangerous because they can be involved in food deterioration (Franz et al. 1999), in food poisoning (Gardini et al. 2001), in nosocomial infections (Kayser 2003) and in the spreading of antibiotic resistance through the food chain (Giraffa 2002).

On the other hand, the presence and growth of enterococci in cheeses contribute to the ripening and results in organoleptically unique products, which contribute to the local cuisine and the region's heritage (Giraffa 2003; Foulquie-Moreno et al. 2006). Due to interlinked European and worldwide markets, these cheeses are widely distributed and are internationally considered as delicacies (Franz et al. 1999). In addition to these technological properties, numerous strains of enterococci associated with cheeses, mainly *E. faecalis* and *E. faecium*, produce one or more bacteriocins, which may be considered as protection against spoilage and pathogenic bacteria (De Vuyst 1994; Giraffa et al. 1995). Different enterocins possess activity against *Listeria monocytogenes, Staphylococcus aureus, Clostridium* spp, and Vibrio cholerae (Giraffa et al. 1995; Maisnier-Patin et al. 1996; Nunez et al. 1997; Simonetta et al. 1997; Ennanhar et al. 1998; Lauková et Czikková 1999; Sarantinoupoulos et al. 2002; Foulquié-Moreno et al. 2003). Therefore, we studied the antibiotic resistance, virulence determinants and anti-microbial activity of enterococci in Bryndza cheese. We proved a relatively low level of enterococcal resistance against anti-microbials in comparison to data concerning most European cheeses (Belicová et al. 2007). We also detected virulence determinants in low numbers of Bryndza cheese isolates identified as *E. faecalis*. Bryndza enteroccoci have various enterocin genes and show an anti-microbial activity against potential bacterial pathogens (Belicová et al. in press). Since food enterococci do not seem to be associated with the potentially high virulence profiles, when compared with clinical strains, it seems that their presence in traditional cheeses results in a low health risk (Eaton et Gasson 2001; Semedo et al. 2003). Nevertheless, the interaction of such strains with susceptible hosts seems to be a concern mainly in high-risk population groups, i.e. immunocompromised patients. However, Bryndza cheese has been consumed safely for more than 200 years and was never associated with foodborne diseases (Kereteš et Selecký 2003).

In addition to enterococci, other microorganisms in Bryndza cheese were identified, especially genus *Lactobacillus*. *Lactobacillus brevis, Lb. parabuchneri, Lb. fermentum, Lb. helveticus, Lb. paracasei, Lb. pentosus, Lb. plantarum* were found by Berta et al. (2009) using RAMP and 16SrDNA sequencing, and the presence of *Lb. plantarum, Lb. rhamnosus, Lb. fermentum and Lb. paracasei* in Bryndza cheese were confirmed also by us using repPCR (Mikulášová et al. 2010). Cocci like *Lactococcus lactis* and *Pediococcus pentosaceus* were also identified (Berta et al. 2009). Microscopic fungi *Geotrichum sp., Kluyveromyces (K. lactis/K. marxianus)* are the most abundant yeasts and *Mucor circinelloides* is the predominant filamentous fungus. Occasionally other yeasts, such as *Candida inconspicua, Candida silvae, Pichia fermentans* and *Trichosporon domesticum* were found (Laurenčík et al. 2008).

NUTRITION AND HEALTH-BENEFITS

Long term tradition, as well as scientific knowledge, shows that the consumption of fermented milk products is beneficial for human health. For instance, longevity in some Mediterranean areas is attributed to an increased consumption of sheep cheese and fermented milk. More than hundred years ago, Russian biologist Ilya Mechnikov already mentioned health effects of fermented milk.

Bryndza, as a fermented milk product, is a rich source of quality proteins, minerals and vitamins. The protein and fat content of Bryndza cheese varies considerably depending on the milk composition and the method of lump cheese production and kind of Bryndza used. The average fat content (in dry matter) in the traditional Bryndza made from ewes' milk cheese is 48-53%, in Bryndza made from a mixture of sheep and cow cheeses, it is 38-43%. Milk lipids are also fermented by some lactic acid bacteria to free fatty acids. Production of conjugated linoleic acid (CLA) is especially important because of its health and nutrition benefit.

The contents of approximately 70 fatty acids in Bryndza cheese were determined by gas chromatography (Meľuchová et al. 2009; Ostrovský et al. 2009; Soják et al. 2009). The relatively high content of health affecting fatty acids was analyzed in Bryndza fat. Conjugated linoleic acid – CLA (*cis-9, trans-11* C18:2) reaches up to 3.2 %, vaccenic acid – VA (*trans-11* C18:1) up to 7.2 %, and α-linolenic acid – ALA (C18:3 n-3) up to 2 % of total fatty acids. Vaccenic acid is a physiological precursor of rumenic acid – the main isomer of CLA.

Data from *in vitro* studies and animal models have been used to suggest that CLA exerts anti-carcinogenic and anti-atherogenic properties, as well as a multiplicity of potentially beneficial effects on human health (Rainer et Heiss 2004; Lee et al. 2005; Mac Rae et al. 2005; Bhatacharya et al. 2006). Daily consumption of thirty grams of Bryndza cheese can lead to an intake of about 300 mg of CLA. Such amount of CLA corresponds to a minimum daily intake that has been shown to be effective in reducing the incidence of cancer in animal models (Dhiman et al. 2005). The relatively high contents of beneficial fatty acids in Bryndza cheese are linked to grazing the pasture with a high content of precursors including α-linolenic acid (ALA) during the summer months (May – September) season.

Oleic acid (C18:1) is the single unsaturated fatty acid at the highest concentration in Bryndza cheese, reaching up to 20 % of total fatty acids. Monounsaturated oleic acid is considered to be favorable for health because it lowers both plasma cholesterol, LDL cholesterol and triacylglycerols and thus, it reduces the risk of coronary artery disease (Mensink et al. 2003). Also, the content of medium-chain saturated fatty acids is relatively high; reaching up to 7 % of the total fatty acids. The beneficial effects of caproic (C6:0), caprylic (C8:0) and capric (C10:0) acids are of special interest from a health-promoting activity. Medium-chain fatty acids reduce body weight and body fat because they are hydrolyzed from triglycerides and are transferred directly from the intestine to the portal circulation without resynthesis of triglycerides. They are a preferred source of energy (β-oxidation) (Marten et al. 2006). Because of their particular metabolism, they are of special interest from a therapeutic point of view (Babayan 1981; Alférez et al. 2001; Sanz Sampelayo et al. 2007; Ebringer et al. 2008).

Milk, cheeses and especially fermented milk products are an important source of calcium and they play a considerable role in human nutrition and the prevention of some civilization diseases including osteoporosis. Bryndza can make an important contribution to the daily intake of minerals, especially of calcium. The mean value for calcium in 100 grams of Bryndza is up to 800 mg.

Assumption of health benefit effects of Bryndza is confirmed by results of historically first clinical tests performed at the Comenius University in Bratislava. A group of 30 volunteers consumed 100 g of Bryndza daily, made by a traditional procedure during eight weeks. A statistically significant decrease of total cholesterol and LDL-cholesterol was observed. In probands with a low level of serum HDL-cholesterol, its significant increase was documented. Values of glucose, serum creatinine, C-reactive protein and blood pressure were decreased as well. Decrease of the C-reactive protein was interesting because this protein is an inflammation marker considered as the risk factor for cardiovascular diseases and colorectal carcinoma (Mikeš et al. 2005).

The traditional production of the Slovak Bryndza cheese is a sophisticated process, which substitutes pasteurization, but with a difference that only risk pathogenic bacteria are eliminated and useful bacteria can proliferate. Bryndza cheese represents a unique microbial phenomenon in terms of a rich mixture of living microorganisms with positive effects on human health and vitality.

OTHER TRADITIONAL SLOVAK EWES' MILK PRODUCTS

Slovak Bryndza cheese and other products from ewes' milk are, in a way, symbols of Slovakia. A multi-functional role of the sheep tradition in Slovakia can be seen in the production of especially tasty delicatessens for gourmets. "Oštiepok" and "Parenica" have been protected under the EU agricultural quality policy and received the Protected Geographical Indication (PGI) status.

- *"Oštiepok"* is a cheese with an oval shape made by using wooden forms with simple folk ornaments, cheese is slightly steamed and smoked.
- *"Parenica"* is a semi-firm, non-ripening, steamed cheese (smoked or non-smoked). The cheese is produced in strips, which are woven into snail-like spirals.
- Another kind of the steamed cheese interwoven into fine strings is „Korbáčik" (roughly translated to "little whip") from the Orava region of Slovakia.
- „Ovčí salašnícky údený syr" – traditional loaf-shaped "smoked sheep cheese from the sheepfold" was recently included to the EU's list of Traditional Specialities Guaranteed (TSG).

In Slovakia, there is a long tradition to use whey, a by-product of cheese and curd manufacturing, for a preparation of a popular fermented drink called "**Žinčica**". The discovery of whey as a functional food with nutritional applications proved whey to a important co-product in the manufacturing of cheese. Milk contains two primary sources of protein, the caseins and whey. After processing occurs, the caseins are the proteins responsible for making curds, while whey remains in an aqueous environment. The components of whey include beta-lactoglobulin, alpha-lactalbumin, bovine serum albumin, lactoferrin, immunoglobulins, lactoperoxidase enzymes, glycomacropeptides, lactose, and minerals. Today, whey is a popular dietary protein supplement supposed to provide anti-microbial activity, immune modulation, improved muscle strength and body composition, and to prevent cardiovascular disease and osteoporosis (Marshall 2004). A characteristic feature of the "Žincica" production has been carving of special wooden mugs for its drinking called "črpáky.

CONSUMPTION

The fresh Bryndza cheese, called "májová" (from May), is very similar in its butter consistency and taste to French cheese. The older one gets spicy. Typical (and very often described as "most favorite") Slovak food *"bryndzové halušky" (Bryndza cheese dumplings)* was cooked mainly in the villages in the north and east, consumed more times a week in order to get energy before hard work on land. Bryndza cheese dumplings, in the form we eat them today, are very similar (and have not changed) for the last 200-250 years. For foreign tourists, except historical and cultural sightseeing, it is important to taste gastronomic specialities of a visited country. Bryndza cheese dumplings are typical Slovak food, which can not be found in any other place. Bryndza cheese gives a unique flavor to the meal on itself, but it is even tastier with small pieces of bacon greaves and chives or dill, usually served with a glass of sour milk called žinčica.

Bryndza cheese is used to preparation of many other foods. The most typical are:

- "*Bryndza spreads*" – Bryndza cheese is usually used spread on a piece of bread or as a compound of more complex spreads. Bryndza cheese mixed with butter, paprika and onion spreadable on the bread is a very popular dish. Many of national names in different parts of Slovakia like bryndzová nátierka, šmirkas, kerezet, byrhunt affirm the long history of use.
- "*Bryndzové pirohy*" – a traditional Eastern Slovak dish which resembles large crescent-shaped ravioli. They are made from rolled pastry (using a cup or glass to cut out circles) filled with Bryndza cheese-potato mixture, closed and boiled. "Bryndzové pirohy" are served with garnish of fried onions and a spoonful of sour cream.
- "*Demikát*" – healthy and typical Slovak soup with Bryndza cheese, potatoes and acid cream.
- "*Bryndzovníky*" – rising dough cakes filled with sliced potatoes, sour cream and Bryndza cheese.
- "*Zemiaková haruľa s bryndzou*" – potato pancakes fried in oil. The dough prepared from potatoes, flour, eggs, garlic, salt, majorant sprinkle with Bryndza cheese and fried.

THE IMPACT ON BRYNDZA CHEESE ON FOLK CULTURE A RURAL DEVELOPMENT

Shepherding is connected to the original lifestyle of people living in the mountains and valleys. Since the 14th century, during the Wallachian colonization, a typical way of sheep breeding has spread. Under the strong influence of the original pastoral culture, the typical Slovak folk culture has profiled itself. Typical Slovak folk hero Juraj Jánošík, the Slovak Robin Hood, the outlaw, is usually portrayed in the shepherd uniform, with a large leather belt with brass brackles, with leather boots "krpce" and typical axe "valaška" (the wallach axe). Slovak dance "odzemok", as well as some music instruments such as "fujara", are also based in pastoral/Wallachian culture. A drink "Žinčica" was responsible for the creation of a brand new craft; "črpáky" are usually beautifully carved with figurative motifs adorning their handles.

Sheep farming and Bryndza cheese as a part of unique and specific Slovak folk culture tradition influenced and boosted tourism, including various annual festivals. There is the World Championship of Cooking and Eating Bryndza Cheese Dumplings, where fans from all over the world meet, cook, taste and enjoy the taste of halušky. An all-day-long program focuses on shepherds' work, competitions of milk products and performances of folklore ensembles. Similar local competitions of "Eating Bryndza Cheese Dumplings" are organized in different places of Slovakia. Another shepherds' festival with a presentation and competitions of milk products "Ovenalie" (Shepherd's Sunday) is organized yearly in a nice open air museum near the High Tatras Mountains.

Production of Bryndza cheese and other ewes' milk products also promotes rural development and an ecological use of grasslands especially in foothill and mountain areas. In addition, it makes a positive contribution in human health and nutrition offering healthy food without preservatives, in enrichment of the consumer market for cheese and fermented-milk specialties.

ACKNOWLEDGMENT

This work was supported by VEGA grants No. 1/1269/04, 1/0132/08 and 1/0114/08 of the Ministry of Education of the Slovak Republic and is the result of the project implementation: "Centre of excellence for exploitation of informational biomacromolecules in the disease prevention and improvement of quality of life", ITMS 26240120003, supported by the Research and Development Operational Programme funded by the ERDF.

REFERENCES

Alférez, M. J. M.; Barrionuevo, M.; López Aliagua, I.; Sanz Sampelayo, M. R.; Lisbona, F. and Campos, M. S. (2001). The digestive utilization of goat and cow milk fat in malabsorption syndrome. *J. Dairy Sci.*, *68*, 451-461.

Babayan, B. K. (1981). Medium chain length fatty acid esters and their medical and nutritional applications. *J. Am.Oil Chem. Soc.*, *59*, 49A-52A.

Belicová, A.; Križková, L.; Krajčovič, J.; Jurkovič, D.; Sojka, M. and Dušinský, R. (2007). Anti-microbial Susceptibility of *Enterococcus* Species Isolated from Slovak Bryndza Cheese. *Folia Microbiol.*, *52*, 115-119.

Belicová, A.; Mikulášová, M.; Krajčovič, J. and Dušinský, R. (2011). Anti-bacterial activity and enterocin genes in enterococci isolated from Bryndza cheese. *J. Food Nutr. Res.*, *50*, in press.

Berta, G.; Chebeňová, V.; Brežná, B.; Pangallo, D.; Valík, L. and Kuchta, T. (2009). Identification of lactic acid bacteria in Slovakian bryndza cheese. *J. Food Nutr. Res.*, *48*, 65-71.

Bhattacharya, A.; Banu, J.; Rahman, M.; Causey, J. and Fernandes, G. (2006). Biological effects of conjugated linoleic acid in health and diseases. *J. Nutr. Chem.*, *17*, 789-810.

Codex Alimentarius Austriacus – cited in: Publication of an application pursuant to Article 6(2) of Council Regulation (EC) No 510/2006 on the protection of geographical indications and designations of origin for agricultural products and foodstuffs. Official Journal C 232, 04/10/2007 P. 0017-0022.

De Vuyst, L.; Avonts, L. and Makras, E. (2004). Probotics, prebiotics and gut health Chap. 17. In: C. Remacle, and B. Reusens (eds.), *Functional Foods, Aging and Degenerative Disease* (pp. 416-484). Cambridge, United Kingdom: Woodhead Publishing Ltd.

Dhiman, T. R.; Nam, S-H. N. and Ure, A. L. (2005). Factors affecting conjugated linoleic acid content in milk and meat. *Crit. Rev. Food Sci. Nutr.*, *45*, 463-482.

Dušinský, R.; Belicová, A.; Ebringer, L.; Jurkovič, D.; Križková, L.; Mikulášová, M. and Krajčovič, J. (2010). Genetic diversity of enterococci in Bryndza cheese. In: M. V.

Magni, (Ed.), *Detection of bacteria, viruses, parasites and fungi. NATO Science for Peace and Security Series A: Chemistry and Biology* (pp. 87-124). Dordrecht: Springer Netherlands.

Eaton, T. J. and Gasson, M. J. (2001). Molecular screening of *Enterococcus* virulence determinants and potential for genetic exchange between food and medical isolates. *Appl. Environ. Microbiol., 67,* 1628-1635.

Ebringer, L.; Ferenčík, M. and Krajčovič, J. (2008). Beneficial health effects of milk and fermented dairy products – review. *Folia Microbiol., 53,* 378-394.

Ennahar, S.; Aoude-Werner, D.; Assobhei, O. and Hasselmann, C. (1998). Anti-listerial activity of enterocin 81, a bacteriocin produced by *Enterococcus faecium* WHE 81 isolated from cheese. *J. Appl. Microbiol., 85,* 521-526.

Foulquie-Moreno, M. R.; Callewaert, R.; Devreese, B.; Van Beeumen, J. and De Vuyst, L. (2003). Isolation and biochemical characterization of enterocins produced by enterococci from different sources. *J. Appl. Microbiol., 94,* 214-229.

Foulquie-Moreno, M. R.; Sarantinopoulos, P.; Tsakalidou, E. and De Vuyst, L. (2006). The role and application of enterococci in food and health. *Int. J. Food Microbiol., 106,* 1-24.

Franz, C. M. A. P.; Holzapfel, W. H. and Stiles, M. E. (1999). Enterococci at the crossroads of food safety? *Int. J. Food Microbiol., 47,* 1-24.

Gardini, F.; Martuscelli, M.; Caruso, M. C.; Galgano, F.; Crudele, M. A.; Favati, F.; Guerzoni, M. E. and Suzzi, G. (2001). Effects of pH, temperature and NaCl concentration on growth kinetics, proteolytic activity and biogenic amine production of *Enterococcus faecalis. Int. J. Food Microbiol., 64,* 105-117.

Giraffa, G. (2002). Enterococci from food. *FEMS Microbiol. Lett., 26,* 163-171.

Giraffa, G. (2003). Functionality of enterococci in dairy products. *Int. J. Food Microbiol., 88,* 215-222.

Giraffa, G.; Carminati, D. and Neviani, E. (1997). Enterococci isolated from dairy products: a review of risks and potential technological use. *J. Food Prot., 60,* 732-738.

Giraffa, G.; Picchioni, N.; Neviani, E. and Carminati, D. (1995). Production and stability of an *Enterococcus faecium* bacteriocin during Taleggio cheesemaking and ripening. *Food Microbiol., 12,* 301-307.

Jurkovič, D.; Križková, L.; Dušinský, R.; Belicová, A.; Sojka, M.; Krajčovič, J. and Ebringer, L. (2006a). Identification and characterization of enterococci from bryndza cheese. *Lett. Appl. Microbiol., 42,* 553-559.

Jurkovič, D.; Križková, L.; Sojka, M.; Belicová, A.; Dušinský, R.; Krajčovič, J.; Snauwaert, C.; Naser, S.; Vandamme, P. and Vancanneyt, M. (2006b). Molecular identification and diversity of enterococci isolated from Slovak Bryndza cheese. *J. Gen. Appl. Microbiol., 52,* 329-337.

Jurkovič, D.; Križková, L.; Sojka, M.; Takáčová, M.; Dušinský, R.; Krajčovič, J.; Vandamme, P. and Vancanneyt, M. (2007). Genetic diversity of *Enterococcus faecium* isolated from Bryndza cheese. *Int. J. Food Microbiol., 116,* 82-87.

Kayser, F. H. (2003). Safety aspects of enterococci from the medical point of view. *Int. J. Food Microbiol., 88,* 255-262.

Keresteš, J. and Selecký, J. (2003). Slovak bryndza cheese. In: Keresteš, J. (Ed.), *Dairy Industry in Middle Slovakia* (pp. 109-122). Považská Bystrica: Eminent (in Slovak).

Lauková, A. and Czikková, S. (1999). The use of enterocin CCM 4231 in soy milk to control the growth of *Listeria monocytogenes* and *Staphylococcus aureus. J. Appl. Microbiol.*, *87*, 182-186.

Laurenčík, M.; Sulo, P.; Sláviková, E.; Piecková, E.; Seman, M. and Ebringer, L. (2008). The diversity of eukaryotic microbiota in the traditional Slovak sheep cheese-Bryndza. *Int. J. Food Microbiol.*, *127*, 176-179.

Lee, K. W.; Lee, H. J.; Cho, H.Y. and Kim Y.J. (2005). Role of conjugated linoleic acid in the prevention of cancer. *Crit. Reviews Food Sci. Nutr.*, *45*, 135-144.

Maisnier-Patin, S.; Forni, E. and Richard, J. (1996). Purification, partial characterization and mode of action of enterococcin EFS2, an anti-listerial bacteriocin produced by a strain of *Enterococcus faecalis* isolated from a cheese. *Int. J. Food Microbiol.*, *30*, 255-270.

Marshall, K. (2004). Therapeutic applications of whey protein. Altern. Med. Rev., *9*, 136-156.

Marten, B.; Pfeuffer, M. and Schrezenmeir, J. (2006). Medium-chain triglycerides. *Int. Dairy J.*, *16*, 1374-1382.

Meľuchová, B.; Blaško, J.; Kubinec, R.; Górová, R.; Dúbravská, J.; Margetín, M. and Soják, L. (2008). Seasonal variations in fatty acid composition of pasture forage plants and CLA content in ewe milk fat. *Small Rum. Res.*, *78*, 56-65.

Mensink, R. P.; Zock, P. L.; Kester, A. D. and Atan, M. B. (2003). Effects of dietary fatty acids and carbohydrates on the ration of serum total to HDL cholesterol and on serum lipids and apolipoproteins: a meta-analysis of 60 controled trials. *Am. J. Clin. Nutr.*, *77*, 1146-1155.

Mikeš, Z.; Ebringer, L.; Boča, M.; Dušinský, R. and Jahnová, E. (2005). Some cardiovascular factors after consumption of the traditional Slovak bryndza cheese – pilot study (in Slovak). *Geriatria*, *1*, 29-36.

Mikulášová, M.; Dušinský, R. and Belicová, A. (2010). Identification of bacteria isolated from food by rep-PCR. *Common protection of human and animal health* (Spoločná ochrana zdravia ľudí a zdravia zvierat), 139-142, (in Slovak).

Núñez, M.; Rodríguez, J. L.; García, E.; Gaya, P. and Medina, M. (1997). Inhibition of *Listeria monocytogenes* by enterocin 4 during the manufacturing and ripening of Manchego cheese. *J. Appl. Microbiol.*, *83*, 671-677.

Ostrovský, I.; Paulíková, E.; Blaško, J.; Górová, R.; Kubinec, R.; Margetín, M. and Soják, L. (2009). Variation of fatty acid composition of ewe´s milk during continuous transition from dry winter to natural pasture diet. *Int. Dairy J.*, *19*, 545-549.

Sanz Sampelayo, M. R.; Chilliard, Y.; Schmidely, P. and Boza, J. (2007). Influence of type of diet on the fat constituents of goat and sheep milk. *Small Rum. Res.*, *68*, 42-63.

Sarantinopoulos, P.; Leroy, F.; Leontopoulou, E.; Georgalaki, M. D.; Kalantzopoulos, G.; Tsakalidou, E. and De, V. L. (2002). Bacteriocin production by *Enterococcus faecium* FAIR-E 198 in view of its application as adjunct starter in Greek Feta cheese making. *Int. J. Food Microbiol.*, *72*, 125-136.

Semedo, T.; Santos, M. A.; Lopes, M. F. S.; Marques, J. J. F.; Crespo, M. T. B. and Tenreiro, R. (2003). Virulence factors in food, clinical and reference enterococci: a common trait in the genus? *Syst. Appl. Microbiol.*, *26*, 13-22.

Simonetta, A. C.; Moragues de Velasco, L. G. and Frisón, L. N. (1997). Anti-bacterial activity of enterococci strains against *Vibrio cholera. Lett. Appl. Microbiol.*, *24*, 139-143.

Soják, L.; Pavlíková, E.; Blaško, J.; Meľuchová, B.; Górová, R.; Kubinec, R.; Ebringer, L.; Michalec, M. and Margetín, M. (2009). The quality of Slovak and alpine milk products based on fatty acid health affecting compounds. *Slovak J. Anim. Sci.*, 42, 62-69.

APPENDIX

Recipes for Preparation of Traditional Bryndza Cheese Food

Bryndza Cheese Dumplings

Ingredients: 3 potatoes, 5 tablespoons (tbsp) flour, one egg, salt, bacon, Bryndza cheese
Instructions:

1) First, peel potatoes and shred them.
2) Add egg and flour. Make a dough that is not too tough but not too watery. You may use more or less flour or add little bit of water if it is too tough. Add 1 tsp (teaspoon) of salt.
3) Boil water with 2 tbsp of salt (the water has to boil all the time during the preparation).
4) Toss pieces about 2.5 cm (an inch) long into the boiled water, using kitchen knife and cutting board. Besides this original procedure a special stainless steel mesh can be used as a "halušky maker".
5) Cook them for few minutes until they float on the water level. Take them out with a strainer and halušky are ready.
6) Cut bacon into small pieces and fry them.
7) Put Bryndza on top of halušky and heat them together. It is very difficult or many times impossible to buy Bryndza outside Slovakia, but you can use other cheese instead, for example feta cheese mixed with cream cheese and milk, however, the taste is different.
8) Put the fried bacon on the top of halušky (with a bit of grease) before serving.

Bryndzové Pirohy

Ingredients: about 2 potatoes, 2 cups flour, one egg, salt, bacon, Bryndza cheese
Instructions:

1) Cook potatoes until they are quite soft and mash them by hand. Add about a cup of flour, egg and about a tablespoon of salt. Mix everything together by hand. Then add more flour until you get a fairly stiff mixture. Also, place a large pot full of salted water onto the stove.
2) Form the dough into a loaf and place it onto a dusted board. Dust top with flour to prevent the pin from sticking. Roll out to about 3 millimeters thick pancake.
3) Cut out circles by a drinking glass. Do this by pushing down with the glass and twisting your wrist left and right few times. The dough will come out with the glass. Top each circle with a teaspoon worth of Bryndza cheese.
4) Fold the circle over and pinch the seal closed with the tip of your fingers.

5) Place pirohy into the pot of boiling water. Scoop them up with a wooden spoon to keep them from sticking to the bottom. Cook them for few minutes until they float on the water level. Take them out with a large strainer.
6) Cut bacon into small pieces and fry them.
7) Put the fried bacon on the top of pirohy (with a bit of grease) and finally top with sour cream before serving.

Demikát

Ingredients: 150 g Bryndza cheese, 100 ml cream, 1500 ml water, 2 onions, one tablespoon lard, one teaspoon paprika, half teaspoon ground cumin, 2 slices of black bread, salt, chives or dill.

Instructions:

1) Add chopped onions to boiling water and cook. Season with salt, add ground red pepper, ground cumin and cook until onion is tender.
2) In the soup tureen, mix the Bryndza with cream and pour with the broth of onions. Cut black bread into small cubes, fry in warm lard and serve up the soup. The finished soup can be flavored by chopped chives or chopped dill.

Bryndza Spread

Ingredients: Bryndza cheese, butter, paprika, onion, bread or rolls

Instructions:

1) Finely slice onions and combine them with about equal amounts of Bryndza cheese and butter. Add a spoonful of paprika and mix together.
2) Serve the spread on bread or rolls.

Bryndzovníky

Ingredients: Dough - one pkg yeast, one teaspoon sugar, 100 ml milk, one kg flour, salt. Filling - 1.5 kg potatoes, one big onion, 250 g Bryndza cheese, salt, oil, butter, milk

Instructions:

1) Make dough like you do for a pizza.
2) Cook the potatoes in salty water, smash them and mix with Bryndza cheese and a finely sliced onion.
3) Place the dough on an oily tray (it should be possible to fill 3 big trays) and spread the top with filling. Bake for 15-20 min at 180 °C.

In: Cheese: Types, Nutrition and Consumption
Editor: Richard D. Foster, pp. 157-169
ISBN 978-1-61209-828-9
© 2011 Nova Science Publishers, Inc.

Chapter 8

PROCESSED CHEESE: RELEVANCE FOR LOW SODIUM CHEESE DEVELOPMENT

Adriano G. Cruz[1], Adriane E.C. Antunes[2], Renata M.S. Celeguini[1], Jose A.F. Faria[1] and Marise Aparecida Rodrigues Pollonio[1]

[1] FEA/UNICAMP- Faculdade de Engenharia de Alimentos (Faculty of Food Engineering)/ Universidade de Campinas (UNICAMP)
[2] FCA/UNICAMP – Faculdade de Ciências Aplicadas (School of Applied Sciences) / Universidade Estadual de Campinas (University of Campinas)

1. SODIUM AND HEALTH

1.1. Introduction

Sodium is a mineral widely consumed in human diets, bestowing pleasant sensory characteristics when added to foods at certain concentrations.

Besides, salt was a precious commodity and was also an emblem of immortality and a symbol of immutable loyalty. This is reflected for instance by the act of sharing bread and salt with a guest—still practised in Slavic countries (Ritz, 2006). Sodium consumption is even quoted in the Holy Bible in three of the four Gospels (Matthew 5: 13-14, Mark 9, 50 and Luke 14, 34): "You are the salt of the earth. But if the salt loses its saltiness, how it be made salty again?". Certainly, the motivation of biblical quotations were using elements of daily life to explain the religious values and not properly discuss salt consumption in the population.

It has been recommended by government-appointed bodies and nutrition experts a reduction in salt intake from the current average consumption of 10–12 g to an expected intake of 5–6 g/day (Abbott et al., 1994). The amount of sodium chloride in the diet of industrialized nations far exceeds physical requirements. The deliberate addition of salt to food only began 5,000 – 10,000 years ago at the beginning of agriculture and farming so that the present consumption of 10 g/day on average is, in evolutionary terms, relatively recent (Meneton et al., 2005).

Greater consumption of sodium is due to the increase of salt to food and increasing consumption of processed foods, which tend to have high amounts of the mineral due to its sensory properties and property salt that act as a helper for food conservation. We stress that the human diet without sodium chloride already present naturally a percentage of this mineral, because many food items have intrinsic sodium. In the past, food consumed by terrestrial mammals, including primates, never contained a lot of salt. Indeed, except for rare cases, plants contain only traces of salt, and the consumption of very large amounts of fruits, roots, leaves, or seeds does not bring much salt in the organism (Meneton et al., 2005). For omnivorous and carnivorous species, the occasional or regular absorption of meat increases salt intake, but in limited proportions because the eaten meat corresponds most often to the sodium-poor intracellular medium and not to the sodium-rich extracellular medium that is generally lost when the animal is killed or cooked (Meneton et al., 2005).

Under healthy conditions almost 90% of sodium ingested is excreted through urine, thus, the urinary sodium represents a reliable biochemical marker of dietary intake of this mineral (Dawson-Hughes, 2009). Although the human body in health status is able to efficiently eliminate sodium from dietary source, the high consumption of that macromineral may have two important adverse effects: (1) raising systemic blood pressure and (2) causing an increase in renal calcium excretion, which may contribute to long-term osteoporosis.

1.2. Sodium Intake versus Osteoporosis

Osteoporosis is a massive community problem that affects many millions of people around the world. It is characterized by low bone mass and microarchitectural deterioration of bone tissue, leading to enhanced bone fragility and consequent increase in fracture risk (Prentice, 1997).

Bone depends upon dietary intake to supply the bulk materials needed for synthesis of the extracellular material which composes more than 95% of the substance of bone and which is largely responsible for its structural and mechanical properties. These bulk materials are mainly calcium, phosphorus and protein. Roughly half the volume of the extracellular material of bone consists of protein and the other half of calcium phosphate crystals (Heaney, 2000). Vitamin D also plays a fundamental role in bone health, since it acts by optimizing the absorption of dietary calcium.

On the other hand, a high sodium intake is considered deleterious to bone health. Sodium have been reported to affect calcium balance, because increased urinary sodium excretion produces an increase in urinary calcium excretion and raised biochemical markers of bone turnover (Devine et al., 1995). Sodium and calcium share some of these transport systems in the proximal tubule (Itoh and Suyama, 1996). When dietary sodium chloride is increased, the fractional reabsorption of sodium is decreased, leading to a parallel reduction in calcium reabsorption. Approximately 1 mmol calcium is excreted for every 100 mmol of sodium excreted (Nordin et al., 1993).

Calcium is lost through shed skin, hair, nails, sweat, urine and digestive secretions, with total daily losses in adults today, by these routes combined, in the range of 4 to 8 mmol, depending upon extent of physical activity and the levels of other dietary constituents, such as sodium (Heaney, 2000).

Longitudinal study of Devine et al. (1995) followed women after menopause. The authors reported significant effect of sodium excretion and bone loss in the population assessed. A significant positive correlation was found between the average dietary calcium intake with change in bone density at the total hip, intertrochanter, femoral neck, and ultra distal site of the ankle. On the other hand, urinary sodium excretion was a significant negative correlate of change in bone density at the total hip site and ultra distal site of the ankle. The higher the urinary sodium excretion the greater the bone loss. According to them, these effect can be reversed by salt restriction.

Sellmeyer et al. (2002) examined the effect of increased dietary sodium chloride on urine calcium excretion and bone turnover markers in postmenopausal women and, further, whether potassium citrate attenuates the effects of increased dietary salt. Increased intake of dietary sources of potassium alkaline salts, namely fruit and vegetables, may be beneficial for postmenopausal women at risk for osteoporosis, particularly those consuming a diet generous in sodium chloride. Sixty postmenopausal women were recruited to participate of the randomized, double blind, placebo-controlled trial. The results obtained suggest that increased dietary salt not only enhances urinary calcium excretion, but also results in increased excretion of bone resorption biomarkers.

The promotion of dietary guidelines to prevent osteoporosis focuses on increased consumption of dairy products and other calcium-rich foods. Devine et al. (1995) suggest that dietary information encouraging postmenopausal women to increase their consumption of calcium-rich foods should be coupled with messages to reduce their sodium intake, promoting a twofold dietary strategy for prevention of osteoporosis. A reduction in sodium-rich foods may enhance the effect of the calcium intake by preventing raised concentrations of urinary calcium. The amount of potassium that reduced urine calcium excretion could be ingested by consuming 7-8 serving of potassium-rich fruit and vegetables each day, that correspond to 90 mmol/d of potassium citrate.

It should be emphasized that the protein and sodium contents of dairy foods do not adversely affect the bone benefit of the dairy package of calcium, phosphorus, protein, and vitamin D. Their effects on bone health are likely more than can be accounted for by any single constituent, and, indeed, the totality of their effects may more than the sum of the parts (Heaney, 2000).

There is a questionable theory, which stands that the consumption of animal proteins would result in a substantial metabolic acid load which in turn would cause the dissolution of bone mineral due to increased calciuria, that result in an accelerated loss of bone mineral mass. The calciuria would increase (in the long term) the risk of osteoporotic fracture in a population consuming a relatively high amount of animal proteins (sulfur-containing amino acids), including those from dairy sources (Bonjour, 2005). However, there is no consistent evidence for superiority of vegetal over animal proteins on calcium metabolism, bone loss prevention and risk reduction of fragility fractures (Bonjour, 2005).

1.3. Sodium Intake versus Hypertension

The understanding of hypertension and cardiovascular diseases is very difficult to achieve. These are multifactorial diseases, meaning that they cannot be ascribed to a single gene or environmental factor (Meneton et al, 2005). Part of the confusion surrounding the relationship between sodium intake and blood pressure between individuals results from the interplay of other determinants: genetics (family history), weight, body mass index and Na/K ratio (Altschul et al., 1981). The extent of lowering the blood pressure is clearly a major determinant of risk of stroke, other hypertensive complications, and atherosclerotic diseases, such as myocardial infarction (Kuller, 1997).

This is far known that salt increase blood pressure. When salt is ingested, increased thirst and water intake cause expansion of the plasma and extracellular volumes, raising cardiac output and tending to increase blood pressure. In the long run, through poorly understood mechanisms of autoregulation, peripheral resistance would increase, thus increasing blood pressure further (Ritz, 2006).

A century of epidemiological and clinical research and one decade of genetic investigation in humans and animals have provided remarkable insights on the relationships existing between dietary salt, renal salt handling, and blood pressure (Meneton et al, 2005). The evidence points to a causal link between a chronically high salt intake and the development of hypertension when the kidneys have a reduced ability to excrete salt (Meneton et al, 2005). From an evolutionary viewpoint, the human species is adapted to ingest and excrete <1 g of salt per day, at least 10 times less than the average values currently observed in industrialized and urbanized countries (Meneton et al, 2005).

Cailar et al. (2002), hypothesized that sodium intake may amplify the effect of arterial pressure on target organ damage (ie, left ventricular mass and microalbuminuria) in a large group of normotensive subjects and patients with never-treated uncomplicated essential hypertension. The results obtained suggest that sodium intake may amplify the effect of arterial pressure on both the left ventricle and the kidney, and thus suggest that dietary sodium may be an independent factor of cardiovascular risk.

Campaigns to reduce salt in the diet intended to cooperate with public health of the population by reducing systemic blood pressure and comorbidities associated with it. For hypertensive patients, the combination of nonpharmacological treatments and drugs may be better than drug therapy alone (Kuller, 1997).

It was demonstrated that with the decrease of only 1.3 g in the amount of sodium consumed per day among the population group of 25 to 55 year old, the estimated decrease in systolic arterial pressure would be of 5 mmHg or 20% in the prevalence of arterial hypertension. Therefore, it would also cause a reduction in mortality by 14% caused by vasculocerebral accidents and by 19% by coronary disease, resulting in an annual saving of approximately 150,000 lives worldwide (Dickinson and Havas, 2007).

2. SODIUM REDUCTION IN PROCESSED CHEESES

2.1. General Considerations

Process cheese is a dairy product which differs from natural cheese in the fact that process cheese is not made directly from milk. They are manufactured by grinding, melting, and emulsifying one or more varieties of pieces of cheese with different degrees for maturation in the presence of emulsifying salts and other optional ingredients using continual heat and agitation to form a homogeneous product with an extended shelf life (GUINEE et al. 2002).

The emulsifying salts do not act as emulsifying agents themselves; their role is to react with proteins, making their properties to ensure that such proteins act as emulsifiers of oil-water dispersion (ZEHREN and NUSBAUM, 1992). The emulsifying salt acts by breaking down the bridges of calcium phosphate between the micellae and submicelae. When the calcium caseinate is removed, there is an ion exchange between calcium and sodium, turning calcium caseinate, which is insoluble, into soluble sodium caseinate (BRICKLEY et al. 2008), with the consequent formation of homogeneous sol (Meyer, 1973), forming a protein structure more open and detailed and also more susceptible to a greater volume of water of hydration in the hydrophilic portions (BERGER et al. 1989), as shown in Figure 1. Casein, more hydrated, can remain dispersed in a colloidal suspension, exposing its polar and nonpolar groups, which allows it to act as an emulsifier in oil-water interface (ZEHREN and NUSBAUM, 1992). The solubilized casein is able to bind water and fat under stirring and heating and form a gel during cooling. The casein network formation in a stable colloidal dispersion is accompanied by an increase in melt viscosity, and such increase in viscosity is known as creaminess (GUINEE et al. 2004).

The major steps in process cheese manufacture can be divided into 2 stages (Zehren and Nusbaum, 2000): (1)Ingredient selection and formulation: covers the selection and grinding of natural cheese (on the basis of age, pH, flavor, and intact casein content), the selection of appropriate emulsifying salt and formulation and computation of other ingredients (in order to meet the targeted moisture, fat, salt, and pH values of the final product as per government regulations) and (b)Process cheese processing and storage which cover the Cooking (heat and mixing), packaging, cooling, and storage.

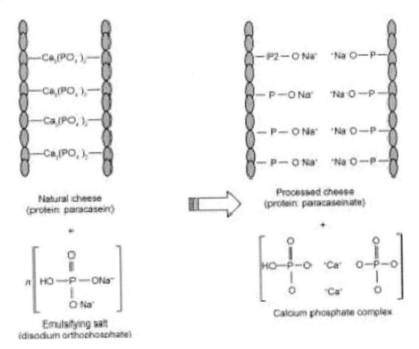

Figure 1. Action of the emulsifying salts in the processed cheese manufacture.

The major principles for the manufacture of processed cheese involve calcium sequestration, pH displacement and stabilization, para-casein dispersion, water binding, and emulsification (Henning, Baer, Hassan, and Dave, 2006).

2.2. Sodium Reduction in Processed Cheeses

Reducing the amount of sodium chloride in cheese represents a great challenge for the industry, since salt exerts specific functions such as taste, body, texture and shelf life extension and its consumption is directly related to lifestyle, psychological, social, economical, cultural, sensory and technological factors (Purdy and Armstrong, 2007). Moreover, consumers desire the amount of salt as a characteristic of each type of cheese, but they are also concerned about having varied options of cheese with lower amounts of sodium (Johnson and Paulus, 2008).

The three main ingredients that contribute to sodium level in processed cheeses are the emulsifiers based on sodium (from 44 to 48%), natural cheese (from 28 to 37%) and added salt (from 15 to 24%). Consequently, a reduction of sodium in processed cheeses involves mainly the modification of one of the three ingredients during formulation and production (Johson *et al.*, 2009)

While industry and researchers are joining forces to produce table cheeses with low sodium content, it is possible that the best alternative would be to produce cheese with reduced sodium content for use as an ingredient (Johson *et al.*, 2009). Metzger and Kapoor (2007) were successful in developing Cheddar type cheese (ingredient) with reduced sodium and fat contents. This type of cheese after one week of maturation was used in the production of processed cheese, which resulted in a product with reduced sodium (140 mg per 50 g) and fat (reduction of 67%) contents, with no significant changes in the sensory or functional properties, although the study did not show any results regarding the acceptance of the product.

Euston *et al.* (2002) demonstrated an interactive effect between the level of salt and the pH on the microstructure and rheology of skim-milk cheese; when the content of NaCl increased from 1.5 to 3.5% at pH 4.6, there was an increase in the degree of dilation of protein structures (indicating an increase in the level of hydration), which reduced the elasticity of cheese, making it more brittle (increase in the plastic property). A similar effect was observed on increasing the pH from 4.6 to 5.2 and maintaining the concentration of salt at 1.5%.

Reps *et al.* (1998) studied the possibility to increase the K content in processed cheeses. In laboratory scale, potassium chloride was added to cheese mass before melting in such quantitities as to obtain a K content of 25; 50; 75 and 100%, respectively, of the sodium level. It was found that potassium chloride may be added in a quantity to reach a K content equal to 50 % of the Na content without affecting in a negative way the organoleptic properties of the processed cheese. Good quality processed cheeses with a potassium content of 75-80% of that of sodium content were produced on an industrial scale.

The influence of salt on functionality of cheese can be observed in studies with Muenster type cheese which is originally salt-free and is submitted to brine injections (20% of sodium) until a soft concentration of 2.7% is acquired. In salt concentrations up to 0.5% of salt, the influence on functionality was more dominant, yielding increase in hardness and viscosity. In salt concentrations over 0.5%, an additional increase in hardness and a decrease in adhesiveness occurred, although there was no change in melting characteristic. Moreover, the increase in salt content did not cause exchanges between ions of calcium and sodium, which maintained a constant solubility of calcium (Pastorino, Hansen, and McMahon, 2003).

Reps, Wisniewska, and Kuzmicka (2009) evaluated the possibility of incorporating more potassium in processed cheese type spread, and demonstrated that it was feasible to produce such type of cheese with good quality with the addition of KCl, use of viscosity reducing agents with increased concentration of potassium salts or diet salt containing KCl. The product required a proportion of Na:K, that is very similar to that recommended and the flavor, aroma and texture were considered acceptable. Furthermore, the results of the sensory analyses showed an increase in acceptance due to the addition of KCl.

Cervantes, Lund, and Olson (1983), Mistry and Kasperson (1998), Olson (1982) and Pastorino et al. (2003) reported that decreasing the salt content of cheese decreases cheese hardness. According to Cervantes et al. (1983), salt affects cheese hardness by promoting interactions between proteins. However, proteins in cheese not only interact among themselves, but also with water, fat, and salts, the nature and extend of these interactions depending on the ionic environment of cheese and processing conditions. Adding sodium chloride to protein suspensions or cheese increases the ionic strength of the system (Floury et al., 2009)

When considering the influence of salt content on cheese texture, data from the literature appears to be conflicting. Most of the authors observed that raising the salt level increased firmness and decreased springiness of several cheese products (Mistry and Kasperson, 1998; Stampanoni and Noble, 1991). An explanation for this is that a salt increase could induce a pH decrease, leading to an aggregation of casein fractions and, thus, firmer cheeses. However, some studies reported that salt had no influence on the texture of cream cheese (Wendin, Langton, Caous, and Hall, 2000).

2.2.1. Reduction of Emulsifying Salts

During the production of processed cheeses, emulsifying salts play an important role and ensure that homogeneous products with desired consistency are made. The actual effect of emulsifying salts lies in the exchange of calcium cations of insoluble calcium paracaseinate for sodium ions, which leads to the formation of more soluble sodium paracaseinate (Mizuno and Lucey, 2007).

The omission of emulsifying salts in processed cheese reduces the levels of sodium (from 20 to 40%) significantly, depending on the amount and type added. However, during the processing of cheese without an emulsifying salts, the application of heat and cutting in the mixture normally results in a heterogeneous mass, excessive viscosity, with exudation oil and separation of water in cooking (Guinee and O'Kennedy, 2007).

The production of processed cheese based on Cheddar with low sodium content and substitution of NaCl (75% of reduction of Na) using combinations of emulsifiers with potassium salts (citrates and phosphates) exhibited acceptable results regarding quality (Karahadian and Lindsay, 1984).

Cerníková' et al. (2010), examined different hydrocolloids as replacements for traditional citrate-and phosphatebased emulsifying salts in processed cheese production. The products were assessed by sensory analysis, microscopic image analysis and dynamic oscillatory rheometry. Modified starch, locust bean gum and low methoxyl pectin could not be recommended as replacements for traditional emulsifying salts. Model processed cheeses without traditional emulsifying salts of 40% (w/w) dry matter and 55% (w/w) fat-in-dry matter containing 1.0% (w/w) k-carrageenan or i-carrageenan were found to be homogeneous, however the products were hard with fracturable texture.

Another approach to reduce the utilization of sodium-based emulsifying salts in a processed cheese formula may involve utilization of different traditional emulsifiers such as mono- and diglycerides at various levels (Lucey 2008; Paulus 2008). Lucey (2008) formulated a reduced fat mozzarella-type product using mono- and diglycerides at various levels and showed improved meltability and stretching-ability of the final product produced when compared to the control.

3. SENSORY IMPACT

The studies covering sensory aspects of low sodium processed cheeses are scarce what it means the sensory aspects of low sodium processed cheese should be faced in a global context, as other processed food. Recently, a study was conducted to identify and define the flavor lexicon of processed and imitation cheese available in United States (Drake, Yates, and Drake, 2010). It was being observed that the amount of natural cheese used in the manufacturing of the processed product, as well as operational parameters used in their processing, as the heat treatment applied and the presence or absence of other ingredients.

When consuming a product, multiple sensations originating from flavor, aroma, texture, and temperature are experienced. The sensations may interact either at perceptible levels (smell, palate, chewing) or at physico-chemical levels (Guichard, 2002; Kilcast and Rider, 2007; Saint-Eve *et al.*, 2009). The final perception results due to integration of all sensory information identified during consumption (Floury *et al.*, 2009).

Other substances may promote salty taste, but only NaCl offers what is really recognized as pure salty taste. Additionally, one of the most important functions of salt is to create a base for the perception of other flavors, that is, it works as an enhancer of taste in some cases and inhibitor in other, in addition to promoting higher perception of aromas (Kilcast and Rider, 2007).

Saint-Eve *et al.* (2009) evaluated the consumer perception regarding cheeses with low salt and fat contents and reported that alterations in texture had no impact on the saltiness perception, although the reduction in salt did have an impact on the smell perception and, in this case, the smell sensation influenced the texture perception. Moreover, they also concluded that only in cheeses with reduction of fat and/or salt, the results showed interaction of sensations, differently from the results of standard cheeses.

Lawrence *et al.* (2009) demonstrated that in solutions with low salt content, the smell may increase the perception of saltiness. However, they also observed that the influence of smell only occurs when the smell has some chemical association with salt, while for smells when not associated with salt, the case is reversed and thus decreasing the perception of saltiness.

In a recent study, Phan *et al.* (2008) concluded that the release of sodium during chewing is mainly influenced by structure and composition of cheese, particularly by the moisture content, whereas the perception of saltiness is limited by the presence of fat. Another alternative would be to decrease the concentration of salt and increase the saltiness perception with other flavoring compounds. Knowing about diffusion coefficients may help predict the salting time and identify the amount of aroma lost during the conservation of products, exerting an impact directly in the formulations and release of these substances during chewing (Lauvejat et al., 2009). Zorrilla and Rubiolo (1999) identified that the redistribution of salt in Fynbo type cheese suffered alterations during the maturation process, as saltiness increased in the centre of the product and decreased at the external areas.

Saint-Eve et al. (2009), evaluated the impact of texture and composition (salt, fat and dry matter) of a model cheese: (i) on salt and flavour perception, and; (ii) on profile texture and flavour release. Variations of salt, fat and dry matter highly influenced texture perception and instrumental texture parameters. Differences in aroma release and olfactory perception ("blue cheese" odour perception) between different model cheeses were highlighted when salt and fat content varied. However, a major result of this study showed that salty perception was not influenced by texture characteristics of model cheeses. Furthermore, olfactory perception modified texture perception but only for model cheeses with low fat and low-dry matter contents. Variations in salt content and sensory interactions therefore seem to have a greater impact on products with low fat content than on those with high-fat content.

Gupta, Karahadian and Lindsay (1984) evaluated the effects on flavor and texture of emulsifying salts in processed cheese and concluded that potassium based emulsifiers may work properly. Nevertheless, emulsifying systems, based only on potassium orthophosphates in order to reduce the concentration of sodium, did not produce cheese with high levels of acceptance.

Moreover, the incorporation of autolytic fermented extracts in processed cheese with reduced sodium content (0.4%) resulted in a cheese with unsuitable flavors (ex.: burning taste) and low acceptance by consumers. The addition of glucono-delta lactone increased the perception of salt in processed cheese with low sodium content, but does not affect the taste effectively. Other materials including citrate and ammonium phosphate, and monosodium glutamate increased the salty flavor in processed cheese with low sodium content, but caused residual sour flavor (Karahadian and Lindsay, 1984).

4. PERSPECTIVES

The effective implementation of all changes in the production process of cheese will need a high level of control in the production process and further studies regarding the quality and level of salt acceptable for the marketing of cheese with reduced salt content in the market are required. Efforts have also been directed at the development of novel formulations in order to utilize potassium-based emulsifying salts, various salt replacers, and other flavor enhancers without causing a detrimental effect on the flavor, sensory, and functional properties of the final processed cheese.

With the improvements of rheological, structural and sensory parameters, associated with campaigns aimed at the consumer on the value addition to the product, the expected success regarding the benefits of sodium reduction in cheese can be achieved with establishment of new products with health benefits.

REFERENCES

Abbott, D., Campbell N., Carruthers-Czyzewski P., Chockalingam A., David M., Dunkley G., Ellis E., Fodor J. G., McKay D., Ramsden V. R. (1994). Guidelines for measurement of blood pressure, follow-up, and lifestyle counselling. *Canadian.*

Berger, W., Klostermeyer, H., Merkenich, K., Uhlmann, G. (1989) Processed cheese manufacture. *A joha Guide. BK Landenburg*, 238.

Bonjour, Jean-Philippe. (2005) Dietary protein: an essential nutrient for bone health. *Journal of the American College of Nutrition*, 24, 526S–536S.

Brickley, C. A.; Govindasamy-Lucey, S., Jaeggi, J.J., Johnson, M.E., McSweeney, L.H., and Lucey, J.A. (2008). Influence of Emulsifying Salts on the Textural Properties of Nonfat Process Cheese Made from Direct Acid Cheese Bases. *Journal of Dairy Science*, 91, 39-48.

Cailar, G., Ribstein, J. and Mimran, Albert (2002). Dietary sodium and target organ damage in essential hypertension. *American Journal of Hypertension,* 15, 222–229.

Cernikova, M., Bunka, F., Pospiech, M., Tremlova, B., Hladka, K., Vladimír Pavlínek, V., and Brezina, P.(2010). Replacement of traditional emulsifying salts by selected hydrocolloids in processed cheese production. *International Dairy Journal*, 20, 336–343.

Cervantes, M. A., Lund, D. B., and Olson, N. F. (1983). Effects of salt concentration and freezing on Mozzarella cheese texture. *Journal of Dairy Science*, 66, 204–213.

Coalition for High Blood Pressure Prevention and Control. *Canadian Journal of Public Health, 85*, S29–S43.

Dawson-Hughes, B. Osteoporose. In: Shils, M. E., Shike, M., Ross, A. C., Caballero, B., Cousins, R. J. (2009) (Eds) *Nutrição Moderana na Saúde e na Doença*, 10th edition. *Manole*, Barueri, 1435-1449.

Devine, A., Criddle, R. A., Dick, I. M., Kerr, D. A. and Prince, R. L. A. (1995). longitudinal study of the effect of sodium and calcium intakes on regional bone density in postmenopausal women. *American Journal of Clinical Nutrition*, 62, 740-745.

Dickinson, B. D. and Havas, S. (2007). Reducing the population burden of cardiovascular disease by reducing sodium intake. *Archive of International Medicine,* 167, 1460-1468.

Drake, S.L., Yates, M.D. and Drake, M.A. (2010). Development of a flavor lexicon for processed and imitation cheeses. *Journal of Sensory Studies*, 25, 720-739.

Euston, S. R., Piska, I., Wium, H. and Qvist, K. B. (2002). Controlling the structure and rheological properties of model cheeses systems. Australian *Journal of Dairy Technology*, 57, 145 -152.

Floury, J., Camier, B., Rousseau,F., Lopez, C., Tissier, J-P. and Famelart, M.-H. (2009). Reducing salt level in food: Part 1. Factors affecting the manufacture of model cheese systems and their structure–texture relationships. LWT - *Food Science and Technology*, 42, 1611–1620.

Floury, J., Rouaud, O., Le Poullennec, M., and Famelart, M. H. (2009). Reducing salt level in food: Part 2: Modelling salt diffusion in model cheese systems with regards to their composition. LWT - *Food Science and Technology, 42, 1621-1628.*

Guichard, E. (2002). Interations between flavor compounds and food ingredients and their influence on flavor perception. *Food Reviews International*, 18, 1, 49-70.

Guinee, T. P. and O'Kennedy, B. T. (2007). Mechanisms of taste perception and physiological controls. In: Guinee, T. P. and O'Kennedy, B. T., (Eds.), Reducing salt in foods: Practical strategies. *Boca Raton LA, USA: CRC Press* 246-287.

Guinee, T. P.(2002) The functionality of cheese as an ingredient: a review. *The Australian Journal of Dairy Technology*, v. 57, n. 2, 79-91.

Guinee, T. P; Caric, M.; Kaláb, M. (2004). Pasteurized processed cheese and substitute/imitation cheese products. In: FOX, P. F.; McWEENEY, P. L. H.;COGAM, T. P. (Eds.) Cheese: Chemistry, Physics and Microbiology Volume 2: Major cheese groups. 3rd. London: Elsevier Ltd.,349-394

Gupta, S. K., Karahadian, C. and Lindsay, R. C. (1984). Effect of emulsifier salts on textural and flavor properties of processed cheese. *Journal of Dairy Science*, 67, 764-778.

Heaney, R. P. (2000). Calcium, dairy products and osteoporosis. *Journal of the American College of Nutrition, 19*, 83S–99S.

Henning, D.R., Baer, R.J., Hassan, A. N. and Dave, R. (2006). Major Advances in Concentrated and Dry Milk Products, Cheese, and Milk Fat-Based Spreads. *Journal of Dairy Science*, 89, 1179–1188

Itoh, R. and Suyama, Y. (1996). Sodium excretion in relation to calcium and hydroxyproline excretion in a healthy Japanese population. *American Journal of Clinical Nutrition, 63*, 735-740.

Johnson, M. E., Kapoor, R., McMahon, D. J., McCoy, D. R. and Narasimmon, R. G. (2009). Reduction of sodium and fat levels in natural and processed cheese: Scientific and technological aspects. *Comprehensive Reviews in Food Science and Food Safety*, 8, 252-268.

Johnson, M., and Paulus, K. (2008). Confronting the challenge of low salt cheese. *Dairy Pipeline*, 20, 4.

Karahadian, C. and Lindsay, R. (1984). Flavour and textural properties of reduced-sodium process American cheeses. *Journal of Dairy Science*, 67, 1892-1904.

Kilcast, D. and Rider, C. (2007). Sensory issues in reducing salt in food products. In: Guinee, T. P. and O'Kennedy, B. T., (Eds.), Reducing salt in foods: Practical strategies (pp 201-220). *Boca Raton LA, USA: CRC Press*.

Kuller, L. H. (1997). Salt and blood pressure population and individual perspectives. *American Journal of Hypertension, 10*, 29S–36S.

Lauverjat, C., Loubens C., Déléris, I., Tréléa, I. C. and Souchon, I. (2009). Rapid determination of participation and diffusion properties for salt and aroma compounds in complex food matrices. *Journal of Food Engineering*, 93, 407-415.

Lawrence, G., Salles, C., Septier, C., Busch, J. and Thomas-Danguin, T. (2009). Odour-taste interactions: A way to enhance saltiness in low-salt content solutions. *Food Quality and Preference*, 20, 241-248.

Lucey, J. A., Johnson, M. E., and Horne, D. S. (2003). Perspectives on the basis of therheology and texture properties of cheese. *Journal of Dairy Science*, 86, 2725–2743

Meneton, P., Jeunemaitre, X., Wardener, H. and Macgregor, G.A. (2005). Links between dietary salt intake, renal salt handling, blood pressure, and cardiovascular diseases. *Physiological Reviews, 85,* 679 – 715.

Metzger, L. E. and Kapoor, R. (2007). Novel approach for producing with reduced-fat and reducedsodium content. *Journal Dairy Science*, 86, 1, 198.

Meyer, A. Process cheese manufacture (1973). *London: Food Trade Press*, 360. Mistry, V.V., and Kasperson, K.M. (1998). Influence of salt on the quality of reduced fat Cheddar cheese. *Journal of Dairy Science*, 81, 1214–1221.

Mizuno, R., and Lucey, J. A. (2007). Properties of milk protein gels formed by phosphates. *Journal of Dairy Science*, 90, 4524 – 4531.

Nordin, B.E.C., Need, A. G., Morris, H.A. and Horowitz, M. (1993). The nature and significance of the relationship between urinary sodium and urinary calcium in women. *Journal of Nutrition, 123,* 1615–1622.

Olson, N. F. (1982). Salt affects cheese characteristics. *Dairy Field* , 72–73.

Pastorino, A.J., Hansen, C.L. and Mcmahon, D.J. (2003). Effect of salt on structure-function relationships of cheese. *Journal of Dairy Science*, 86, 60 - 69.

Paulus K. (2008). New mozzarella breaks lowfat impasse. Dairy Pipeline. *Wisconsin Center for Dairy Research.* 2 (2).

Phan,V. A., Yven, C., Lawrence, G., Chabanet, C., Reparet, J. M. and Salles, C. (2008). In vivo sodium release related to salty perception during eating model cheeses of different textures. *International Dairy Journal*, 18, 956 - 963.

Prentice A. (2004). Diet, nutrition and the prevention of osteoporosis. *Public Health Nutrition, 7,* 227-243.

Prentice A. (1997). Is nutrition important in osteoporosis? *Proceedings of the Nutrition Society, 56,* 357–67.

Purdy, J. and Armstrong, G. (2007). Dietary salt and the consumer: reported consumption and awareness of associated healthy risks. In:Guinee, T. P. and O'Kennedy, B. T., (Eds.), Reducing salt in foods:Practical strategies. *Boca Raton LA, USA: CRC Press*. 99-123

Reps, A., Wisniewska, K. and Kuzmicka, M. (2009). Possibilities of increasing the potassium content of processed cheese spread. *Milchwissenschaft,* 64, 2, 176-179.

Reps, A, Iwanczak, M., Wisniewska, K., and Dajnowiec. (1998) F. Processed cheeses with an increased potassium content. *Milchwissenschaft*, 53, 690-693

Rickley, C.A., Govindasamy-Lucey, S., Jaeggi, J.J., Johnson, M. E., McSweeney, L.H., and Lucey, J.A. (2008) Influence of Emulsifying Salts on the Textural Properties of Nonfat Process Cheese Made from Direct Acid Cheese Bases. *Journal of Dairy Science*, v. 91, p. 39-48.

Ritz, Eberhard (2006). Salt—friend or foe? *Nephrology Dialysis and Transplantation, 21,* 2052–2056.

Saint-Eve, A., Lauverjat, C., Magnan, C., Déléris, I., and Souchon, I. (2009). Reducing salt and fat content: Impact of composition, texture and cognitive interactions on the perception of flavored model cheeses. *Food Chemistry*, 116, 167-175.

Sellmeyer, D.E., Schloetter, M., and Sebastian, A. (2002). Potassium citrate prevents increased urine calcium excretion and bone resorption induced by a high sodium chloride diet. *The Journal of Clinical Endocrinology and Metabolims, 87,* 2008-2012.

Stampanoni, C.R., and Noble, A.C. (1991). The influence of fat, acid and salt on thetemporal perception of firmness, saltiness and sourness of cheese analogs. *Journal of Texture Studies*, 22, 381–392.

Wendin, K., Langton, M., Caous, L., and Hall, G. (2000). Dynamic analyses of sensory and microstructural properties of cream cheese. *Food Chemistry*, 71, 363–378.

Zehren, V.L., and Nusbaum, D.D. (1992). Process cheese. Madison: Cheese *Reporter. Publishing Company*, 363 p.

Zorrilla, S.E. and Rubiolo, A.C. (1997). Kinectics of casein degradation during ripening of Fynbo cheese salted with NaCl/KCl brine. *Journal of Food Science*, 62, 386-389.

In: Cheese: Types, Nutrition and Consumption
Editor: Richard D. Foster, pp. 171-182

ISBN 978-1-61209-828-9
© 2011 Nova Science Publishers, Inc.

Chapter 9

ITALIAN CHEESE TYPES AND INNOVATIONS OF TRADITIONAL CHEESES

Palmiro Poltronieri, Maria Stella Cappello, Federico Baruzzi, and Maria Morea

National Research Council of Italy, CNR-ISPA, Institute of Sciences of Food Productions, Lecce, Italy

ABSTRACT

Dairy productions in the Italian area are rich in fresh soft cheeses, spreadable cheese, like Crescenza and Gorgonzola, fresh type cheeses, like Primo sale and Cacioricotta, and ripened cream types, such as Ricotta forte.

Manufacturing trends and consumer novel products influenced the development of different innovative dairy products such as cheeses containing probiotic microorganisms. These cheese productions help the sustainable development and growth of local producers increasing the economy of dairy factories through the development of products dedicated to individuals with special dietary requirements.

INTRODUCTION

In recent years a positive sustainable increase in the marketing of traditional foods resulted from the introduction of guarantee quality labels. After France (48 PDO cheeses), Italy is the second country with 39 out of 170 PDO cheeses registered in European Community (source: http://ec.europa.eu/agriculture/quality/door/list.html). The Italian Ministry of Agriculture, in addition to PDO designed cheese, listed more than 400 'regional' cheeses [1].

In this way, consumers request their PDO products of choice trusting the local manufacturing processes based on traditional manufacturing and healthy milk material. Normative on nutritional value labels introduced on packaged cheese the information on the recommended dose of calcium/day and the Kcal/KJoule content.

Table 1. Yearly Production of PDO italian cheeses in Tons (Date: 01-09-2010)

Production of PDO italian cheeses, Tons							
	2004	2005	2006	2007	2008	2009	± variations
Grana Padano	C 149.153	159.607	158.243	158.017	163.341	158.326	*-3,07%*
Parmigiano Reggiano	C 116.855	118.979	117.410	117.044	116.064	113.436	*-2,26%*
Gorgonzola	C 47.623	48.480	48.134	48.860	48.721	47.644	*-2,21%*
Provolone Valpadana	C 13.470	12.745	9.630	9.637	9.615	8.799	*-8,49%*
Asiago	C 22.851	23.621	23.330	22.649	23.318	23.528	*+0,90%*
Taleggio	C 9.547	9.196	8.766	8.814	8.800	8.497	*-3,44%*
Montasio	C 7.821	8.190	7.325	7.144	7.349	7.691	*+4,65%*
Fontina	C 3.523	3.606	3.735	4.535	4.473	3.820	*-14,60%*
Quartirolo Lombardo	C 3.462	3.428	3.654	3.747	3.693	3.700	*+0,19%*
Valtellina Casera	C 1.500	1.464	1.400	1.280	1.360	1.400	*+2,94%*
Toma Piemontese	C 1.288	1.234	1.116	1.128	1.078	1.067	*-0,99%*
Bra	C 832	1.028	816	758	762	731	*-4,16%*
Raschera	C 811	994	686	793	780	734	*-5,87%*
Caciocavallo Silano	C 993	1.119	1.050	1.008	750	750	*+0,03%*
Monte Veronese	C 461	537	482	496	589	655	*+11,19%*
Castelmagno	C 167	201	201	201	197	215	*+9,36%*
Ragusano [3]	C 131	169	155	137	131	165	*+25,95%*
Formai de Mut	C 55,1	60,9	58,6	67,1	71,0	72,0	*+1,41%*
Fromadzo	C 3,0	4,0	6,0	5,1	4,2	4,6	*+10,58%*
Spressa delle Giudicarie	C (p) 88,1	137	46,1	98,4	150	58,0	*-61,28%*
Stelvio	C n.p.	n.p.	n.p.	n.p.	1.112	1.186	*+6,61%*
Casatella Trevigiana	C n.p.	n.p.	n.p.	n.p.	n.p.	467	-
Provolone del Monaco	C n.p.	n.p.	n.p.	n.p.	n.p.	40,0	-
Casciotta d'Urbino (70% P)	M 240	240	250	245	229	220	*-3,93%*
Bitto (10% C)	M 350	332	310	275	290	264	*-8,97%*
Robiola di Roccaverano	M 81,8	76,4	104	78,5	84,2	88,3	*+4,87%*

Murazzano (60% P)	M 34,4	26,0	24,6	22,9	21,5	15,8	-26,62%
Castelmagno	M 167	201	201	201	197	215	+9,36%
Total		381.341	395.473	386.931	387.041	392.982	383.573 -2,39%*
		2004	2005	2006	2007	2008	2009 ± su 2008
Mozzarella di bufala campana	B	27.632	29.645	33.805	35.640	31.960	33.900 +6,07%
Total		27.632	29.645	33.805	35.640	31.960	33.900 +6,07%*
		2004	2005	2006	2007	2008	2009 ± of 2008
Pecorino Romano [1]	E	38.138	23.855	24.470	33.425	29.461	25.581 -13,17%
Pecorino Siciliano [3]	E	14,3	13,1	8,9	15,6	35,0	21,0 -40,00%
Pecorino Toscano	E	1.880	1.869	1.965	1.943	2.816	2.933 +4,15%
Fiore Sardo [2]	E	518	466	620	600	650	(e) 712 +9,54%
Pecorino Sardo	E	1.579	1.600	1.800	1.800	1.960	1.860 -5,10%
Canestrato Pugliese	E	129	107	107	104	106	83,7 -21,37%
Pecorino di Filiano	E	n.p.	n.p.	n.p.	n.p.	8,0	8,0 0,00%
Total		42.258	27.910	28.971	37.888	35.036	31.199 -10,95%*

(e): estimated Value.
(p): start of production PDO: May 2004.
* variation calculated on the total of the same products in the previous year
1) *Dairy production October-July*
2) *Dairy production November-May*
3) *Dairy production November-December*
B: buffalo milk; C: cow's milk; E: ewe's milk; M: mixed type milks
Source: CLAL Italy and CSQA - Thiene, INOQ - Cuneo, CORFILAC - Ragusa, ISMECERT, Bioagricoop – Bologna.

One important aspect contributing to a great diversification of cheeses is flavour development process and the type of livestock feeding, herbs at different altitudes of the pasture lands and specified silage feeds.

Producing specific milks for speciality cheeses is an objective that may support local economic development [2]. On the basis of quality of the milk, cheeses are differentiated in those from cow's cheese (80,7% of total), buffalo's milk (6,8%) ewe's cheese (12,5%), or mixed types. In Italy and Spain ewe's milk is abundant, as mixed types with many herds consisting in sheep and goats grown together. Nowadays, customers visiting local farms or ordering cheeses from dealers have large choices of dairy products.

Concerning the milk quality, factors of typicality are species and/or breed, pedoclimatic conditions, animal management system and feeding. Other factors that influence cheese quality are milk treatments (raw milk is treated with at 72°C differently from pasteurised milk), curd processing and the ripening method.

In addition, also when these factors are the same or very similar each other, such as the case of dairies located in the same area, microflora used to ferment milk and ripen cheese, make the difference.

Principally the categories of cheese may be classified according to the structure, flavour, and ageing /ripening time [3].

Hard cheeses are the main productions, with Grana Padano, Parmigiano Reggiano and Pecorino being the most representative products. Soft cheeses cover the remaining 30% of the total production. Considering that soft cheese production reaches 300 tons, Gorgonzola production is 1/3 of this total, the other main products are Taleggio, Italico, Quartirolo, Crescenza, and Caciotta, followed by Brie, Provola and Scamorza, two pasta filata cheeses with short ripening time. Italy is the third country in Europe for cheese production, reaching 12,5% of the 8.200.000 ton/year produced in the European Community countries in recent years (Table 1).

In 2009, 250.000 tons of the Italian production were exported. Grana Padano and Parmigiano Reggiano were the main exported products, followed by Gorgonzola, Provolone, Montasio, Caciocavallo, Ragusano and Asiago.

The disciplinary for the production of PDO cheeses such as "Parmigiano Reggiano" [4] has set established standards in the animal feed based on selected silage together with flowering herbs forage, in the manufacturing process using whey starters propagated day by day using a whey inoculum [5].

The ewe's cheese types are Pecorino Romano [6], Siciliano [7], Toscano [8], Abruzzese [9] and from central Italy [10], Fiore Sardo [11, 12], Canestrato, either Pugliese [13, 14] and the Sicilian type, Caciotta, Murazzano and Calcagno, produced in several variable sizes, from kilograms to 8-10 kilograms, and other different types, from fresh cheeses such as Tuma, Vastedda, or Primo Sale, softly brined with the highest water content, to semi hard forms such as Caciotta, to well ripened hard types.

Product specification of PDO cheeses states a minimum moisture content, but generally moisture content for cheeses is not legally defined. Cheese consistency depends not only on moisture, but also on other parameters, such as fat content and the duration of ripening. On the basis of consistency, depending on moisture content, Italian cheeses may be classified in:

- soft cheeses: moisture content over 45% (as Robiola, Quartirolo, Stracchino, Crescenza, Mozzarella, Burrata, Gorgonzola, Caprini, Casatella, Squacquerone). These cheeses may have a rind (Taleggio) or not (Pannerone)
- semi-hard cheeses: moisture content varying between 35 and 45% (as Ragusano, Asiago, Bitto, Fontina, Bra, Castelmagno, Italico)
- hard cheeses: moisture content below 35% (as Grana Padano, Parmigiano-Reggiano, Pecorino Romano, Montasio, Pecorino Sardo, Fiore Sardo, Canestrato.

On the basis of processing technology and the temperature at which the curd is cooked, cheeses are classified as follows:

- raw cheeses: obtained without applying any heat-treatment to the curd after coagulation (as Robiola, Mozzarella, Crescenza, Gorgonzola)

- semi-cooked cheeses: curd is cooked at temperatures up to 48°C (as Asiago, Fontina, Italico)
- cooked cheeses: curd is cooked at temperatures over 48°C (as Grana Padano, Parmigiano-Reggiano, Montasio, Bitto)
- "pasta filata" cheeses: characterized by a treatment of the curd with water at 70-90°C (as Mozzarella, Fiordilatte, Caciocavallo, Provolone)

On the basis of duration of ripening, cheeses are classified as follows:

- fresh cheeses: no ripening occurs; cheeses devoid of rind or superficial microflora, which must be consumed shortly after production (as Mozzarella, Fiordilatte, Crescenza, Casatella, Giuncata). The field of fresh type cheeses are present in the territory in several productions characterised in their mild flavours and wateriness, to be consumed in weeks for their high moisture content. In this group: Primo Sale, made by addition of starters into renneted milk, Casatella, made with presamic curd, cottage cheeses made by acid coagulation, and Cacioricotta, obtained from renneted milk coagulated by the combined effect of high temperature and low pH
- short-ripened cheeses: ripening period up to 30 days (as Taleggio, Murazzano, Bra, Quartirolo Lombardo, Asiago, Monte Veronese, Casciotta d'Urbino, Scamorza)
- medium-ripened cheeses: ripening period up to 6 months, such as Fontina, Castelmagno, Raschera, Toma Piemontese, Valtellina Casera, Provolone Valpadana, Caciocavallo Silano, Canestrato Pugliese, Pecorino Siciliano, Pecorino Sardo, Bitto
- long-ripened cheeses: ripened over 6 months, as Grana Padano, Parmigiano-Reggiano, Fiore Sardo, Ricotta Forte

On the basis of manufacturing technology and structure formation, cheeses may be classified on the type of curd treatment, the type of brining, the surface treatment, the addition of surface microflora and the development of a rind:

- the "pasta filata" category of stretched cheeses groups several different types of cheese, such as "Mozzarella", made with cow's or buffalo's milk, with the highest water content corresponding to a "low fat" cheese, and other cheeses as "Scamorza" and "Provola", to be consumed in weeks or months, or more ripened such as Provolone and the Kashkaval-type "Caciocavallo" with semihard to hard characteristics. The loss of weight due to water evaporation translates in a higher content of proteins and fat compared to unripened cheese.
- **Pressed Cheese:** the curds of these types of cheese are hand or mechanically pressed to remove the maximum amount of water during production. After pressing the cheese may be **cooked** to remove even more moisture from the curd. This cooking process creates a very firm inner paste and a hard outer rind. If the cheese remains **uncooked** its inner paste and outer rind will remain partially firm. Uncooked cheeses tend to be sweet and fruity when they are young, developing a much more complex flavour as they age. After further drying the young cheeses are subjected to a salt bath and are then allowed to age in cool rooms or caves. Natural rind cheeses tend to have hard outer rinds and are for the most part not edible. Examples of **cooked**

pressed cheeses include Parmigiano Reggiano, Asiago, Fontina, Piave. Examples of **uncooked pressed cheeses** include Pecorino and Castelmagno.
- **Washed Rind Cheese: in** these cheeses when the rind is removed an exquisitely flavoured inner paste is revealed. An example is Taleggio.
- **Soft Ripened Cheeses or** Bloomy **Rind Cheeses: with** a white or light beige velvety layer covering the entire outer rind. The outer rinds are edible but it is a matter of individual taste. As these cheeses age or "ripen" they become melting or completely runny. Examples of **soft ripened cheeses** include Toma, Alpino and Brie-like types.

The type of rennet (calf, lamb or pig rennet) used influences the rate of lipolysis and is directly involved in the formation and release of flavour. In some small dairies, milk is also still curdled by using rennet of plant or fungi origin.

MICROBIOLOGY AND ORGANOLEPTIC QUALITY OF TRADITIONAL DAIRY PRODUCTS: ISOLATION OF STRAINS OF NON STARTER LACTIC ACID BACTERIA (NSLAB)

Texture and structure formation rely on the manufacturing technology and on the survival of the starters and original microflora. A great part of the microbiological studies performed on traditional cheeses were directed to understand the microbial community dynamics during various stages of cheese production and storage. These studies, carried out on "pasta filata cheeses", such as Fiordilatte di Agerola PDO [15], Mozzarella cheeses [16], Caciocavallo Pugliese [17], Scamorza [18], or on hard and semi-hard cheeses such as Canestrato Pugliese [14] and Pecorino [19, 7, 9, 10] or on several ewe's type cheeses [20-22], showed an amazing microbial biodiversity well represented by NSLAB such as *Lactobacillus acetotolerans, Lb. alimentarius, Lb. brevis, Lb. casei/paracasei* species group, *Lb. curvatus, Lb. gasseri, Lb. hilgardii, Lb. kefiri, Lb. plantarum* species group, *Lb. fermentum*, enterococci (mainly *E. faecalis* and *E. faecium*) and sporadically by *Lactococcus garviae, Lc. lactis, Leuconostoc mesenteroides* subsp. *mesenteroides, Pediococcus pentosaceus* and *Streptococcus macedonicus*.

Considering cheese microbiology, the addition of NSLAB strains as adjunct cultures was monitored in several cheese products, ewe's cheese [21], Caciocavallo [23]; Roncal ewe's cheese [24], Fiore Sardo cheese [12] and "high moisture" Mozzarella [25]. In other countries, similar studies are carried on adjunct strains in Swiss cheeses using microfiltered milk [26]. Selection and use of autochthonous multiple strain cultures were performed to obtain improved cheese products with extended shelf-life maintaining the flavours and texture requirements. More often in addition to microbial characterisation, other factors linked to typicality of cheeses are analysed and linked to the microbial profile, as the compositional, biochemical, volatile profile and sensory characteristics [20], biochemical and textural characteristics [17], lipolytic and proteolytic patterns [27] and flavour analysis [28, 29]. Most of these studies showed the importance of milk as a source of technologically interesting strains that could be used to ensure a higher quality of artisanal cheese productions. Innovative molecular methods for monitoring Lactic Acid Bacteria associated to dairy products have been applied [30] in analysis of food processing and origin traceability.

ADVANCEMENTS IN THE MANUFACTURING OF INNOVATIVE AND TRADITIONAL CHEESES

Probiotic Cheeses

The addition of probiotic strains in cheeses is an established technique, and nowadays several types of soft cheeses are marketed with the "probiotic cheese" label.

Examples of cheeses studied for the addition of probiotic strains are the stracchino type of soft cheeses Certosa and Crescenza [31, 32], Cheddar cheese [33-36], Fresh Minas cheese [37], White Turkish cheese [38], Argentinian semi-hard [39] and Fresco cheeses [40], semi-hard goat cheese [41, 42], a smear-ripened, semisoft cheese "Pikantne" cheese [43] and Requeijão, a Portuguese whey cheese [44].

Generally, these cheeses at the marketing stage present a content of probiotics sufficient to assure the introduction of millions of bacteria and the presence in the gut for several days after cheese ingestion. The principal aspects that researchers investigate using probiotics are: adherence to intestinal tissue or gut-derived cell lines, antagonism to pathogens or antimicrobial activity, stimulation of immune system to produce anti-inflammatory cytokines and anti-inflammatory activity, stimulation of beneficial bacteria, and clinical effect on volunteers. Many of the studies conducted on cheeses enriched with probiotics have been made using probiotic strains whose probiotic activity was already assessed, other studies have been focused on bacteria isolated from milk or the environment that shows survival in the gut (resistance to low pH, to biliary salts) [44] and that could produce any of the beneficial effects required.

IMPROVEMENT OF MICROBIOLOGICAL, TECHNOLOGICAL AND NUTRITIONAL ASPECTS OF TRADITIONAL CHEESES

The main directions of the PDO studies are the characterization of compounds involved in the sensory quality (texture, flavours) and the assessment of quality traits useful in defining the typicality of PDO and traditional Italian cheeses. Several aspects from microbiology to chemical analysis are combined together, as the characterization of bacterial population dynamics, compounds that confer flavours, organoleptic quality and requirements of standard textures and structures.

CHEESE FORTIFICATION AND INNOVATIVE CHEESES WITH ADDED INGREDIENTS

Cheeses may be enriched with minerals as calcium, proteins as Lactoferricin and other beneficial peptides, vitamins, and prebiotic fibres. One of these ingredients is vitamin D, with several milk products available on the market. Other studies provided evidence for great health benefit of cheeses with added omega-3 fatty acids. These products may have a good acceptance, as the established products such as the pasta added with flax seeds or canola oil. A different approach has been used by increasing the conjugated linoleic acid (CLA) content in milk through feeding of the livestock with CLA rich seeds, thus increasing the content in cheeses. This CLA rich dairy product is addressing low cholesterol diets for specific disease treatments. This field is highly promising for the development of innovative products for specific groups of individuals with health problems or with specific nutrient requirements.

STRATEGIES TO REDUCE FAT AND SALT CONTENT

Dairy products with reduced fat are already available especially for the industrial products. Several studies showed the effects of lower fat content in cheese models [45]. An excessive reduction in fat content may produce changes in texture and structure, so that other hydrocolloids must replace fat. Fat reduction in cheese is known to provide firmer, springier and less meltable products, since fat inhibits the formation of crosslinks in the protein network [46-48]. In industrial low-moisture mozzarella produced with different fat contents [46], as fat percentage was reduced, there was a significant decrease in the moisture, in pizza baking performance, meltability, and free oil release, with good results obtained for a cheese with 2 g of fat/100 g of cheese.

So far, the most economically interesting field is low salt cheese, keeping in consideration that more dried cheeses are more salty [49]. One limit for an excessive salt reduction is for *Lactococcus lactis sbsp. cremoris* starters used in cheddar cheese [50]. The replacement of sodium chloride with other salts could be a solution, but these compounds could be responsible for off-flavour and bitterness. Sodium chloride affects flavour by regulating the growth of certain microbes and the activity of particular enzymes. Salt concentrations significantly impact activities of proteolytic and lipolytic enzymes during ripening of cheese. Growth and metabolic activities of cheese starter cultures may be stimulated or depressed by specific sodium chloride levels, affecting flavour and aroma compounds synthesized by the microflora [51].

Another possibility is to tailor food matrix in order to increase salty perception without increasing salt content. Many studies evidence the interactions between food structure and texture and aroma or taste perception [48, 52].

Combined NaCl and KCl experiments were carried out and data were analysed and showed that in combination KCl is a direct 1:1 molar replacement for the antimicrobial effect of common salt. If this is a general finding then, where salt is used to help to preserve a product, partial or complete replacement with KCl is possible [53, 54]. Studies on partial replacement of salt (2.6% NaCl) using a mixture of 1.0% NaCl, 0.55% KCl and 0.74% $CaCl_2$ in food products have been made evaluating an antagonistic activity on food pathogens similar to the original NaCl based product [55].

Novel salt formulations have been made in certain cheese types, such as a 33% salt reduction in processed cheese [56], and a reduction from 1602 mg to 63 mg/100 g in Parmigiano cheese (data from http://www.nal.usda.gov/fnic/foodcomp/search/).

CONCLUSION

Cheese productions may support the sustainable economical growth both through the survival of traditional cheeses made at local dairies and also through the manufacturing of novel cheeses dedicated to individuals with special dietary requirements.

REFERENCES

[1] Council Regulation (EC) No 510/2006 of 20 March 2006, on the protection of geographical indications and designations of origin for agricultural products and foodstuffs.

[2] Bertoni G, Calamari L, Maianti MG. Producing specific milks for specialty cheeses. *Proc. Nutr. Soc.* 2001, 60:231-246.

[3] Fox P.F., Mc Sweeney P.L.H., Cogan T.M. and Guinee T.P. Eds., Cheese: Chemistry, Physics and Microbiology. Major Cheese groups. IVth Edition, Chapman and Hall, 2004. ISBN: 0-1226-3653-8.

[4] Battistotti B., Corradini C. Italian cheese. 221-242. In: Fox P.F. Ed., Cheese: Chemistry, Physics and Microbiology. Volume 2. Chapman and Hall, 1998.

[5] Bottari B, Santarelli M, Neviani E, Gatti M. Natural whey starter for Parmigiano Reggiano: culture- independent approach. *J. Appl. Microbiol.* 2010, 108:1676-1684.

[6] Mannu L., Riu G., Comunian R., Fozzi MC and Scintu MF. A preliminary study of lactic acid bacteria in whey starter culture and industrial Pecorino Sardo ewes' milk cheese: PCR-identification and evolution during ripening. *Int. Dairy J.* 2002 12:17-26

[7] Randazzo CL, Pitino I, De Luca S, Scifò GO, Caggia C. Effect of wild strains used as starter cultures and adjunct cultures on the volatile compounds of the Pecorino Siciliano cheese. *Int. J. Food Microbiol.* 2008, 122:269-278.

[8] Bizzarro R., Torri Tarelli G., Giraffa G., Neviani E. Phenotypic and genotypic characterization of lactic acid bacteria isolated from pecorino toscano cheese. *Italian J. Food Sci.* 2000, 12:303-316.

[9] Serio, A., Chaves-Lòpez, C., Paparella, A., Corsetti, A., Martino, G., Suzzi, G. (2006) Microbiological and physico-chemical characterization of Pecorino Abruzzese cheese during ripening. In: Proceedings of Technological Innovation and Enhancement of Marginal Products, Foggia, Italy, 6–8 April 2005.

[10] Aquilanti L., Silvestri G., Zannini E., Osimani A., Santarelli S., Clementi F. Phenotypic, genotypic and technological characterization of predominant lactic acid bacteria in Pecorino cheese from central Italy. *J. Appl. Microbiol.* 2007, 103:948-960.

[11] Pisano B, Fadda E, Deplano M., Corda A., Cosentino S. Microbiological and chemical characterization of Fiore Sardo, a traditional Sardinian cheese made from ewe's milk. *Int. J. Dairy Technol.* 2006, 59: 171-180.

[12] Pisano MB, Elisabetta Fadda M, Deplano M, Corda A, Casula M, Cosentino S. Characterization of Fiore Sardo cheese manufactured with the addition of autochthonous cultures. *J. Dairy Res.* 2007, 74:255-261.

[13] Albenzio M, Corbo MR, Rehman SU, Fox, De Angelis M, Corsetti A, Sevi A, Gobbetti M. Microbiological and biochemical characteristics of Canestrato Pugliese cheese made

from raw milk, pasteurized milk or by heating the curd in hot whey. *Int J Food Microbiol.* 2001, 67(1-2):35-48.
[14] Aquilanti L., Zannini E., Zocchetti A., Osimani A., Clementi F. Polyphasic characterization of indigenous lactobacilli and lactococci from PDO Canestrato Pugliese cheese. *LWT - Food Science and Technology*, 2007b, 40: 1146-1155.
[15] Coppola S, Fusco V, Andolfi R, Aponte M, Blaiotta G, Ercolini D, Moschetti G. Evaluation *J. Dairy Res.* 2006, 73:264-72.
[16] Morea M, Baruzzi F, Cocconcelli PS. Molecular and physiological characterization of dominant bacterial populations in traditional mozzarella cheese. *J. Appl. Microbiol.* 1999, 87:574-582.
[17] Gobbetti M., Morea M., Baruzzi F., Corbo M. R., Matarante A., Considine T., Di Cagno R., Guinee T., Fox P.F. Microbiological, compositional, biochemical and textural characterisation of Caciocavallo Pugliese cheese during ripening. *Int. Dairy J.* 2002, 12:511–523.
[18] Baruzzi F, Matarante A, Morea M, Cocconcelli PS. Microbial community *J Dairy Sci.* 2002, 85:1390-1397.
[19] Cappello MS, Laddomada B, Poltronieri P, Zacheo G. Characterisation of LAB in typical Salento Pecorino cheese Meded *Rijksuniv Gent Fak Landbouwkd Toegep Biol Wet.* 2001, 66(3b):569-72.
[20] Di Cagno R., Banks J., Sheehan L., Fox P.F., Brechany E.Y., Corsetti A., Gobbetti M. Comparison of the microbiological, compositional, biochemical, volatile profile and sensory characteristics of three Italian PDO ewes' milk cheeses. *Int. Dairy J.* 2003, 13:961–972.
[21] De Angelis M., Corsetti A., Tosti N., Rossi J., Corbo M.R., Gobbetti M. Characterization of non-starter lactic acid bacteria from Italian ewe cheeses based on phenotypic, genotypic, and cell wall protein analysis. *Appl. Environ. Microbiol.* 2001, 67:2011–2020.
[22] Baruzzi F., Morea M., Matarante A., Cocconcelli P. S. Changes in the Lactobacillus community during Ricotta forte cheese natural fermentation. *J. Appl. Microbiol.* 2000, .89: 807–814.
[23] Morea M., Matarante A.,. Di Cagno R, Baruzzi F., Minervini F.. Contribution of autochthonous non-starter lactobacilli to proteolysis in Caciocavallo Pugliese cheese. *Int. Dairy J.*, 2007, 17: 525-534.
[24] Ortigosa M, Arizcun C, Irigoyen A, Oneca M, Torre P. Effect of lactobacillus adjunct cultures on the microbiological and physicochemical characteristics of Roncal-type ewes'-milk cheese. *Food Microbiol.* 2006, 23:591-598.
[25] De Angelis M, de Candia S, Calasso MP, Faccia M, Guinee TP, Simonetti MC, Gobbetti M. Selection and use of autochthonous multiple strain cultures for the manufacture of high-moisture traditional Mozzarella cheese. *Int. J. Food Microbiol.* 2008, 125:123-132.
[26] Bouton Y, Buchin S, Duboz G, Pochet S, Beuvier E. Effect of mesophilic lactobacilli and enterococci adjunct cultures on the final characteristics of a microfiltered milk Swiss-type cheese. *Food Microbiol.* 2009, 26:183-191.
[27] Vannini L., Patrignani F., Iucci L., Ndagijimana M., Vallicelli M., Panciotti R., Guerzoni M.E. Effect of a pre-treatment of milk with high pressure homogenization on

yield as well as on microbiological, lipolytic and proteolytic patterns of "Pecorino" cheese. *Int. J. Food Microbiol.* 2008, 128:329-335.

[28] Smit G., Smit B.A., Engels W.J.M.. Flavour formation by lactic acid bacteria and biochemical flavour profiling of cheese products. *FEMS Microbiol. Rev.* 2005, 29:591–610.

[29] Randazzo CL, Pitino I, Ribbera A, Caggia C. Pecorino Crotonese cheese: study of bacterial population and flavour compounds. *Food Microbiol.* 2010, 27(3):363-374.

[30] Poltronieri P., D'Urso OF, Blaiotta G, Morea M. DNA arrays and membrane hybridization methods for screening six Lactobacillus species common in food. *Food Analyt. Meth.* 2008. 1(3): 171-180.

[31] Gobbetti, M, Corsetti A, Smacchi E, Zocchetti A, De Angelis M. Production of Crescenza cheese by incorporation of bifidobacteria. *J. Dairy Sci.* 1998; 81:37–47.

[32] Burns P, Patrignani F, Serrazanetti D, Vinderola GC, Reinheimer JA, Lanciotti R, Guerzoni ME. Probiotic Crescenza cheese containing *Lactobacillus casei* and *Lactobacillus acidophilus* manufactured with high-pressure homogenized milk. *J. Dairy Sci.* 2008, 91, 500-512.

[33] Ong L, Shah NP. Probiotic cheddar cheese: influence of ripening temperatures on proteolysis and sensory characteristics of cheddar cheeses. *J. Food Sci.* 2009, 74:S182-91.

[34] Gardiner GE, Bouchier P, O'Sullivan E, Kelly J, Collins JK, Fitzgerald G, Ross RP, Stanton C. A spray-dried culture for probiotic Cheddar cheese manufacture. *Int. Dairy J.* 2002, 12:749–56.

[35] Phillips M, Kailasapathy K, Tran L. Viability of commercial probiotic cultures (*L. acidophilus*, *Bifidobacterium sp.*, *L. casei*, *L. paracasei* and *L. rhamnosus*) in cheddar cheese. *Int. J. Food Microbiol.* 2006, 108:276-80.

[36] Daigle A, Roy D, Belanger G, Vuillemard JC. Production of probiotic cheese (cheddar-like cheese) using enriched cream fermented by *Bifidobacterium infantis*. *J Dairy Sci.* 1999, 82:1081-1091.

[37] Buriti FCA, da Rocha JS, Assis EG, Saad SMI. Probiotic potential of Minas fresh cheese prepared with the addition of *Lactobacillus paracasei*. *LWT- Food Sci. Technol.* 2005, 38:173–180.

[38] Kasımoglu A, Goncuoglu M, Akgun S. Probiotic white cheese with *Lactobacillus acidophilus*. *Int. Dairy J.* 2004,14:1067–1073.

[39] Bergamini CV, Hynes ER, Quiberoni A, Suarez VB, Zalazar CA. Probiotic bacteria as adjunct starters: influence of the addition methodology on their survival in a semi-hard Argentinean cheese. *Food Res. Int.* 2005, 38:597–604.

[40] Vinderola, CG, Prosello W, Ghiberto TD, Reinheimer JA. Viability of probiotic (*Bifidobacterium*, *Lactobacillus acidophilus* and *Lactobacillus casei*) and non probiotic microflora in Argentinian Fresco cheese. *J. Dairy Sci.* 2000; 83:1905–1911.

[41] Gomes AM, Malcata FX. Development of probiotic cheese manufactured from goat milk: response surface analysis via technological manipulation. *J. Dairy Sci.* 1998; 81:1492–1507.

[42] Kalavrouzioti I., Hatzikamari M., Litopoulou-Tzanetaki E., Tzanetakis N. "Production of hard cheese from caprine milk by the use of two types of probiotic cultures as adjuncts" *Int. J. Dairy Technol.* 2005, 58:30-38.

[43] Songisepp E., Kullisaar T., Hutt P., Elias P., Brilene T., Zilmer M., Mikelsaar M. "A new probiotic cheese with antioxidative and antimicrobial activity" *J. Dairy Sci.* 2004, 87:2017-2023.

[44] Madureira AR, Pereira CI, Truszkowska K, Gomes AM, Pintado ME, Malcata FX. Survival of probiotic bacteria in a whey cheese vector submitted to environmental conditions prevailing in the gastrointestinal tract. *Int. Dairy J.* 2005, 15:921−7.

[45] Saint-Eve A, Lauverjat C, Magnan C, Deleris I, Souchon I. Reducing salt and fat content: impact of composition, texture and cognitive interactions on the perception of flavoured model cheeses. *Food Chem.* 2009, 116:167–75.

[46] Rudan MA, Barbano DM, Yun JJ, Kindstedt PS. Effect of fat reduction on chemical composition, proteolysis, functionality, and yield of Mozzarella cheese. *J. Dairy Sci.* 1999, 82:661-672.

[47] Gunasekaran S, Ak MM. Cheese rheology and texture. CRC Press, 2003. ISBN: 9781587160219.

[48] Madadlou A, KhosroshahiA, Mousavi ME. Rheology, microstructure, and functionality of low-fat iranian white cheese made with different concentrations of rennet. *J. Dairy Sci.* 2005, 8:3052-3062.

[49] Guinee TP, O'Kennedy BT. Reducing salt in cheese and dairy spreads. p 316–57. In: Kilcast D, Angus F, Eds. Reducing salt in foods. CRC Press, Boca Raton, FL, 2007.

[50] Reddy AK; Elmer MH. Lactic Acid Bacteria in Cheddar Cheese Made with Sodium Chloride, Potassium Chloride or Mixtures of the Two Salts. *J. Food Prot.* 1995, 58:62-69.

[51] Man CMD. Technological functions of salt in food products, p. 157–173. In: Kilcast D and Angus F Eds., Reducing salt in foods. CRC Press LLC, Boca Raton, FL, 2007.

[52] Panouillé M, Saint-Eve A, de Loubens C, Déléris I, Souchon I. Understanding of the influence of composition, structure and texture on salty perception in model dairy products, Food Hydrocolloids 2010, doi: 10.1016/j.foodhyd.2010.08.021.

[53] Bidlasa E, Lambert RJW. Comparing the antimicrobial effectiveness of NaCl and KCl with a view to salt/sodium replacement. *Int .J. Food Microbiol.* 2008, 124:98-102.

[54] Lambert RJW, and Lambert R. A model for the efficacy of combined inhibitors. *J. Applied Microbiol.* 2003, 95:734–743.

[55] Gimeno O., Astiasaran I., Bello J. Influence of partial replacement of NaCl with KCl and CaCl2 on microbiological evolution of dry fermented sausages. *Food Microbiol.* 2001, 18:329-334.

[56] Kilcast D, den Ridder C. 2007. Sensory issues in reducing salt in food products. In: Kilcast D, Angus F, editors. Reducing salt in foods. Boca Raton, Fla.: CRC Press. p 201–20.

In: Cheese: Types, Nutrition and Consumption
Editors: Richard D. Foster, pp. 183-206

ISBN 978-1-61209-828-9
©2011 Nova Science Publishers, Inc.

Chapter 10

NMR Spectroscopy in Dairy Products Characterization

Elvino Brosio and Raffaella Gianferri*
Department of Chemistry (*V. Cagliolti Building*),
University of Rome *La Sapienza*

Abstract

A low- and high-resolution nuclear magnetic resonance spectroscopy based protocol to characterise traditional Italian cheese as *Mozzarella di Bufala Campana* and *Grana Padano* is reported. Low-resolution relaxometry was used for studying the state and distribution of water in different structural elements of cheese resulting from the production process. High-resolution NMR allowed definition of the "chemical fingerprint", the cheese complex matrix profile of low molecular weight metabolites extracted from *Mozzarella* and *Grana Padano*. Both low-resolution and high-resolution NMR seem to provide useful parameters that could be used for monitoring structure and evolution of PDO Italian cheese.

Introduction

Nuclear Magnetic Resonance (NMR) is a spectroscopic technique based on interaction between a magnetic field oscillating at an appropriate frequency and net macroscopic magnetization originating from magnetic moments of nuclei inside a sample (i.e., ^{1}H, ^{13}C, ^{31}P, ^{23}Na, etc.), polarized by an intense static magnetic field, B_0, (typically B_0 = 1-16 Tesla).

Due to low energy difference between energy states allowed for the nuclear magnetic moments, NMR spectroscopy is a low sensitivity technique compared to other forms of spectroscopy. This could limit the utility of NMR as an analytical tool. However, the wealth of detailed information that can be obtained by NMR, largely compensate for low sensitivity

---

* P.le Aldo Moro, 5 – 00185 Roma, Italy. Telephone: #39 06 49913307, fax: #39 06 490324, e-mail: elvino.brosio@uniroma1.it.

of the technique. In particular, the fact that NMR is totally non-invasive and that in some cases does not even need any pre-treatment of the sample, largely extend applicability of NMR methods for analysis of intact systems, especially materials, living systems and foods. The inherent insensitivity of NMR is the reason why ^{1}H is the most used nucleus for the analysis of food systems, even if in some cases less sensitive nuclei like ^{13}C, ^{31}P, ^{17}O and ^{23}Na are used.

Depending on different experimental equipment employed, we distinguish a variety of NMR techniques: *low-resolution NMR*, *high-resolution NMR*, *solid-state high-resolution NMR*, and *NMR imaging*. For field homogeneity, $\Delta B_0/B_0$ of about 10^{-6}, we refer to *low-resolution* NMR. In *high-resolution* NMR experiments, instead, magnetic field must be highly homogeneous, $\Delta B_0/B_0 < 10^{-9}$. Finally, localization or *imaging* techniques constitute a particular case where magnetic field is made inhomogeneous by superimposition of controlled linear field gradients in one or more directions so to encode spatial information of nuclei in resonance frequency or phase of the signals.

Low-resolution NMR is concerned with quantitative determination and characterization of the most abundant components of foods – water, lipids, proteins, and carbohydrates – through the analysis of amplitudes and decay rates of NMR signal. That is why this technique has been extensively used for food analysis, mainly because of the possibility of studying the properties of water – a very abundant probe, whose amount, dynamic state, and interaction with solid matrixes affect many of the properties of food products. Furthermore, it has to be pointed out that, once developed, the standard protocols based on rapid measurements obtained by low-cost NMR instruments can be easily transferred to on-line quality control applications.

High-resolution NMR mono- and multi-dimensional is the area of NMR which chemists are most familiar with and is concerned with the elucidation of the chemical structure of molecules in solution by the analysis of spectrum parameters: chemical shift, δ, coupling constant, J, relaxation times, T_1 and T_2, nuclear Overhauser effect, NOE. High-resolution NMR is widely employed for the elucidation of molecular and supra-molecular structures and for quantitative analysis of different components in mixtures.

Solid-state high-resolution NMR is concerned with elucidation of chemical structure and conformation of solid components (proteins and carbohydrates) in the sample and, differing from high-resolution NMR of liquid samples, does not require any time consuming extraction or dissolving procedure.

Finally, *NMR Imaging* enables the internal morphology of materials to be described and investigated with a one-plane resolution of up to 10 mm and slice thickness of about 1 mm. Its potential lies in the possibility of obtaining resolved signals from different regions within the image and of monitoring dynamic events, such as migration of water, during processing, ripening and storage of foods.

In this paper we reported some illustrative examples of typical Italian cheese characterization by NMR spectroscopy: *Mozzarella di Bufala* and *Grana Padano*, which represent, with a turn over of about 1,400 million euro of year production (year 2008), more than one third of DPO/PGI Italian productions. The aim is to outline how dairy industry would benefit from rapid and non-destructive characterization of moisture content and texture of cheese products. The characterization was carried out by low-resolution NMR, particularly by measuring and analyzing of proton relaxation curves, to characterize fat and water states in soft and hard cheese cheeses. NMR relaxometry was able to provide information on water behaviour (i.e. the quantity and level of interactions with proteins) in the cheese. Further, the analysis was deepened by high-resolution NMR by ^{1}H-NMR spectra interpretation in order to describe metabolic profile of cheese examined.

Finally, in Appendix I and II a brief description of NMR experiment, details of involved NMR pulsed techniques and the magnetic site exchange model used to interpret NMR relaxation data are given.

CHEESE CHARACTERIZATION BY NMR: SOME EXAMPLES

We report some illustrative examples of cheese characterization by NMR methods.

Relaxation measurements represent most widespread application among of the low-resolution NMR methods. In heterogeneous food systems different NMR relaxation times can be measured for the more abundant components, i.e. water and lipids, as well as for presence of different structural elements such as pores or fat globules. Furthermore, water relaxation is affected by a food network structure as a result of water-macromolecules interactions. Therefore, not only translation and rotation of water molecules affect relaxation, but also diffusive and chemical exchange processes between water molecules and biopolymers strongly contribute to T_2 and T_1 values. Varied compositional and structural information can be gained. Furthermore, in some cases, the variation in the value of those parameters can be correlated with the system evolution due to the product aging as derived from product processing as is the case of *Mozzarella di Bufala Campana* cheese, or derived from ripening process of a cheese, as is the case of *Grana Padano*. Some more the T_2 and T_1 values variation can be correlated with the system modification due to temperature processing or water sorption as is the case of products storage.

As already said, generally in foods proton relaxation curves show a multi-exponential behaviour [1, 2] and their measurement and interpretation is not so obvious. The experimental strategies used to optimise the analysis of relaxation curves are represented by Curr Purcell Meiboom Gill (CPMG) measuring parameters and Inversion Recovery (IR) sequences chosen properly in order to correctly sample the experimental curve to be fitted, further a correct fitting procedure should to be selected to avoid any unreliable deconvolution of the exponential functions. The obtained relaxation time values can then be reliably attributed to the different chemical and physical components in the sample.

The main features of water proton NMR relaxation measurements in foods are: i) a multi-exponential of relaxation curves; ii) an enhanced relaxation rate of water with respect to the one measured in pure water; iii) the observation of transverse proton relaxation dispersions as a function of CPMG, pulse spacing. These experimental findings cannot be accounted for the presence of the so-called 'bound' water molecules, more or less immobilized. In fact, should they be present, because structured polysaccharides and proteins influence the state of water around them, the dominant role in determining relaxation time T_1 and T_2 values is played by diffusive and chemical exchange of water molecules and/or water protons. In particular, water protons transverse T_2 values, being not influenced by a cross-relaxation with protein and polysaccharides protons, have been quantitatively interpreted in terms of fast chemical exchange between water and protein or polysaccharides and of diffusive exchange of water molecules within different spatially separated regions of one heterogeneous system.

Unfortunately, in complex multi-compartmental heterogeneous systems, as foods, the effect of chemical and/or diffusive exchange prevent the exact solution of the Bloch equations and even the numerical analytical solutions of the Bloch equations leads to extremely complicated series expansions for the magnetization density [3, 4, 5]

However, for various model situations analytical solutions of the generalized Bloch equations have been derived to quantitatively rationalize the effect of diffusive and chemical exchange of water molecules in foods.

In order to make it easier to understand examples of characterization by the measurement and analysis of proton NMR relaxation curves of cheeses discusses below, a brief outline of the chemical and diffusive exchange model underlying the interpretation of NMR relaxation curves is given in Appendix II.

MOZZARELLA DI BUFALA CAMPANA CHEESE CHARACTERIZATION

As already outlined, one of the most valuable applications of NMR relaxation measurements is to study heterogeneous food systems. In particular, water protons T_1 and T_2 measurements can give information about water dynamics, which proved to be valuable in the understanding of hydration of macromolecules in foods, as well as of the interplay of morphology and dynamics in compartmentalized systems.

As a first example, we report herewith the results obtained from samples of a traditional Italian cheese, one of the most highly valued, the *Mozzarella di Bufala Campana* cheese. It has obtained the protected designation of origin (PDO) trademark, which the European Community assigns to high quality traditional products, hence the interest of setting up methods to determine the authenticity of the product.

Mozzarella di Bufala cheese is a "pasta filata" (fresh and stretched curd) cheese, obtained only from buffalo (*Bubalus bubalus*) milk in Southern Italy. It is an unripened soft cheese, of a milk-white colour, with a fresh and slightly acid taste and a pleasant aroma. The *Mozzarella di Bufala* is high in moisture (55-60%) and in fat (24-25% on a dry matter basis [6]); it is very rich in whey (which is released under pressure) and is normally stored at 4-7°C in packages containing liquid (diluted whey, water from the stretcher-moulder or aqueous solution of sodium chloride). *Mozzarella* must be eaten right away; otherwise the fermentation process spoils the cheese as its shelf-life is < 7 days [7, 8]. Furthermore, *Mozzarella* cheese is a very complex system and its water distribution differs from most other cheeses due to micro-structural differences resulting from the curd stretching process, which creates an elastic network of oriented parallel protein fibres [9]. Changes in microstructure of *Mozzarella* cheese during storage and the short shelf-life, suggest that the proteins are not in a quiescent state immediately after stretching and moulding, but undergo a continuous structural rearrangement [10].

LOW-RESOLUTION NMR MEASUREMENTS OF PDO *MOZZARELLA DI BUFALA CAMPANA* CHEESE

As expected, the *Mozzarella di Bufala Campana* cheese relaxation curves, measured by the CPMG sequence, show a multi-exponential behaviour because of the presence of different components, i.e. water and lipids, as well as of different structural elements in the sample. The transverse magnetization decay curves of *Mozzarella* cheese were analyzed using distributed exponential fitting analysis according to the regularized inverse Laplace transform, based on the CONTIN program developed by Provencher [11, 12] to determine the number of relaxation components, because it does not require any assumption of their number. The continuous analysis provides evidence to the presence of four components, characterised by different T_2 values and amplitudes. The obtained T_2 values, reported as logarithmically distributed transverse relaxation times, are shown in Figure 1.

Assuming the models validated by continuous analysis (to four pure exponential components), the data were also analysed by using a discrete exponential fit to determine the mean T_2 relaxation times of the different water populations. The discrete fits to the imposed number of the pure exponential components were evaluated by direct comparison between estimated and experimental points and statistical analysis of regression results. The T_2 time constants from discrete exponential fitting correspond with the peaks maxima resulting from continuous analysis for each sample (Figure 1). In Table 1 the different components T_2 values and their relative percentages are reported.

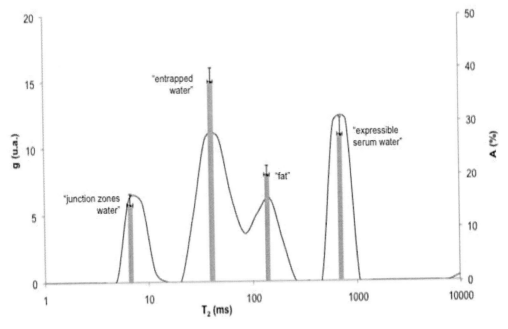

Figure 1. Distributed transverse relaxation times (normalised amplitudes vs. logarithmically distributed relaxation times) and T_2 values from discrete exponential fitting (relative components amplitudes vs. relaxation time values) for *Mozzarella di Bufala Campnana* cheese (Fratelli Francia cheese-maker).

Table 1. Proton transverse relaxation times and signal percentages at day 1 after manufacturing (fresh Mozzarella) of the four components in the relaxation curve of Mozzarella di Bufala Campana (Fratelli Francia cheese-maker).

component	T_2 (ms)	%
serum water	951 ± 40	28 ± 6
fat	160 ± 15	20 ± 3
entrapped water	47 ± 3	37 ± 1
junctions zones-bound water	7.3 ± 0.3	15 ± 4

Data are the averages of four samples from a single *Mozzarella di Bufala Campana* cheese loaf and sampling three loaves, errors represent the standard deviations of the twelve values.

According to reported relaxation data for heterogeneous systems [13, 14, 15, 16, 17, 2, 18] and on the account of the generally reported composition of *Mozzarella* cheese (water 54-60%, lipids 20-25%, proteins 16-20%, sugars 0.4-2% [6]), the following assignments to the four components were made. The slow relaxation component, $T_2 = 951 \pm 40$ ms, was ascribed to water molecules remote from the casein network whose motion is unaffected by the presence of the protein. This is the water accumulated in the large open channels formed by protein fibres ('serum water'), with essentially the same properties as water in a solution, *i.e.* characterised by an isotropic motion. The fast relaxation component, $T_2 = 7.3 \pm 0.3$ ms, was attributed to water molecules trapped within casein junction zones ('junction zone water'). This water can be seen as an integral part of the protein structure, trapped within the casein matrix in an interstitial form. Its transverse relaxation time is essentially dominated by a fast chemical exchange with protein exchangeable protons, which have a shorter T_2 than water. Of the remaining two components one was assigned to protons of the lipid phase of *Mozzarella* cheese ($T_2 = 160 \pm 15$ ms), on the basis of the lipid content in the water plus the fat phase of *Mozzarella* samples. The last component in the relaxation curve, whose relaxation T_2 value is of the order of few tens milliseconds ($T_2 = 47 \pm 3$ ms) can be ascribed to water molecules inside the meshes of the gel network made by casein molecules ('entrapped water'). This water can interact with the protein structure by diffusion from the bulk to the biopolymer interface, and its T_2 value is controlled by a diffusive exchange.

For assignment of the different components in the relaxation curve of *Mozzarella* cheese samples, the difference in T_2 values for the different types of water molecules can be accounted for only by considering the effect of the chemical and diffusive exchange between water and the protein network. A systematic approach to proton NMR relaxation, based on the understanding of the effects of the diffusive and chemical exchange (described in the Appendix II), can provide valuable information about water dynamic state and morphology of *Mozzarella* cheese sample, thus allowing for a thorough insight into the cheese physical structure and for NMR dynamic parameters to be related to the evolution of samples.

Now, even though the slow diffusive exchange regime explains the multi-exponential relaxation in the *Mozzarella* cheese casein network compartment, in itself it doesn't explain why the relaxation rates of the entrapped water and junction zone water are faster than those in bulk water. As far as the measured entrapped water relaxation is concerned, it is essentially controlled by a diffusive exchange from the bulk to the biopolymer interface, which acts as a relaxation surface sink, and surface relaxation will become significant. If relaxation on the surface is faster compared with diffusion to the surface – 'diffusion limited relaxation' regime

– the observed water transverse relaxation rate is independent of the effective surface relaxation strength and given, for spherical geometry, by the equation [19]

$$\frac{1}{T_{2,obs}} = \frac{1}{T_{2,w}} + \frac{\pi^2 \cdot D}{2a^2} \qquad (1)$$

where $T_{2,obs}$ and $T_{2,w}$ are the intrinsic relaxation times of water molecules inside meshes of casein network ('entrapped water') and water protons, respectively, a is the characteristic dimension of a spatial heterogeneity, and D is the water self-diffusion coefficient. $T_{2,w}$ value (2.50 ± 0.01 s) was measured by an independent CPMG experiment on conservation liquid of *Mozzarella di Bufala Campana* (Fratelli Francia cheese-maker). Assuming that water diffusion is in the order of that for bulk water, the equation (1) gives a maximum diffusive distance [19] a = 26 μm.

Now, let us consider T_2 value of water molecules in junction zones of casein network, which is dominated by the fast chemical exchange of water protons with exchangeable protons of casein molecules, according to the equation [20]

$$\frac{1}{T_{2,obs}} = \frac{1}{T_{2,w}} + \frac{P_{exch}}{T_{2,exch} + k_{exch}^{-1}} \qquad (2)$$

where, now, $T_{2,obs}$ is the intrinsic relaxation times of water molecules water molecules trapped within casein junction zones ('junction zones water'). P_{exch} is given by the number of exchangeable protons in casein and can be estimated as about 0,02 [21], $T_{2,exch}$ is in the order of few tens of microseconds and it can be neglected compared to k_{exch}^{-1} [17], then from the measured T_2 = 7.3 ± 0.3 ms, a value of $k_{exch} \approx 10^4$ s^{-1} can be derived. Clearly, this is only a rough estimation by assuming casein as the unique protein in the sample.

In order to get information on *Mozzarella* aging process, T_2 values of serum water, entrapped water, junction zone water and fat droplets as a function of aging time (from day 1 to 14) of *Mozzarella di Bufala Campana* (Fratelli Francia cheese-maker) were measured. The obtained results are shown in Figure 2. Inspection of the data of relaxation measurements in aged *Mozzarella di Bufala Campana* cheese shows a nearly constant value for T_2 transverse relaxation time of entrapped water and junction zone water, indicating that water in a like-gel casein structure, as far as it concerns its microscopic interactions, experiences no substantial differences, at least in the sampled time (days 1 – 14).

On the contrary, serum water T_2 values show a notable and gradual lowering from day 1 to day 7, until a constant limiting value is obtained.

In conclusion, even if it has to be emphasized that the relationship among various physical-chemical characteristics and shelf-life (meant as the time before that cheese is considered unsuitable for consumption) of *Mozzarella* is not obvious, we think it is very relevant to have identified a reliable physical-chemical parameter – the serum water T_2 – whose value is useful to monitor the evolution of *Mozzarella* samples.

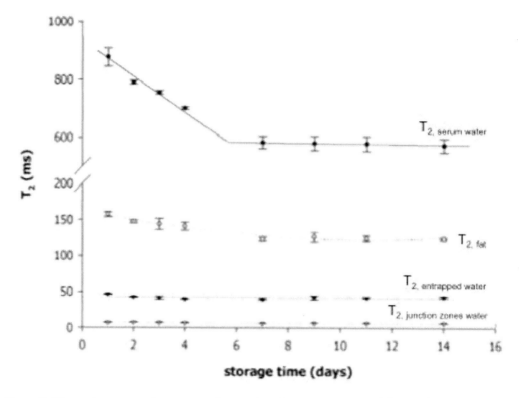

Figure 2. Change in serum water, entrapped water, junction zones water, and fat T_2 values of *Mozzarella di Bufala Campana* (Fratelli Francia cheese-maker) during storage time at 8°C. Lines are guide to eyes only.

HIGH-RESOLUTION NMR MEASUREMENTS OF PDO *MOZZARELLA DI BUFALA CAMPANA* CHEESE

Analysis of the NMR spectrum was carried out to define the profile of water-soluble metabolites in *Mozzarella di Bufala Campana*, such as major organic acids and carbohydrates, minor amino acids, aromatic compounds, and other components. A deep knowledge of *Mozzarella* composition assists in providing a solid and informed control of PDO foods. The 400 MHz proton spectrum of one aqueous extract from *Mozzarella di Bufala Campana* cheese sample (at day 1 after manufacture) is shown in Figure 3. As expected, the NMR spectrum reveals the predominance of lactate resonance signals. Lactate is the most abundant component because it is the main product of fermentation of lactose during cheese making.

In addition, several tens of signals from many metabolites are readily and easily detectable in the spectrum. To perform a full spectral assignment to specific compounds, expanded regions of the mono-dimensional NMR spectrum, and bi-dimensional COSY (Correlated Spectroscopy) and TOCSY (Total Correlated Spectroscopy) experiments were performed and analysed. The combined connectivity information gathered from COSY and TOCSY experiments, taking advantage of the spread of complex resonances into the extra dimensions, and the use, as guidelines, of chemical shift data from the literature [22, 23, 24, 25] allowed an almost complete and unambiguous assignment of the resonance signals.

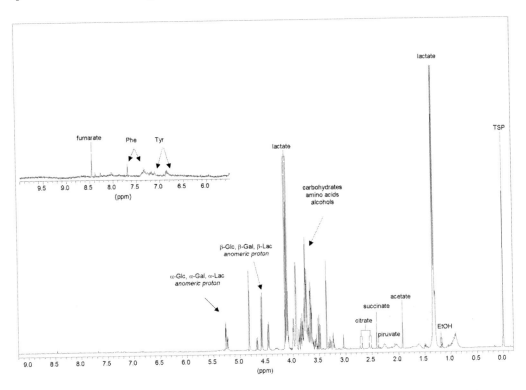

Figure 3. 400 MHz ^{1}H-NMR spectrum of an aqueous extract of *Mozzarella di Bufala Campana* cheese (Fratelli Francia cheese-maker), in phosphate/D$_2$O buffer with 3-(trimethylsilyl)-tetradeuterium sodium propionate (TSP). Vertical expansion is shown for the downfield aromatic spectrum region (from 9.0 to 6.0 ppm). Some assignments are indicated.

The high-field region (0.0 – 3.0 ppm) of the NMR spectrum shows the resonance signals arising from aliphatic groups of amino acids, organic acids belonging to the lactose and galactose glycolytic pathways and Krebs (or citric acid) cycle, as well as from alcohols. In particular, the signals arising from leucine (Leu), isoleucine (Ile), valine (Val), threonine (Thr), alanine (Ala), glutamate (Glu), lactate, acetate, pyruvate, succinate, citrate, ethanol (EtOH), and iso-butanol were clearly identified. The resonance signal at 1.30 ppm, assigned to the Ile methylene group, partially overlaps the doublet of the lactate methyl group. It was assigned according to 2D spectra correlations of this peak with the multiplets at 2.04 ppm (COSY and TOCSY) and 3.69 ppm (TOCSY).

The overlapping signals at 0.8 – 1.2 ppm arise from methyl or methylene groups of Leu, Ile, Val and Thr, and alcohols (ethanol and *iso*-buthanol) derived from the fermentation processes. These assignments were made according to COSY and TOCSY correlations and data from the literature [22, 24]. The same can be said for overlapping resonances and unresolved multiples between 1.4 and 2.2 ppm due to several amino acids.

The singlets at 2.05, 2.38 and 2.41 ppm arise from methyl groups of acetate, pyruvate and succinate, respectively, whereas the typical doublet of doublets at 2.62 ppm arises from the methyl group of citrate [22, 23]. In *Mozzarella di Bufala Campana* cheese, citrate and acetate are involved in the Krebs cycle where they act both as a substrate and a product. Pyruvate is readily formed through the glycolytic pathway, but it also acts as a substrate of several metabolic reactions such the formation of formate and ethanol [26].

In the mid-field region (3.0 – 5.5 ppm) of the proton spectrum, the main contributions arise from the three principal carbohydrates of *Mozzarella* cheese (lactose, glucose and galactose) and overlapped contributions from amino acids and derivates, organic acids (principally lactate), ethanol, methanol and glycerol. Again, the 2D NMR spectrum allows the unequivocal assignment of the resonances of the metabolites present in those spectral regions characterized by strong overlapping of signals (in particular, the region between 3.3 and 4.6 ppm is rich in overlapping signals due to glycosidic moieties and CH-α of amino acids). The α- and β-lactose, α- and β-galactose and α- and β-glucose peaks, as well as the signals from glycerol, were clearly identified by COSY and TOCSY correlations.

The signals in the low-field region (5.5 – 10.0 ppm) are the weakest in the spectrum and arise from the aromatic groups of amino acids and phenolic compounds. Formate, tyrosine (Tyr) and phenylalanine (Phe) can be readily identified, whereas some difficulties arise in the assignment of the remaining spin systems which seem to originate from olefin or ring protons [27]. The broad lines between 6.6 and 7.2 ppm remained unassigned. Although it is rational to hypothesize the presence of polyphenolic compounds [28], the TOCSY experiment showed no correlation with these spectral lines.

GRANA PADANO CHEESE CHARACTERIZATION

Grana Padano is one of the most popular PDO cheeses of Italy and is one of hard cheeses most consumed in the world. *Grana Padano* cheese contains about 32% water, 33% proteins and 28% fat, which correspond to 42% by weight of dry product [29]. Its protein content has a high biological value and the amino acids profile is unique. The distinctively grainy texture of the cheese is due to a specific processing technique, a long ripening, and the quality of milk. *Grana Padano* is a semi-fat hard cheese which is cooked and ripened slowly (for at least 9 months, then, if it passes the quality tests, it will be fire-branded with the *Grana Padano* trademark). The final and critical step in the production of *Grana Padano* cheese is the natural ripening which requires the cheese to be stored at a fixed temperature and humidity (15-22°C and 85-88%, respectively). The ripening time can be from 9 to over 24 months; generally is at least 12-14 months. The ripening process implies many modifications of high complexity, which take place simultaneously or successively, for that cheese components undergo physico-chemical and enzymatic modifications. The biochemical transformation gives to *Grana Padano* new characteristics: the paste of cheese is modified in its composition and structure and, consequently, in its appearance, consistency and colour. The ripening process is affected by various factors: the state of water, the structure of casein micelles and fat. In particular, water plays an essential role in determining structure of proteins and lipid aggregates, influencing the texture and stability of final product. This is why it is important to investigate water dynamic properties and water interactions with other components in the system [30].

LOW-RESOLUTION NMR MEASUREMENTS OF PDO *GRANA PADANO* CHEESE

As expected, also the *Grana Padano* cheese relaxation curves, measured by the CPMG sequence, show a multi-exponential behaviour due to presence of different components (water and lipids) and structural elements in the sample. The transverse magnetization decay curves of *Grana Padano* cheese at different ripening times were analyzed using distributed exponential fitting analysis according to the regularized inverse Laplace transform and provided evidence to the presence of four components, characterised by different T_2 values and amplitudes.

As an example, the obtained T_2 distribution of 12 months ripening *Grana Padano* cheese samples, reported as logarithmically distributed transverse relaxation times, are shown in Figure 4.

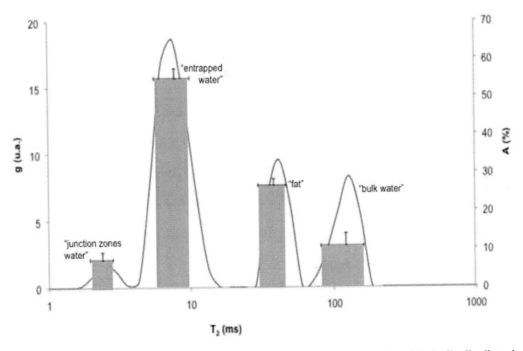

Figure 4. Distributed transverse relaxation times (normalised amplitudes vs. logarithmically distributed relaxation times) and T_2 values from discrete exponential fitting (relative components amplitudes vs. relaxation time values) for *Grana Padano* cheese (winter season 1998-99) aged 12 months.

The T_2 time constants from discrete exponential fitting, to the imposed number of the pure exponential components as validated by continuous analysis (to four pure exponential components for *Grana Padano* cheese at all different ripening states), and their relative percentages at three ripening stages are reported in Table 2.

The assignment of the relaxation components, characterized by different intrinsic T_2 relaxation times, to several sub-populations of water and fat within *Grana Padano* samples were made as described previously for *Mozzarella* cheese and on the account of the generally reported composition of *Grana Padano* cheese (water 32%, lipids 28%, proteins 33% [29]).

Table 2 – Proton transverse relaxation times and signal percentages at different ripening stages (6, 12 and 18 months) of the four components in the relaxation curve of *Grana Padano* (winter season 1998-99).

ripening time (months)	"bulk" water T$_2$ (ms)	%	fat T$_2$ (ms)	%	entrapped water T$_2$ (ms)	%	junctions zones water T$_2$ (ms)	%
6	110 ± 1	8.6 ± 0.1	35.8 ± 0.4	22.5 ± 0.1	8.6 ± 0.1	62.4 ± 0.4	2.5 ± 0.1	6.5 ± 0.2
12	124 ± 1	10.9 ± 0.1	39.1 ± 0.4	26.8 ± 0.4	8.1 ± 0.1	55.0 ± 0.3	2.5 ± 0.1	7.3 ± 0.3
18	104 ± 1	11.0 ± 0.4	33.3 ± 0.3	26 ± 1	7.3 ± 0.1	54 ± 2	2.6 ± 0.1	9.0 ± 0.1

Data are the averages of 30 samples of different points from a single *Grana Padano* cheese loaf; errors represent the standard deviations of the 30 values.

Hence, with reference to the data, reported in Table 2, for 12 months ripening *Grana Padano* cheese samples the following assignments to the four components were made. The slow relaxation component, $T_2 = 124 \pm 1$ ms, was ascribed to water molecules remote from the casein network whose motion is slightly affected by the presence of the protein; this is the water accumulated in the finely grained pores formed by protein fibres ('bulk water'). The fast relaxation component, $T_2 = 2.5 \pm 0.1$ ms, was attributed to water molecules trapped within casein junction zones ('junction zone water'); this water can be seen as an integral part of the protein structure, trapped within the casein matrix in an interstitial form. Its transverse relaxation time is essentially dominated by a fast chemical exchange with protein exchangeable protons, which have a shorter T_2 than water. The component in the relaxation curve, whose relaxation T_2 value is of the order of tens milliseconds ($T_2 = 8.1 \pm 0.1$ ms) can be ascribed to water molecules inside the meshes of the gel network made by casein molecules, i.e. the water inside the micelles themselves ('entrapped water'). This water can interact with the protein structure by diffusion from the bulk to the biopolymer interface, and its T_2 value is controlled by a diffusive exchange. Finally, the last transverse relaxation component, $T_2 = 39.1 \pm 0.4$ ms, was assigned to protons of the lipid phase of *Grana Padano* cheese, on the basis of the lipid content in the water plus the fat phase of *Grana Padano* samples.

As seen for *Mozzarella* cheese, the *Grana Padano* relaxation data interpretation based on the effects of the diffusive and chemical exchange (described in the Appendix II) between water and the protein network can provide valuable information about water dynamic state and morphology of *Grana Padano* cheese sample, thus allowing for a thorough insight into the cheese physical structure and for NMR dynamic parameters to be related to the evolution of samples.

As far as the measured entrapped water relaxation is concerned, it is essentially controlled by a diffusive exchange from the bulk to the biopolymer interface, which acts as a relaxation surface sink. If relaxation on the surface is faster compared with diffusion to the surface – 'diffusion limited relaxation' regime – the observed water transverse relaxation rate is independent of the effective surface relaxation strength and for spherical geometry given by the equation (1) [19]. Assuming that water diffusion is in the order of that for bulk water, the characteristic dimension of a spatial heterogeneity of meshes of the casein gel network (maximum diffusive distance for entrapped water obtained by equation (1)) is ca. 5 µm, as expected for *Grana Padano* cheese that is characterized by a finely grained texture, cheese more crumbly of *Mozzarella*.

The T_2 value of water molecules in junction zones of casein network is dominated by the fast chemical exchange of water protons with exchangeable protons of casein molecules, according to the equation (2) [20]. Assuming that P_{exch} about 0,02 [21], then from the measured $T_2 = 2.5 \pm 0.1$ ms, a rough estimation of k_{exch} value of about $2 \; 10^4 \; s^{-1}$ can be derived.

In order to get information on *Grana Padano* ripening process, T_2 values of bulk water, entrapped water, junction zone water and fat droplets of *Grana Padano* samples at three different ripening stage (6, 12 and 18 months) were measured. The obtained results are reported in Table 2 and shown in Figure 5.

Now, the *Grana Padano* ripening correlates directly to the cheese's taste and texture. In fact, variance in maturity leads to dramatic differences in the texture (and flavour) of the cheese: during the ripening processes its paste is modified in composition and structure and, consequently, in appearance, consistency and colour. The younger wheels will have a sweeter flavour with a noticeable tang, the older ones have a deeper straw-yellow colour, many more protein crystals, a more complex nutty flavour, and a much longer finish. In particular, during the ripening process the total amount of water decreases. This is due to a migration–evaporation process, much stronger at the periphery of the wheel, and water distribution is influenced by various parameters (evaporation, diffusion, proteolysis) [31].

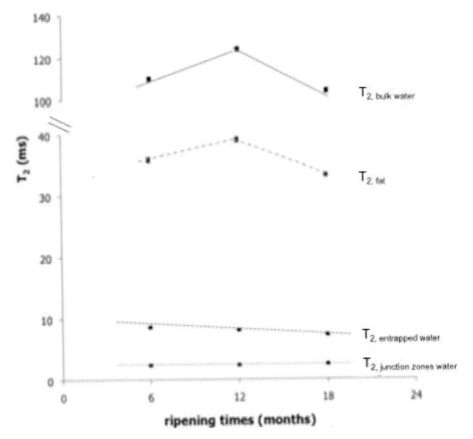

Figure 5. Change in "bulk" water, entrapped water, junction zones water, and fat T_2 values of *Grana Padano* (winter season 1998-99) during ripening time at 8°C. Lines are guide to eyes only.

Inspection of the data of relaxation measurements in *Grana Padano* cheese as function to ripening storage (Fig. 5) shows a similar behaviour of T_2 transverse relaxation times of bulk water and fat, while entrapped water T_2 values show a gradual lowering from month 6 to month 18, indicating that water and fat molecules in cheese system, as far as it concerns their microscopic interactions, experiences differences in the sampled ripening times. On the contrary, T_2 transverse relaxation time of junction zone water shows a nearly constant value, then water molecules trapped within junction zones of the like-gel casein structure – as an integral part of the protein structure –, experiences no substantial differences, at least in the sampled stage.

As concerning transverse relaxation signal percentages during the *Grana* Padano cheese ripening process, Table 2 data show a increasing of the junction zones water amounts and a decreasing of that entrapped water, indicating that casein micelles shrinkage and lets out water molecules (entrapped water) that, in turn, becomes "interstitial" water (junction zones water).

In conclusion, low-resolution NMR measurements and diffusive and chemical exchange approach have been providing information about water distribution in *Grana Padano* cheese system and ripening processes. Even if it has to be emphasized that the ripening processes implies many modifications of high complexity, the present approach provide a way to verify the effect of the ripening process on foodstuffs.

HIGH-RESOLUTION NMR MEASUREMENTS OF PDO *GRANA PADANO* CHEESE

High-resolution NMR experiments have allowed to define the profile of water-soluble metabolites in *Grana Padano* cheese, such as amino acids, major organic acids and carbohydrates, aromatic compounds, and other components. All amino acids present in the spectrum were quantitatively and qualitatively evaluated.

The 500 MHz proton spectrum of one aqueous extract from *Grana Padano* cheese sample (at 12 months of ripening) is shown in Figure 6. The assignments were performed on the basis of chemical shift, comparison with model compounds and pH variation and the use, as guidelines, as well chemical shift data from the literature [22, 23, 24]. ^{1}H NMR spectra are very complex and a strong overlap of the resonance occurs. The unequivocal assignment was obtained by 2D NMR COSY experiments where scalar interactions between adjacent groups of the same molecules are revealed.

The NMR spectrum reveals, as seen in the *Mozzarella di Bufala* cheese spectrum, the intense lactate resonance signals, with a quartet at 4.05 ppm (α-CH) and a doublet at 1.30 ppm (-CH$_3$).

The high-field region (0.0 – 3.0 ppm) of the NMR spectrum shows the resonance signals arising from aliphatic groups of amino acids, organic acids belonging to the lactose and galactose glycolytic pathways and Krebs (or citric acid) cycle, as well as from alcohols. The overlapping signals at 0.8 – 1.2 ppm arise from methyl or methylene groups of Leu, Ile, Val and Thr, and other amino acids. These assignments were made according to COSY and TOCSY correlations and data from the literature [22, 24]. The same can be said for overlapping resonances and unresolved multiples between 1.4 and 2.2 ppm due to several amino acids.

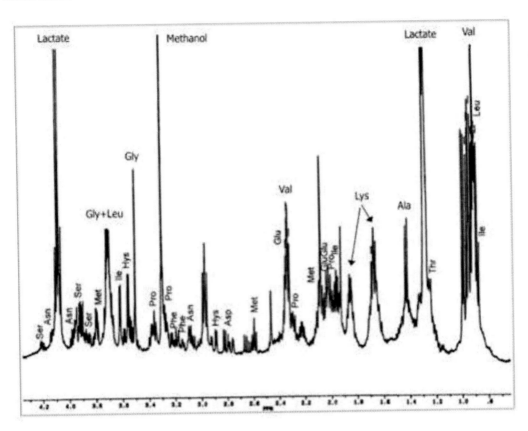

Figure 6. 500 MHz ^{1}H-NMR spectrum of an aqueous extract of *Grana Padano* cheese (winter season 1998-99), at 12 months of ripening, in D$_2$O with 3-(trimethylsilyl)-tetradeuterium sodium propionate (TSP). Some free amino acids assignments are indicated.

In particular, the signals arising from several amino acids: Leu (doublets at 0.98 and 0.96 ppm of δ- and δ'-CH$_3$, respectively, and multiplets at 1.90 and 1.70 ppm of β-CH$_2$), Ile (doublet at 1.0-0.9 ppm of -CH$_3$ and multiplet at 1.95 ppm of β-CH), Val (doublets at 1.0-0.9 ppm of γ- and γ'-CH$_3$), Thr (multiplet at 2.37 ppm of β-CH), Ala (doublet at 1.4 ppm), Glu (triplets at 2.05 ppm of β- and β'-CH), Aspartate (Asp with double-doublet at 2.75 ppm of α-CH), Histidine (His with multiplet at 1.70 ppm of γ-CH), Lysine (Lys with multiplets at 1.70 and 1.50 ppm of δ-CH$_2$ and γ-CH$_2$, respectively), Methionine (Met with singlet at 2.15 of – CH$_3$ and triplet at 2.60 of γ-CH$_2$), Proline (Pro with multiplets at 2.20 and 2.05 of β-CH and γ-CH$_2$, respectively), Serine (Ser with the doublet at 1.30 ppm of -CH$_3$).

In the mid-field region (3.0 – 5.5 ppm) of the proton spectrum, the main contributions arise from the three principal carbohydrates of *Grana Padano* cheese (lactose, glucose and galactose) and overlapped contributions from amino acids and derivates, organic acids (principally lactate), ethanol, methanol and glycerol. Again, the unequivocal assignment of the resonances of the metabolites present in those spectral regions characterized by strong overlapping of signals has been allowed by 2D NMR spectrum. The amino acids resonance signals present in this region were: Asp (double-doublets at 4.20 and 3.02 ppm of α-CH and β,β'-CH, respectively), Phenylalanine (Phe with double-doublets at 3.25 and 3.15 ppm of β- and β'-CH, respectively), Glycine (Gly wit singlet at 3.50 ppm of α-CH), Gln (triplet at 3.70 ppm of α-CH), Ile (multiplet at 3.62 ppm of α-CH), His (double-doublets at 3.60 and 3.00 ppm of α-CH and β-CH, respectively, and triplet at 3.70 ppm of α-CH), Lys (triplet at 3.80 ppm of α-CH), Met (triplet at 3.38 ppm of δ-CH), Pro (triplet at 3.25 ppm of δ'-CH and double-doublet at 4.25 ppm of α-CH), Ser (double-doublet at 3.90-3.95 ppm of β-CH) and Thr (doublet at 3.50 ppm of α-CH and multiplet at 4.25 ppm of β-CH).

A quantitative analysis of the ^{1}H-NMR spectra of *Grana Padano* cheese aqueous extract at different ripening stages was performed from signal areas. The free amino acid content can be expressed as a percentage of the total proteins, which is an index of the solubilisation of caseins and of the digestibility of the cheese product [32, 33]. The free amino acid contents (as percentage of total amino acids) in a cheese sample (at sample point E14: 8 centimetre from the base and 14 centimetre from the rind side of the wheel, respectively) at different ripening stages (6, 12 and 18 months) are reported in Table 3.

Now, the chemical modifications during *Grana Padano* ripening are, principally, due to proteolysis and lipolysis. Then, free amino acid contents change are associated to ripening process; in particular, β-casein is the primary source of free amino acid production in *Grana Padano* cheese [33, 31]. Then, during the ripening processes its chemical composition is modified and, consequently, significant variations in the free amino acids levels due to ripening are found as a function both aging time and distance from the centre of wheel.

Table 3. Free amino acid contents as a percentage of total amino acids in Grana Padano cheese (winter season 1998-99) at different ripening stages (6, 12 and 18 months), at the same sampled point of the wheel*, determined by quantitative analysis of 500 MHz 1H-NMR spectra.

ripening time (months):	6	12	18
free amino acid	percentage of total amino acids (%)		
Ala	3.5 ± 0.2	4.1 ± 0.3	4.2 ± 0.2
Asn	4.2 ± 0.2	3.9 ± 0.2	4.1 ± 0.3
Asp	3.2 ± 0.2	3.4 ± 0.3	3.8 ± 0.2
Glu	16.9 ± 0.6	16.8 ± 0.7	15.3 ± 0.9
Gly	3.3 ± 0.1	2.6 ± 0.2	3.1 ± 0.1
His	3.3 ± 0.1	3.8 ± 0.2	3.6 ± 0.3
Ile	4.8 ± 0.2	4.2 ± 0.2	4.7 ± 0.4
Leu	9.8 ± 0.5	7.5 ± 0.5	9.2 ± 0.8
Lys	13.6 ± 0.7	13.4 ± 0.8	13.6 ± 0.8
Met	2.9 ± 0.1	3.4 ± 0.3	3.5 ± 0.1
Phe	4.9 ± 0.2	5.5 ± 0.3	5.6 ± 0.2
Pro	8.7 ± 0.4	8.2 ± 0.2	8.4 ± 0.3
Ser	4.9 ± 0.3	5.9 ± 0.3	5.7 ± 0.4
Thr	4.2 ± 0.3	3.6 ± 0.3	4.1 ± 0.3
Tyr	2.6 ± 0.1	2.8 ± 0.1	2.8 ± 0.2
Val	8.9 ± 0.3	8.1 ± 0.6	8.5 ± 0.5

*E14: sample point at 8 cm from the base and 14 cm from the rind side of the wheel, respectively.

The quantitative ^{1}H-NMR spectra analysis of *Grana Padano* cheese as function to ripening storage (Table 3) shows variations in the levels of the free amino acids, indicating that the proteolytic process is substantial in the first months, while the data at 18 months are the same as at 12 months. This confirms the results obtained with different techniques [30, 34]. In particular, inspection of the data shows a free Ala, Met, Phe and Ser content gradual increasing from month 6 to month 18, until a constant limiting value is obtained. On the contrary, a free Glu, Leu and Val content show a lowering from month 6 to month 18. These trends are related to proteolysis and metabolic processes associated to the natural *Grana Padano* ripening and indicate the role played by the enzyme system present in the samples.

The free amino acids are the most important free metabolites of the proteolytic activity. Then, their qualitatively and quantitively determination allows to evaluate all the enzymatic activities, which occur in the course of ripening. So, it is important to utilize a technique capable of detecting amino acid levels that avoids the many steps of analysis. NMR is a non-destructive, multinuclear, multiparametric and often non-invasive technique, successfully employed in plant and mammalian biochemistry [22]. The advantages of this technique are the possibility of detecting all the substances in the sample at the same time, avoiding treatment repetitions and avoiding artefacts due to demolition of macromolecular structures.

EXPERIMENTAL

Materials

Mozzarella di Bufala Campana cheese, freshly prepared (day 1), were produced by artisan Fratelli Francia cheese-maker certified by 'PDO *Mozzarella di Bufala Campana*' consortium (Latina – Italy). Each cheese loaf of about 250 g was individually packaged in its conservation liquid and stored in a cold chamber at 8°C (± 2°C) until tested. The cheese-maker declared shelf-live was of 14 days.

To explore the water relaxation behaviour associated with the age-related changes, measurements began when *Mozzarella* cheese samples were at day 1 after manufacturing (fresh *Mozzarella*) and lasted for the following 14 days.

Grana Padano round cheeses, produced during the winter season (1998-1999) and certified by 'PDO *Grana Padano*', were kindly gifted from Prof. Bruno Battistotti, University Cattolica del Sacro Cuore, Piacenza (Italy) at different stages of ripening (6, 12 and 18 months). Sampling method of *Grana Padano* was described in other paper [31].

LOW-RESOLUTION NMR EXPERIMENTS

For low-resolution NMR measurements on *Mozzarella di Bufala Campana* four samples were prepared by cutting cylindrical-shaped pieces (diameter 8 mm and height 10 mm) out of the central part of the loaf cheese, at a distance of ca. 3 cm from the surface; each measurements set were carried out sampling three different loaves.

For low-resolution NMR measurements on *Grana Padano* thirty samples were prepared by cylindrical form (diameter 8 mm and height 10 mm) extrudes in different points from a single *Grana Padano* cheese loaf.

The different aliquots, of *Mozzarella* or *Grana Padano* cheeses were weighed (approximately 350-400 mg), and then transferred into a NMR tube (outside diameter 10 mm). To prevent water evaporation, a Teflon plug was inserted and the tube was then sealed by a laboratory film.

Measurements on *Mozzarella di Bufala Campana* and *Grana Padano* samples were performed with a Minispec mq 20 pulsed NMR spectrometer (Bruker Spectrospin Company, Milano, Italy) and Minispec PC120 pulsed NMR spectrometer (Bruker Spectrospin Company), respectively, both with an operating frequency of 20 MHz for protons (magnetic field strength: 0.47 T). The NMR spectrometers were equipped with an external thermostat (Julabo F25, Julabo Labortechnik GmbH, Seelbach, Germany) to maintain the desired temperature conditions. Before, the NMR measurements, the tube was kept in the NMR probe as long as needed for thermal equilibration (ca. 15 min).

The measurements on *Mozzarella* cheese were taken at the storage temperature, i.e. 8°C (± 0.8°C), while the measurements on *Grana Padano* cheese were taken at the temperature of 18°C (± 1°C).

The transverse relaxation curves were measured by the CPMG sequence [35] with pulse spacing (τ_{cp}) between two following pulses of 0.04 and 0.45 ms for *Mozzarella* and *Grana Padano* cheese, respectively. The first 200 data points of relaxation curve of *Mozzarella* samples were acquired after each echo signal (to detect the shortest T_2 value), then 6000 data points were acquired after each 10th echo (to detect the longer T_2 values) as an average of 16 repetitions, and with a recycle delay (RD) of 10 s. On the other hand, 6000 data points were acquired after each 10th echo as an average of 16 repetitions, and with a RD of 10 s to measure the relaxation time of Mozzarella conservation liquid samples. Finally, the first 169 data points of relaxation curve of *Grana Padano* samples were acquired after each echo signal (to detect the shortest T_2 value), then ca. 160 data points were acquired after each 10th echo (to detect the longer T_2 values) as an average of 144 repetitions, and with a RD of 1 s.

HIGH-RESOLUTION NMR EXPERIMENTS

For high-resolution NMR measurements of both *Mozzarella* and *Granan Padano* cheese, one slice of about 250 mg was weighed and stored at −20°C prior to extraction procedures by previously described Bligh Dyer method [13, 31].

Phosphate buffer (0.7 mL, ionic strength 600 mM, pH 6.5, in D2O — Merck, Darmstadt, Germany), containing 3-(trimethylsilyl)-tetradeuterium sodium propionate, TSP (0.1mM — Wilmand Lab Glass, Buena, NJ, USA), was added to the precisely weighed samples of water soluble compounds of *Mozzarella* cheese (approximately 25mg) and then placed in an NMR tube (outside diameter 5 mm).

Deuterium oxide (0.4 mL, 99.996%$_D$ — Merck) was added to the precisely weighed samples of water-soluble compounds of *Grana Padano* cheese (approximately 25mg) and then placed in an NMR tube (outside diameter 5 mm).

High-resolution experiments on *Mozzarella di Bufala Campana* samples were performed using a pulse Fourier transform NMR spectrometer AvanceTM 400 (Bruker Spectrospin Company) with an operating frequency of 400.130 MHz for protons (magnetic field strength: ca. 9.40 T) and equipped with a two-channel probe ^{1}H/^{13}C and field gradients.

High-resolution experiments on *Grana Padano* samples were performed using pulse Fourier transform NMR spectrometer AM 500 (Bruker Spectrospin Company) with an operating frequency of 500.137 MHz for protons (magnetic field strength: ca. 11.74 T) and equipped with a two-channel probe ^{1}H/^{13}C.

All ^{1}H-NMR spectra were recorded at the usual working temperature of the instrument, i.e. 25°C. Data were accumulated for 256 scans with a recycle time of 6 s; 32K data points were acquired with spectral widths of 6009 Hz. Water suppression was obtained by water resonance irradiation with a weak radio frequency field; the decoupler was switched off before the radio frequency excitation pulse and acquisition.

Two-dimensional shift ^{1}H–^{1}H correlated spectroscopy (COSY) spectra were acquired using 64 increments into 1024 data points using a spectral width of 5580Hz. Two dimensional ^{1}H–^{1}H total correlation spectroscopy (TOCSY) spectra were acquired in phase sensitive mode using time proportional phase incrementation (TPPI); 64 transients were collected for each of the 40 increments into 512 data points per increment over a spectral width of 6009 Hz in both dimensions, using a mixing time of 120 ms. The spin-locking was achieved using the MLEV-17 sequence. A relaxation delay of 2 s was included and pre-saturation of the water resonance was achieved using solvent pre-saturation (by a pre-saturation pulse sequence present in the instrumental routine) [36]. Experimental data were transferred to a PC and transformed and processed by WIN NMR (mono-dimensional experiments) and TopSpin (2 D experiments) data processing software (both from Bruker Spectrospin Company).

CONCLUSION

The described results, even if preliminary, indicate the potential of NMR to characterise different typical cheese. The NMR protocol based on both low-resolution NMR relaxometry and high-resolution NMR spectra seems to be a useful approach to characterise Mozzarella di Bufala Campana and Grana Padano cheeses.

By the analysis of magnetization decay curves, based on the diffusive and chemical exchange model, detailed information can be obtained about different components in the samples, water and fat, as well as their dynamic state. This allows for some insight in the physical structure of cheese by NMR dynamic parameters. Thence, the application of NMR relaxation data for quality control.

Furthermore, the richness and complexity of information yielded by high-resolution spectra allows this NMR technique to characterise the sample chemical profile. The reported results illustrate the ability of high-resolution NMR to detect differences in the metabolite profile of several cheeses. As a trivial example, the amino acid profile of the Mozzarella di Bufala Campana compared to that of Grana Padano, reported in the following section, allows a prompt visualization of some differences between these two cheeses. In fact, Ala, Arg and Tyr have been found in Mozzarella di Bufala Campana aqueous extracts, but they are not present in Grana Padano aqueous extracts. Others amino acids (aspartate, asparagine, glycine, glutamine, histidine, lysine, methionine, proline and serine) found in Grana Padano have not been detected in Mozzarella di Bufala Campana.

In conclusion, if low-resolution NMR measurements are coupled to information got by high-resolution NMR, a complete food fingerprint can be arranged, that can be used to define a picture of cheese and their traceability.

Obviously, in order to propose NMR protocol as a standard method for authenticity and quality assessment of PDO cheese further methodical work is needed.

APPENDIX I – THE NMR EXPERIMENT [1]

Certain nuclei possess a property that is called spin. Although spin has to be formally described in a quantum mechanical way, it can be thought of as arising from a spinning movement of the nucleus about an axis. Because nuclei carry electric charges, spinning produces a small magnetic field, which is called a magnetic moment. The strength of a magnetic moment of the nucleus is determined by the magnetogyric ratio, γ, a fundamental physical constant for each nuclear species. The proton has the largest magneto-gyric ratio and hence the largest magnetic moment of all stable, non-radioactive nuclei.

When nuclei are placed in an external magnetic field, the associated magnetic moments will respond to the force of the field by lining up with it, similar to the way a compass needle would line up with the earth's magnetic field. Nevertheless, because the orientation of the spin angular momentum is quantized, for nuclei with a spin quantum number of ½, such as protons, two basic orientations are allowed. The spins do not exactly line up parallel or anti-parallel to the field, but they make a precession movement about the direction of the field. The process, known as Larmor precession, from the classical point of view is directly analogous to the motion of a gyroscope or spinning top under the influence of gravity, while for quantomechanics it does not oppose to Heisenberg's uncertainty principle.

In an ensemble of processing magnetic moments that are distributed with spin up and spin down over the energy states, the individual magnetic moments combine to create a vector that is called macroscopic magnetization. In the case of thermal equilibrium, this vector is aligned along the magnetic field, since the phase of the processing spins is randomly distributed.

The equilibrium magnetization ($\mathbf{M_0}$) is proportional to the total number of non zero spin nuclei in the sample and is aligned along the magnetic field direction (z-axis) – this resulting in a longitudinal component of the magnetization $\mathbf{M}_{//}$ coincident with $\mathbf{M_0}$ and in a zero transverse component $\mathbf{M}_\perp$.

Magnetic resonance absorption can only be detected if transverse magnetization, that is, magnetization oriented perpendicular to the external magnetic field, is generated.

The magnetic moments are then excited by a very short pulse of radio frequency (*rf*) satisfying the resonance condition: $\omega_0 = \gamma \mathbf{B_0}$, where ω_0 is the angular frequency of the *rf* radiation and γ is the magnetogyric ratio of nuclei. The *rf* pulse rotates the $\mathbf{M_0}$ vector around an axis normal to the static magnetic field (x-axis), in such a way that the longitudinal and transverse components of the magnetization result as $\mathbf{M}_{//} < \mathbf{M_0}$ and $\mathbf{M}_\perp \neq 0$. After the *rf* pulse is switched off the longitudinal and transverse components of the magnetization return to their equilibrium value by two distinct relaxation mechanisms called spin-lattice and spin-

spin relaxation process characterized by the time constants T_1 (spin-lattice or longitudinal relaxation time) and T_2 (spin-spin or transverse relaxation time), respectively.

The transverse magnetization decays to zero, as does the amplitude of the detected voltage. For this reason, the signal is called the 'free induction decay' (FID), and manifests itself as a damped oscillation, induced in the receiver coil that is situated in the transverse plane. This technique, which is used in almost all NMR spectrometers, is called pulsed NMR, since a short pulse of *rf* radiation is sufficient to rotate the magnetization vector. The NMR spectrum is obtained after a Fourier transformation of the FID. The great advantage of pulsed NMR as compared with continuous-wave NMR is that the FID lasts for about one second for most nuclei, whereas obtaining the spectrum by scanning the frequency would take much longer (~ 200 s). For insensitive nuclei, several thousands of pulsed NMR experiments need to be carried out to obtain a sufficient signal-to-noise ratio, and the free induction decays are accumulated in a computer that also carries out the Fourier transformation. An additional, unique advantage of pulsed NMR is that special pulse sequences can be applied, that offer a large range of new possibilities for the NMR spectroscopist to generate new types of NMR spectra and extract valuable information from them. For example, by suitable pulse sequences T_1 and T_2 relaxation times can be easily measured. In addition, from the pulsed NMR technique, two- and three-dimensional NMR techniques have been developed that provide information about the three-dimensional molecular structure, as well as NMR imaging methods that give a unique overall view inside materials, foods and human body.

APPENDIX II – THE CHEMICAL AND EXCHANGE MAGNETIC SITE MODEL [37]

In order to get easier the understanding of the reported examples to cheese characterization by the measurement and analysis of proton NMR relaxation curves, a brief outline of the chemical and diffusive exchange model will be preliminary given.

As concerns the fast chemical exchange (exchange rates as fast as 10^4 s^{-1}) between water and exchangeable protons of proteins and polysaccharides (–OH, –COOH, –NH, –SH), the major features of NMR water proton transverse relaxation is a strong dispersion in the transverse relaxation rate as the inter-pulse spacing in the CPMG pulse sequence becomes comparable to the exchange rate. In practice, the data multi-parameters fitting of the dispersion is make unreliable because the difficulties in determining, by independent measurements, the experimental values of the unknown parameters in equations that describe dispersion curve [3, 4, 5, 38, 19].

Now, in the limit of very short pulse spacing, the relaxation rate becomes described from [20]

$$\frac{1}{T_{2,obs}(\text{short }\tau_{cp})} = \frac{1}{T_{2,w}} + \frac{P_{exch}}{T_{2,exch} + k_{exch}^{-1}} \qquad \text{(AII-1)}$$

where $T_{2,obs}$ and $T_{2,w}$ are the observed intrinsic relaxation times (measured by CPMG experiment with the inter-pulse spacing very short) of water molecules and bulk water protons, respectively, P_{exch} and $T_{2,exch}$ are the macromolecular exchangeable protons molar fraction and transverse relaxation time, respectively; k$_{exch}$ is the pseudo-first order rate constant of proton chemical exchange between water and biopolymer.

However, T$_{2,w}$ can be independently measured, since the mid-point of the dispersion curves does give us an estimate for the exchange rate, so that the magnitude of this parameter is fixed, sample chemical composition can give an estimate of P$_{exch}$, so that a set of physically reasonable parameters can be derived [18, 39].

The effects of diffusive exchange on NMR relaxation times are of considerable importance in the interpretation of NMR data from heterogeneous systems: for instance, the enhanced relaxation rate as well as the observed multi-exponential character of water protons relaxation curves can be interpreted as ascribable to more than one size and type of diffusive domains. That gives the possibility to get morphological information on sub-compartments within the heterogeneous system by the analysis of water relaxation curves.

Basically, there are two limiting cases in the theoretical description of the relaxation of water filling pores in food compartments[40].

These cases are either slow-diffusion or fast-diffusion (surface-limited) relaxation, provided that bulk diffusion or surface, which acts as a relaxation sink, dominates, respectively[41].

A comparison of the diffusion rate D/2a – where D is water molecular self-diffusion coefficient and a is the characteristic dimension of diffusive domain – and surface relaxivity, ρ, shows that the slowest process limits the relaxation [42, 40].

So that, when D/2a << ρ the relaxation is diffusion limited, and the observed water relaxation rate is given by [19]

$$\frac{1}{T_{2,obs}} = \frac{1}{T_{2,w}} + \frac{\alpha \cdot D}{2a^2} \tag{AII-2}$$

where α = 1, 2 or 3 is a shape factor for planar, cylindrical and spherical geometry of diffusive domain, respectively.

On the other hand when D/2a >> ρ, the relaxation is surface limited, and the observed water relaxation rate holds [43]

$$\frac{1}{T_{2,obs}} = \frac{1}{T_{2,w}} + \rho \cdot \frac{\alpha}{a} \tag{AII-3}$$

The expressions (AII-2) and (AII-3) thus relate water relaxation rate to diffusive domains size (to either a^2 or a) and allow water T$_2$ values in foods to be quantitatively rationalized.

However, while an independent experimental measurement of D in equation (AII-2) is not a problem, an estimate of surface relaxation is less obvious. The efficiency of the surface relaxation is qualified by ρ = ε/T$_{2,s}$ and is referable to an evaluation of the thickness of the water molecules layer near a macromolecule and to T$_{2,s}$ value of macromolecular surface that can be inferred by theoretical data and experimental measurements.

The use of equations (AII-2) and (AII-3) to rationalize water relaxation data enables one to get information on macroporous (a = 1 – 150 μm) as well mesoporous heterogeneous systems (a = 500 Å – 1 mm) [37, 44].

REFERENCES

[1] Brosio, E.; Gianferri, R. In *Basic NMR in foods characterization* Brosio, E.; Research Signpost: Kerala, India, 2009, ISBN: 978-81-308-0303-6, pp. 9-38.

[2] Brosio, E.; Barbieri, R.; Gianferri, R. (2002). In *Recent research developments in polymer science*; Pandalai S. G.; Transworld Research Network: Kerala, India; pp. 177–196.

[3] McConnell, H. M. *J. Chem. Phys.* 1958, *28* (3), 430-431.

[4] Swift, T. J.; Connick, R. E. *J. Chem. Phys.* 1962, 37, 307-320.

[5] Luz, Z.; Meiboom, S. *J. Chem. Phys.* 1964, *40* (9), 2686-2692.

[6] INRAN Authors In *Food database – INRAN Tabelle di Composizione degli Alimenti*; Istituto Nazionale di Ricerca per gli Alimenti e la Nutrizione: Roma, ITALY, 2003.

[7] Romano, P.; Ricciardi, A.; Salzano, G.; Suzzi, G. *Int. J. Food Microbiol.* 2001, 69, 45-51.

[8] Calandrelli, M. In *Technical guidelines*; CIRVAL: Corte, Corsica, France, 1997, pp. 1-36.

[9] Kuo, M. I.; Gunasekaran, S.; Johnson, M.; Chen, C. *J. Dairy Sci.* 2001, 84, 1950-1958.

[10] McMahon, D. J.; Fife, R. L.; Oberg, C. J. *J. Dairy Sci.* 1999, 82, 1361-1369.

[11] Provencher, S. W. *Comput. Phys. Commun.* 1982, 27, 213-216.

[12] Provencher, S. W. *Comput. Phys. Commun.* 1982, 27, 229-242.

[13] Gianferri, R.; Maioli, M.; Delfini, M.; Brosio, E. *Int. Dairy J.* 2007, 17, 167–176.

[14] Brosio, E.; Barbieri, R. *Rev. Anal. Chem.* 1996, 15(4), 273–291.

[15] Le Dean, A.; Mariette, F.; Marin, M. *J. Agric. Food Chem.* 2004, 52, 5449–5455.

[16] Hills, B. P.; Belton, P. S.; Quantin, V. M. *Mol. Phys.* 1993, 78(4), 893–908.

[17] Hills, B. P.; Takacs, S. F.; Belton, P. S. *Food Chem.* 1990, 37, 95–111.

[18] Raffo, A.; Gianferri, R.; Barbieri, R.; Brosio, E. *Food Chem.* 2005, 89 (1), 149–158.

[19] Belton, P. S.; Hills, B. P.; Raimbaud, E. R. *Mol. Phys.* 1988, 63, 825-842.

[20] Hills, B. P.; Wright, K. M.; Belton, P. S. *Mol. Phys.* 1989, 67 (6), 1309-1326.

[21] Gottwald, A.; Creamer, L. K.; Hubbard, P. L.; Callaghan, P. T. *J. Chem. Phys.* 2005, 122, 034506-1-10.

[22] Fan, T. W. M. *Progress NMR Spect.* 1996, 28, 161-219.

[23] Govindaraju, V.; Young, K.; Maudsley, A.A. *NMR in Biomed.* 2000, 13, 129-153.

[24] Sobolev, A.P.; Brosio, E.; Gianferri, R.; Segre, A.L. *Magn. Reson. Chem.* 2005, 43, 625-638.

[25] Brescia, M. A.; Monfreda, M.; Buccolieri, A.; Carrino, C. *Food Chem.* 2005, 89, 139-147.

[26] Califano, A. N.; Bevilacqua, A. E. *Food Chem.* 1999, 64, 193-198.

[27] Gil, A. M.; Duarte, I. F.; Godejohann, M.; Braumann, U.; Maraschin, M.; Spraul, M. *Anal. Chim. Acta* 2003, 488, 35-51.

[28] Balestrieri, M.; Spagnuolo, M. S.; Cagliano, L.; Storti, G.; Ferrara, L.; Abrescia, P.,; Fedele, E. *Food Chem.* 2002, 77, 293-299.

[29] INRAN Authors (2010). Tabelle di Composizione degli Alimenti [E-text type]. http://www.inran.it/646/tabelle_di_composizione_degli_alimenti.html.

[30] Addeo, F.; Chianese, L. In *Grana Padano, un formaggio di qualità*. Consorzio per la tutela del formaggio Grana Padano: Milano, ITALY, 1995, pp. 97-130.

[31] de Angelis Curtis, S.; Curini, R.; Delfini, M.; Brosio, E.; D'Ascenzo, F.; Bocca, B. *Food Chem.* 2000, 71, 495-502.

[32] Choisy, C.; Desmazeaud, M. J.; Gripon, J. C.; Lamberet, G.; Lenoir, J.; Tourner, C.; In *Le Fromage*; Eck, A.; Technique et Documentation (Lavoisier): Paris, 1984.

[33] Hemme, D.; Bouillanne, C.; Metro, F.; Desmazeaud, M. J. *Sci. des Ali.* 1982, 2, 113-123.

[34] Resmini P.; Hogenboom J. A.; Pellegrino L.; Pazzaglia C. In *Grana Padano, un formaggio di qualità*; Consorzio per la tutela del formaggio Grana Padano: Milano, ITALY, 1995, pp. 195-213).

[35] Meiboom, S.; Gill, D. *Rev. Sci. Instr.* 1958, 29, 688-691.

[36] Hull, W. E. *Two Dimensional NMR Spectroscopy. Applications for Chemists and Biochemists*; VCH: New York, NY, 1994 (2nd ed), p. 125.

[37] Brosio, E.; Belotti, M.; Gianferri, R. In *Food Science and Technology: New Research*; Greco, L. V.; Bruno, M. N.; Nova Science Publishers: Hauppauge (NY), 2008, ISBN: 978-1-60456-715-1.

[38] Carver, J. P.; Richards, R. R. *J. Magn. Reson.* 1972, 6 (1), 89-105.

[39] Gianferri, R.; D'Aiuto, V.; Curini, R.; Delfini, M.; Brosio, E. *Food Chem.* 2007, 105 (2), 720-726.

[40] Brownstein, K. R.; Tarr, C. E. *Phys. Rev., A* 1979, 19, 2446-2453.

[41] Korb, J. P.; Godefroy, S.; Fleury, M. *Magn. Reson. Imaging* 2003, 21, 193-199.

[42] Callaghan, P.T.; Godefroy, S.; Ryland, B. N. *J. Magn. Reson.* 2003, 162, 320-327.

[43] Belton, P. S.; Hills, B. P. *Mol. Phys.*, 1987, 61, 999-1018.

[44] Belotti, M.; Martinelli, A.; Gianferri, R.; Brosio, E. *Phys. Chem. Chem. Phys.* 2010, 12, pp. 516-522.

In: Cheese: Types, Nutrition and Consumption
Editor: Richard D. Foster, pp. 207-220

ISBN 978-1-61209-828-9
© 2011 Nova Science Publishers, Inc.

Chapter 11

CHEESE FLAVORS: CHEMICAL ORIGINS AND DETECTION

Michael H. Tunick
Dairy and Functional Foods Research Unit,
Eastern Regional Research Center,
Agricultural Research Service,
U.S. Department of Agriculture,
600 E. Mermaid Lane, Wyndmoor, PA 19038, USA

ABSTRACT

The hundreds of flavor compounds found in cheese arise from the proteins, lipids, and carbohydrates it contains. Flavor compounds are products of diverse reactions that occur in milk during processing, in curd during manufacture, and in cheese during storage, and are detected by a number of methods. Acids, alcohols, aldehydes, esters, ketones, and lactones may all form in cheese depending on the variety. The different pathways of flavor compound formation result from the feed or grass consumed by the animals, enzymes present in the starter culture microorganisms, any adjunct cultures or molds that have been added, the action of the coagulant, and the time and temperature of aging. An assortment of techniques for extracting and identifying flavors has been developed over the years. Gas chromatography and sensory analysis are used to examine these compounds. This chapter will cover the origins of cheese flavors and the ways that scientists can examine them.

INTRODUCTION

The many varieties of cheese in the world generate hundreds of flavors. Microorganisms, coagulation enzymes, and lipolytic enzymes attack the proteins, lipids, and carbohydrates in the milk, leading to typical flavors found in fresh cheese, such as diacetyl. During storage, metabolism of lactate, lactose, and citrate, proteolysis of caseins, and lipolysis of triacylglycerols cause aged flavors to form, including fruity flavors from esters and lactones, and green and fatty flavors from aldehydes. Instrumental analysis of these flavors is performed by extracting compounds from the cheese and passing them through a gas chromatograph equipped with an appropriate detector. Sensory techniques are used to describe flavors and match them with compounds identified instrumentally. These methods enable scientists to evaluate how flavors are formed, their concentrations in the product, and their relative importance.

CHEESEMAKING

The varieties of cheese are distinguished from each other by their production methods. No two varieties have the same flavor, and there are always differences within a variety depending on how it is made. The factors that affect flavor in cheese include the milk itself, pasteurization, homogenization, bacteria and surface microorganisms, coagulant, whey syneresis, salt, and ripening.

Milk

The flavor of milk and thus the flavor of cheese are influenced by the diet of the animal producing the milk. Many cows are consistently fed throughout the year with silage, which consists of alfalfa, barley, corn, vetch, and wheat that has been allowed to ferment anaerobically. In contrast, pasture-fed animals eat the plants they encounter and prefer. Some compounds from grasses, flowers, and other plants ingested by animals on pasture either pass directly into milk or are converted into other compounds [Urbach, 1990]. Many of these compounds impart flowery flavors to cheese [Carpino et al., 2004], which some consumers find desirable. When live pasture plants are consumed by cows, the plants activate the lipoxygenase system, which may be part of an injury response [Gaillard and Chan, 1980]. Lipoxygenase activity breaks down lipids and carotenoids to products that affect cheese flavor [Carpino et al., 2004]. Some of the compounds generated in this way from unsaturated fatty acids in plants are 2,4-decadienal, methyl jasmonate, nonanal, and 2-nonenal. Precursors or degradation products of carotenoids include carvone, citronellol, and geranyl acetate [Carpino et al., 2004]. Artisanal Alpine cheese often contains the terpenes linalool and α-pinene [Curioni and Bosset, 2002]. Many of the cheese varieties in the world are produced from milk from pasture-fed animals, but the flavor origins of these products and their concentrations in cheese are only beginning to be examined [Urbach, 1990]. The health of the animals will also have an effect on cheese, as high somatic cell counts resulting from mastitis and poor nutrition will adversely affect coagulation and proteolysis [Fox et al., 2000].

Pasteurization

Milk is pasteurized to remove potential pathogens. Pasteurization at 63°C for 30 min kills many indigenous microflora while not imparting a cooked flavor to the resulting cheese, but this length of time is longer and thus less economical than the more common 72°C for 15 s

[US Food and Drug Administration, 2009]. Whey proteins, primarily β-lactoglobulin, are denatured when milk is pasteurized above 75°C, causing sulfur-containing amino acids to liberate sulfhydryls and volatile sulfides, especially H_2S [Calvo and de la Hoz, 1992]. These compounds give the milk a cooked flavor that can carry over to the cheese. Heat-induced interactions of whey proteins with casein result when milk is pasteurized at high temperatures, which limits the accessibility of proteases and peptidases to casein micelles and changes the characteristics of proteolysis [Lau, Barbano, and Rasmussen, 1991]. Moreover, pasteurization inactivates microflora and several enzymes normally found in milk. The resulting decreases in proteolysis and lipolysis cause the cheese to contain fewer flavor compounds than raw milk cheese [Grappin and Beauvier, 1997]. A study of seven French cheese varieties made from raw and pasteurized milk showed that pasteurization affects the flavors of different types of cheese in different ways: raw milk cheese tended to have earthy flavors whereas pasteurized milk cheeses had moldy, fermented, and butyric flavors [Chambers, Esteve, and Retiveau, 2010]. Some enzymes such as plasmin survive pasteurization and are present in the milk at the beginning of cheesemaking. Nonstarter lactic acid bacteria may also enter the curd from the environment and produce undesirable levels of proteolysis [Morales, Fernández-García, and Nuñez, M. 2005].

Homogenization

Goats' milk has been described as naturally homogenized since there is a narrow distribution of the sizes of its fat globules [Attaie and Richter, 2000]. Cows' milk is not usually homogenized prior to cheesemaking. Small, homogenized fat globules alter the texture and functionality of the resulting cheese and are subject to a higher level of lipolysis, which may lead to rancid flavors [Fox et al., 2000]. Feta and Blue cheese are often homogenized, however, because increased lipolysis is desirable in these varieties.

Starter and Adjunct Cultures

Starter cultures consist of lactic acid bacteria (LAB), including *Lactococcus lactis, Streptococcus thermophilus, Leuconostoc mesenteroides*, and species of Lactobacillus [Smit, Smit, and Engels, 2005]. LAB, which are added at the start of cheesemaking, lower the pH of the milk before the coagulation step and influence the rate and extent of acid development, which controls the dissociation of colloidal calcium phosphate. Live starter cultures probably contribute little to flavor development once cheesemaking is complete, but the enzymes they release upon cell death are responsible for proteolysis and some lipolysis [Fox et al., 2000].

Nonstarter lactic acid bacteria (NSLAB) are adventitious contaminants that survive pasteurization or are airborne in the cheese plant or present on the equipment. Many NSLAB are species of Lactobacillus, and influence cheese ripening by intensifying development of typical flavors, imparting atypical but desirable flavors, or introducing undesirable off-flavors [Broadbent and Steele, 2007].

Adjunct cultures, which are additional starters intended to produce particular flavors, are added before coagulation. Adjuncts include propionibacteria, which produces the openings in Swiss cheese, and *Penicillium roqueforti* mold, which is used in Blue and Brie manufacture. Lipolysis is enhanced in varieties such as Parmesan and Romano by the addition of lipase enzymes.

Coagulant

Casein, the major protein in milk, consists of α_{s1}-, α_{s2}-, β-, and κ-caseins bundled into micelles [Holt, 1992]. Milk is coagulated by cleaving κ-casein, which destabilizes the micelles and causes them to aggregate into a curd. Unripened cheeses are usually coagulated by the combined action of the starter culture and heat, or by the addition of food-grade acid. Ripened cheeses, which account for the vast majority of the cheese made in the world, are coagulated with the enzyme chymosin, the acid proteinase found in rennet. Chymosin was traditionally extracted from the fourth stomach of calves but nowadays is obtained from microbial sources such as *Rhizomucor miehei, Rhizomucor pusillus,* and *Cryphonectria parasitica*. Some European cheeses are coagulated with proteinases extracted from fruits such as pineapple and papaya [Tejada, Gómez, and Fernández-Salguero, 2007]. The cardoon, also known as artichoke thistle, has been used to coagulate Iberian goat and sheep milk since ancient times [Stepaniak, 2004]. Chymosin and enzymes from microbial sources hydrolyze α_{s1}-casein, which leads to peptide formation [Sousa, Ardö, and McSweeney, 2001]. β-casein is also hydrolyzed, releasing a peptide responsible for bitter flavor [Stepaniak, 2004]. Rennet is inactivated when the curd is cooked at high temperatures, but some chymosin activity remains at lower cooking temperatures, leading to increased proteolysis in the resulting cheese.

Syneresis

The expulsion of whey during cheesemaking is known as syneresis. Around 90% of coagulated milk consists of whey, which imparts a tart flavor that may be objectionable in many cheese varieties. Cheesemakers try to remove most of the whey so they can isolate the curd. They increase syneresis by raising the time and temperature at which the curd is coagulated and cooked, and they also reduce the size of the cubes into which the curd is cut, thus increasing their surface area. Syneresis decreases the moisture in the curd, which slows the growth of bacteria and therefore reduces proteolysis. Whey proteins comprise 20% of milk protein but only 3-6% of the protein in cheese.

Salt and Coloring

Cheese contains 0.5-6% NaCl by weight, depending on the variety. NaCl is a key determinant of water activity, which directly affects biochemical activity, enzyme activity, and microbial growth, all of which influence flavor [Guinee, 2004]. Starter culture activity and metabolism of lactose are inhibited when the salt-in-moisture concentration is above 5%

[Fox et al., 2000]. Of course, NaCl itself is a direct contributor to flavor. NaCl is added in dry form to the curd, or the cheese is immersed in brine. Salt substitutes such as KCl are sometimes used, but impart an uncharacteristic bitter flavor [Fitzgerald and Buckley, 1985]. The addition of coloring agents such as annatto or β-carotene does not affect flavor, although some people believe that cheese tastes better when highly colored [Dunn and Ogden, 1991].

Surface Microorganisms

Cheeses such as Brick, Camembert, and Limburger are aged with the aid of bacteria, fungi, mold, and yeast on the surface. Yeasts such as *Debaryomyces hansenii* and fungi such as *Geotrichum candidum* and *Penicillium camemberti* colonize the cheese surface and metabolize lactic acid [Irlinger and Mounier, 2009]. A series of reactions follows, resulting in the production of NH_3, leading to a pH of around 7.0 on the surface. Less acid tolerant bacteria, including *Arthobacter arilaitensis, Brevibacterium aurantiacum, Brevibacterium linens,* and *Corynebacterium casei* can then grow on the surface [Irlinger and Mounier, 2009]. The pH gradient (the interior of the cheese is initially around pH 4.6) causes migration of calcium phosphate to the surface and stimulates the action of the indigenous milk proteinase plasmin [Fox, Singh, and McSweeney, 1995]. Plasmin is responsible for some proteolysis, and NH_3 imparts an ammonia flavor to cheese. Yeasts such as species of Kluyromyces and Candida, and *G. candidum* fungus metabolize lactate to CO_2 and H_2O, providing an environment in which *B. linens* and *C. casei* flourish [Fox et al., 2001]. *B. linens* and *G. candidum* break down sulfur-containing amino acids, leading to desirable sulfur-type flavors to surface-ripened cheese [Berger et al., 1999]. The microorganisms and the flavor compounds they produce may be present in the residual whey rather than the protein matrix. Mold may be introduced to the interior of blue- and green-veined cheeses by poking holes in the rind and adding mold powder or aerosol.

Ripening

Aging, curing, maturing, and ripening are synonyms for the period between completion of cheesemaking and shipping from the storage room. Various flavors become prominent during ripening and then may strengthen or weaken because of the enzymatic processes taking place. Storage time and temperature depend on the cheese variety -- for example, sharp Cheddar is ripened at 6-8°C for at least 6 mo and Parmesan is stored at 18-20°C for 24-30 mo. Soft cheeses are usually consumed quickly because of bacterial activity, and are often bland.

COMPOUND FORMATION

The flavor compounds in ripened cheese arise from the breakdown of lactate, citrate, protein, and lipids. A list of common flavor compounds in cheese is given in Table 1.

Table 1. Flavor compounds commonly found in cheese

Alcohol	Flavor notes
Ethanol	Mild, ethery
n-Propanol	Pungent
n-Butanol	Floral, fragrant, fruity, sweet
2-Pentanol	Alcoholic, nutty, fruity, sweet
n-Hexanol	Fatty, floral, green
2-Octanol	Green, mushroom, coconut, oil, rancid
1-Octen-3-ol	Mushroom
1,5-Diocten-3-ol	Soil, geranium
Phenol	Floral, medical
2-Phenylethanol	Rose, floral
2-Methylisoborneol	Musty, soil
Citronellol	Rose
Linalool	Floral

Aldehyde	Flavor notes
Acetaldehyde	Sweet, pungent, ethereal
Methional	Boiled potato
2-Methylpropanal	Pungent, chocolate
Butanal	Pungent
2- and 3-Methylbutanal	Dark chocolate, malt, green
Pentanal	Pungent, almond-like
Hexanal	Green, grassy
2-Hexenal	Green, fatty, almond bitter
Heptanal	Green, fatty, oily, sweet, nutty
4-Heptenal	Creamy, biscuit, fatty, oily
Octanal	Green, fatty, soapy, fruity
Nonanal	Green, sweet, floral
2,6-Nonadieneal	Melon, cucumber, fatty, floral
Decanal	Soapy, flowery
2,4-Decadienal	Mayonnaise, bread, fatty, fruity
Phenyl acetaldehyde	Rosy, honey

Ester	Flavor notes
Ethyl acetate	Fruity, sweet, solvent, pineapple
n-Butyl acetate	Pear
3-Methylbutyl acetate	Banana
Isoamylacetate	Pear, banana
Ethyl propionate	Fruity, pineapple
Ethyl butanoate	Fruity, pineapple, bubble gum, sweet
n-Propyl butanoate	Pineapple, banana
Methyl hexanoate	Pineapple
Ethyl hexanoate	Fruity, pineapple, banana
Ethyl octanoate	Fruity, apricot, wine

Ester	Flavor notes
Geranyl acetate	Rose
Methyl jasmonate	Jasmine

Fatty acid	Flavor notes
Acetic and propionic	Pungent, vinegar, rancid
Butanoic	Rancid, cheese, sweaty, sour, putrid
n-Pentanoic	Swiss cheese
3-Methylbutanoic	Swiss cheese, waxy, sweaty, fecal
n-Hexanoic	Pungent, blue cheese, goat
n-Octanoic	Wax, soap, goat, musty, rancid, fruity, stale butter, sweaty
4-Methyloctanoic	Wax, goat, cheese
4-Ethyloctanoic	Goat
Decanoic	Rancid
Dodecanoic	Soapy

Ketone	Flavor notes
2-Butanone	Etheric, acetone
2,3-Butanedione	Buttery, creamy
3-Methyl-2-butanone	Camphor
2-Heptanone	Blue cheese, fruity, musty, soapy, cinnamon
1-Octen-3-one	Mushroom
2-Octanone	Floral, fruity, musty, soapy
2-Nonanone	Green, earthy, blue cheese, fatty, fruity, musty, varnish
2-Undecanone	Floral, fruity, green, musty, tallow
Acetophenone	Orange blossom, almond, musty, glue
Carvone	Herbaceous

Lactone	Flavor notes
δ-Octalactone	Coconut, wine
γ-Octalactone	Fruity, coconut
δ-Decalactone	Peach, coconut, creamy
γ-Decalactone	Peach, apricot, coconut
δ-Dodecalactone	Fresh fruit, peach, pear, plum, coconut
γ-Dodecalactone	Peach

Singh, Drake, and Cadwallader, 2003; Fox et al., 2000; Molimard and Spinnler, 1996; Friedrich and Acree, 1998.

Lactate Metabolism

Although lactose and citrate are present at relatively small concentrations in cheese, their breakdown products are important for flavor in all cheese varieties [Broadbent and Steele, 2007]. The principal carbohydrate found in milk is the disaccharide lactose. Around 98% of the lactose in milk is lost with the whey during the manufacture of most cheeses. Residual lactose is quickly metabolized by LAB, contributing an acidic flavor to cheese. Lactate serves as the primary source of food for LAB that metabolize it to form acetaldehyde, acetate, ethanol, formate, and other compounds that contribute to characteristic cheese flavors [McSweeney and Sousa, 2000]. This process takes as little as 3 wk in Blue and other surface-ripened cheeses, and > 8 mo in Romano and other hard cheeses [Fox, Singh, and McSweeney, 1995]. Lactate metabolism is especially important in surface-ripened cheeses, as mentioned above. In Emmental, Swiss, and related cheeses, lactate is metabolized by propionic acid bacteria to acetate, propionate, water, and CO_2, which forms the eyes in the curd [McSweeney, 2004].

Citrate Metabolism

Around 94% of the citrate in milk is in the soluble phase and is lost in the whey during cheesemaking [Hugenholtz, 1993]. Citrate is a major contributor to flavor despite comprising < 1.0% of the curd. Citrate is metabolized by certain strains of Lactococci and Leuconostoc to 2,3-butanediol, 2,3-butanedione (diacetyl), and 3-hydroxy-2-butanone (acetoin), which are characteristic flavor compounds in cheese [LeBars and Yvon, 2008].

Proteolysis

Approximately 80% of cheese protein is casein, the proteolysis of which is the most complex and perhaps the most important biochemical event during cheese ripening [McSweeney, 2004]. Caseins are hydrolyzed by the coagulant and plasmin to peptides that in turn are hydrolyzed to short peptides and free amino acids by the proteinases and peptidases found in LAB and NSLAB. The process begins when coagulant is added and continues throughout storage. Proteolysis is enhanced by increasing the moisture level and the storage temperature, and by decreasing the salt content. Cheeses that are consumed relatively quickly usually exhibit low levels of proteolysis since the aging time is cut short, but smear-ripened cheeses undergo extensive protein breakdown within weeks. The α_{s1}- and β-casein in blue-veined cheeses are completely hydrolyzed during ripening [McSweeney, 2004].

Amino acids and short peptides contribute to flavor and serve as substrates for reactions that produce other flavor compounds. Amino acid breakdown takes place through transamination, elimination reactions, deamination, and decarboxylation. Aminotransferases convert amino acids by transamination to α-ketoacids while an α-ketoacid acceptor is converted to the corresponding amino acid. Often, α-ketoglutarate is transformed into glutamate in this process [Yvon and Rijnen, 2001]. Acetoin, diacetyl, and 2,3-butanediol may be generated from transamination of alanine and aspartate in the presence of α-ketoglutarate [LeBars and Yvon, 2008]. α-ketoacids are then catabolized through various pathways to alcohols, aldehydes, benzaldehyde, cresol, and esters. Aldehydes are also generated through Strecker degradation, in which an α-amino acid reacts with an α-dicarbonyl [Smit, Smit, and Engels, 2005].

Elimination reactions occur when surface microorganisms such as *B. linens* and yeast cleave the side chains of tyrosine (releasing phenol) and tryptophan (releasing indol) [Yvon and Rijnen, 2001]. These β-eliminations are catalyzed by lyase enzymes, which are also responsible for γ-elimination of methionine to form methanethiol. Sulfur-containing compounds are important for flavors in some cheeses, and these compounds mostly derive from methionine since casein contains low amounts of cysteine [McSweeney, 2004]. Thioesters and di- and trimethyl sulfide are formed by oxidation of methanethiol, and methyl thioesters are formed when methanethiol reacts with free fatty acids [Burbank and Qian, 2008].

Deamination reactions occur when dehydrogenases or oxidases attack amino acids, cleaving off ammonia. Surface-ripened cheeses often have ammonia as part of their flavor profile. Decarboxylation reactions produce amines that generate strong and unpleasant aromas [McSweeney, 2004].

Lipolysis

Lipolytic enzymes hydrolyze triacylglycerols to diacylglycerols, monoacylglycerols, glycerol, and fatty acids (FA). These enzymes are esterases and lipases, and are found in LAB (particularly Lactobacilli) and NSLAB [Malacarne et al., 2009]. Some microorganisms used in surface ripened cheeses exhibit extensive lipolytic activity, as do the rennet pastes that are added during the manufacture of some cheeses. Milk contains lipoprotein lipase, but it is inactivated by heat treatment [Hickey et al., 2007].

Long-chain (> 12 carbon atoms) FA contribute little to cheese flavor because of their high perception thresholds, but short-chain FA impart major flavor notes to cheese and are precursors to the formation of other important flavor compounds [Malacarne et al., 2009]. γ- and δ-hydroxy FA are converted into γ- and δ-lactones, which are responsible for coconut and fruity flavors. Esters, which have flowery and fruity flavors, are produced by reaction of FA with an alcohol, usually ethanol. Thioesters, which have cabbage, cheesy, and rancid flavors, are generated from reactions of FA with thiols, usually methanethiol. Surface microorganisms oxidize FA to 2-methyl ketones. Methyl ketones may then be reduced to secondary alcohols [Collins, McSweeney, and Wilkinson, 2003].

INSTRUMENTAL FLAVOR ANALYSIS

The instrumental analysis of cheese flavors is performed by isolating the compounds from the sample matrix and subjecting them to gas chromatography (GC) [McGorrin, 2007]. Representative samples are obtained by a variety of isolation procedures.

Extraction

Dialysis, steam distillation, and solvent extraction are the classic methods for extracting and isolating flavor compounds. In a comparison of three extraction methods applied to Cheddar cheese [Vandeweghe and Reineccius, 1990], dialysis was found to deliver the most concentrated flavor isolate, but drawbacks included the expense of the membrane and the time required to extract the compounds (3 d, although the setup may be unattended). Distillation and extraction with methylene chloride was tedious (requiring 5 h per sample) and generated methyl ketone artifacts, but yielded a highly concentrated isolate with the most characteristic Cheddar aroma. Solvent extraction was fastest and cheapest, but produced the least concentrated isolate.

Isolation methods may be combined to improve results. Extraction with diethyl ether followed by high vacuum distillation has been used to determine that some aldehydes arising from Strecker degradation are responsible for much of the nutty flavor in Cheddar [Avsar et al., 2004]. A newer technique, solvent-assisted flavor evaporation (SAFE), was developed to reduce extraction time and artifact formation. Samples are dissolved in solvent and flavor compounds are extracted by high vacuum and then condensed with liquid nitrogen [Engel, Barr, and Schieberle, 1999]. The potent odorants in full- and reduced-fat Cheddar were identified after extraction and isolation by SAFE [Carunchia Whetstine et al., 2006].

A solventless extraction method, stir bar sorptive extraction (SBSE, marketed as Twister^{TM}), consists of a stir bar coated with polydimethylsiloxane gum. Flavor compounds are absorbed on the gum during stirring, and are then thermally desorbed and sent through a GC. Eighty-four alcohols, aldehydes, esters, FA, hydrocarbons, ketones, and terpenes were identified in an Italian cheese using SBSE [Panseri et al., 2008].

Headspace Sampling

Volatile compounds may be isolated by sampling the headspace from a vial containing the cheese sample. Equilibrium (or static) sampling, in which a sample is withdrawn using a simple syringe, is fast but lacks sensitivity. An improvement, solid phase dynamic extraction (SPDE), is accomplished by coating the inside wall of a syringe needle with polydimethylsiloxane and activated carbon, which absorbs volatiles [Pillonel, Bosset, and Tabacchi, 2002]. In dynamic headspace (or purge trap) sampling, the volatiles are swept through an adsorbent that traps the compounds. This procedure generates few artifacts and has been applied to measure the differences in flavor of Cantal cheese due to cow diet, pasteurization, and ripening [Cornu et al., 2009].

Solid phase microextraction (SPME) uses a gas-tight syringe that allows compounds to be desorbed into a GC injector port. Volatiles diffuse into the syringe, where they are absorbed onto a fused silica fiber coated with a liquid phase [Chin, Bernhard, and Rosenberg, 1996]. For nonvolatiles, the fiber may be immersed in the sample [Pillonel, Bosset, and Tabacchi, 2002]. Reproducibility is affected by temperature, volatility, and other factors, but has found wide application. For example, the presence of sulfur-containing flavor compounds in cheeses made from heat-shocked or pasteurized milk was determined after SPME extraction [Burbank and Qian, 2002].

Derivatization

Long-chain FA are not volatile and must be derivatized prior to analysis. Acid-catalyzed esterification in methanol with BF_3, CH_3ONa, or H_2SO_4 creates volatile fatty acid methyl esters (FAME), which are injected into the GC. The method, with modifications, was developed almost 50 yr ago [Morrison and Smith, 1964] and is still in use.

GC Analysis

GC is the technique of choice for investigating cheese flavor. GC with flame ionization detection is the primary technique for volatile FA analysis [Collins, McSweeney, and Wilkinson, 2003]. Otherwise, GC is interfaced with mass spectrometry (GC-MS), with compounds being identified by matching the mass spectral data with a library of standards.

Many of the volatiles in food are not odor-active and thus do not contribute to flavor [Friedrich and Acree, 1998]. The most sensitive detector for identifying key odor compounds is a human using his or her nose to characterize their presence and intensity [Pollien et al., 1997].

SENSORY FLAVOR ANALYSIS

Sensory perception is the most important factor in determining consumer acceptance of cheese or any food. Specific methods have been devised to measure human responses to stimuli provided by flavors. These are coupled with instrumental results to provide a complete picture of the flavors found in cheese.

Descriptive Sensory Tests

Analytical sensory tests are conducted with trained panelists and include discrimination tests, threshold tests, and descriptive sensory analysis [Drake, 2007]. The results consist of all the detectable flavors in the cheese. Flavor lexicons with descriptors ("fruity," for example), definitions ("aromatics associated with different fruits"), and specific flavor references ("fresh pineapple, ethyl hexanoate") have been published for Cheddar and Swiss cheeses [Drake, 2007]. The sensory and instrumental results are compared, and compounds are tentatively identified with particular flavors. Some flavors may interact with other components and synergistic effects may be present, so model systems are constructed to evaluate the relationship between perceived flavor and instrumental results [Avsar et al., 2004].

GC-O Analysis

Gas chromatography-olfactometry (GC-O) joins sensory perception and instrumentation. As a compound is eluted from the GC, a panelist sniffs the effluent from the column and describes the odor. GC-O assists in identifying compounds that are present in the sensory threshold range and may screen volatile compounds that play key roles in flavor perception [Avsar et al., 2004].

The sensory contribution of a single compound detected by GC-O is investigated by odor dilution analysis, in which an aroma extract is diluted until no odor is perceived. This method enables the panelist to determine the relative intensity of the odorant and thus its importance [d'Acampora Zellner et al., 2008]. The two most popular techniques for measuring the presence and intensity of odors are CHARM (combined hedonic aroma response method) [Acree, Barnard, and Cunningham, 1984] and AEDA (aroma extraction dilution analysis) [Ullrich and Grosch, 1987]. AEDA panelists evaluate samples as they become more dilute, whereas in CHARM the samples are randomized. An alternative method is nasal impact frequency (NIF), in which one dilution is used but the experiment is replicated many times [Pollien et al., 1997]. Untrained panelists attempt to detect the odor, and its intensity is implied by the number of positive responses.

CONCLUSION

The formation and analysis of flavors arising in cheese are complicated, requiring a great deal of effort and skill to determine the presence, amount, and contribution of each compound. The dairy industry and consumers will benefit if scientists are able to understand the mechanism of flavor production in cheese varieties.

NOTE

Mention of trade names or commercial products in this publication is solely for the purpose of providing specific information and does not imply recommendation or endorsement by the U.S. Department of Agriculture.

REFERENCES

Acree, T.E.; Barnard, J.; Cunningham, D. *Food Chem.* 1984, 14, 273-286.
Attaie, R.; Richter, R.L. *J. Dairy Sci.* 2000, 83, 940-944.
Avsar, Y.K.; Karagul-Yuceer, Y.; Drake, M.A.; Singh, T.K.; Yoon, Y.; Cadwallader, K.R. *J. Dairy Sci.* 2004, 87, 1999–2010.
Berger, C.; Khan, J.A.; Molimard, P.; Martin, N.; Spinnler, H.E. *Appl. Environ. Microbiol.* 1999, 65, 5510-5514.
Broadbent, J.R.; Steele, J.L. In Flavor of Dairy Products; Cadwallader, K.R.; Drake, M.A.; McGorrin, R.J., Ed.; Amer. Chem. Soc.: Washington, DC, 2007, pp 177-192.
Burbank, H.; Qian, M.C. *Int. Dairy J.* 2008, 18, 811-818.
Calvo, M.M.; de la Hoz, L. *Int. Dairy J.* 1992, 2, 69-81.
Carpino, S.; Mallia, S.; La Terra, S.; Melilli, C.; Licitra, G.; Acree, T.E.; Barbano, D.M.; Van Soest, P.J. *J. Dairy Sci.* 2004, 87, 816-830.
Carunchia Whetstine, M.E.; Drake, M.A.; Nelson, B.K.; Barbano, D.M. *J. Dairy Sci.* 2006, 89, 505–517.
Chambers, D.H.; Esteve, E.; Retiveau, A. *J. Sens. Stud.* 2010, 25, 494-511.
Chin, H.W.; Bernhard, R.A.; Rosenberg, M. *J. Food Sci.* 1996, 1118-1112.
Collins, Y.F.; McSweeney, P.L.H.; Wilkinson, M.G. *Int. Dairy J.* 2003, 13, 841-856.

Cornu, A.; Rabiau, N.; Kondjoyan, N.; Verdier-Metz, I.; Pradel, P.; Tournayre, P.; Berdagué, J.L.; Martin, B. *Int. Dairy J.* 2009, 19, 588-594.

Curioni, P.M.G.; Bosset, J.O. *Int. Dairy J.* 2002, 12, 959-984.

d'Acampora Zellner, B.; Dugo, P.; Dugo, G.; Mondello, L. *J. Chromatogr. A* 2008, 1186, 123-143.

Drake, M.A. *J. Dairy Sci.* 2007, 90, 4925–4937.

Dunn, M.L.; Ogden, L.V. *J. Dairy Sci.* 1991, 74, 2042-2047.

Engel, W.; Barr, W.; Schieberle, P. *Eur. Food Res. Technol.* 1999, 209, 237–241.

Fitzgerald, E.; Buckley, J. *J. Dairy Sci.* 1985, 68, 3127-3134.

Fox, P.F.; Guinee, T.P.; Cogan, T.M.; McSweeney, P.L.H. In Fundamentals of Cheese Science; Aspen Publ.: Gaithersburg, MD, 2000, pp 361-371.

Fox, P.F.; Singh, T.K.; McSweeney, P.L.H. In Chemistry of Structure-Function Relationships in Cheese; Malin, E.L.; Tunick, M.H., Ed.; Plenum Press: New York, 1995, pp 59-98.

Friedrich, J.E.; Acree, T.E. *Int. Dairy J.* 1998, 8, 235-241.

Galliard, T.; Chan, H.W.-S. In The Biochemistry of Plants. Lipids: Structure and Function; Stumpf, P.K., Ed.; Academic Press: New York, 1980, Vol. 4, pp 131-161.

Grappin, R.; Beuvier, E. *Int. Dairy J.* 1997, 7, 751-761.

Guinee, T.P. *Int. J. Dairy Technol.* 2004, 57, 99-109.

Hickey, D.K.; Kilcawley, K.N.; Beresford, T.P.; Wilkinson, M.G. *J. Dairy Sci.* 2007, 90, 47-56.

Holt, C. *Adv. Protein Chem.* 1992, 42, 63-151.

Hugenholtz, J. *FEMS Microbiol. Revs.* 1993, 12, 165-178.

Irlinger, F.; Mounier. J. *Curr. Opin. Biotechnol.* 2009, 20, 142-148.

Lau, K.Y.; Barbano, D.M.; Rasmussen, R.R. *J. Dairy Sci.* 1991, 74, 727-740.

LeBars, D.; Yvon, M. *J. Appl. Microbiol.* 2008, 104, 171-177.

Malacarne, M.; Summera, A.; Franceschi, P.; Formaggioni, P.; Pecorari, M.; Panari, G.; Mariani, P. *Int. Dairy J.* 2009, 19, 637-641.

McGorrin, R.J. In Flavor of Dairy Products; Cadwallader, K.R.; Drake, M.A.; McGorrin, R.J., Ed.; Amer. Chem. Soc.: Washington, DC, 2007, pp 23-49.

McSweeney, P.L.H. *Int. J. Dairy Technol.* 2004, 57, 127-144.

McSweeney, P.L.H.; Sousa, M.J. Lait 2000, 80, 293-324.

Molimard, P.; Spinnler, H.P. *J. Dairy Sci.* 1996, 79, 169-184.

Morales, P.; Fernández-García, E.; Nuñez, M. *J. Agric. Food Chem.* 2005, 53, 6835-6843.

Morrison, W.R.; Smith, L.M. *J. Lipid Res.* 1964, 5, 600-608.

Panseri, S.; Giani, I.; Mentasti, T.; Bellagamba, F.; Caprino, F.; Moretti, V.M. *Lebensm. Wiss. Technol.* 2008, 41, 185-192.

Pillonel, L.; Bosset, J.O.; Tabacchi, R. *Lebensm. Wiss. Technol.* 2002, 35, 1-14.

Pollien, P.; Ott, A.; Montigon, F.; Baumgartner; M.; Muñoz-Box, R.; Chaintreau, A. *J. Agric. Food Chem.*, 1997, 45, 2630-2637.

Singh, T.K.; Drake, M.A.; Cadwallader, K.R. *Compr. Revs. Food Sci. Safety* 2003, **2**, 139-162.

Smit, G.; Smit, B.A.; Engels, W.J.M. *FEMS Microbiol. Rev.* 2005, 29, 591-610.

Sousa, M.J.; Ardö, Y.; McSweeney, P.L.H. *Int. Dairy J.* 2001, 11, 327-345.

Stepaniak, L. *Int. J. Dairy Technol.* 2004, 57, 153-171.

Tejada, L.; Gómez, R.; Fernández-Salguero, J. *J. Food Qual.* 2007, 91-103.

Ullrich, F.; Grosch, W. *Z. Lebensm. Unters. Forsch.* 1987, 184, 277-282.
Urbach, G. *J. Dairy Sci.* 1990, 73, 3639-3650.
US Food and Drug Administration. In Grade "A" Pasteurized Milk Ordinance, US FDA: Washington, DC, 2009, p 8.
Vandeweghe, P.; Reineccius, G.A. *J. Agric. Food Chem.* 1990, 38, 1549-1552.
Yvon, M.; Rijnen, L. *Int. Dairy J.* 2001, 11, 185-201.

In: Cheese: Types, Nutrition and Consumption
Editors: Richard D. Foster, pp. 221-245
ISBN 978-1-61209-828-9
©2011 Nova Science Publishers, Inc.

Chapter 12

ANTIHYPERTENSIVE PEPTIDES FOUND IN CHEESE

F. Javier Espejo, M. Carmen Almécija, Antonio Guadix, and Emilia M. Guadix

Department of Chemical Engineering, University of Granada, Spain

ABSTRACT

The production and ripening of cheese involves some biochemical transformations such as the proteolysis of caseins by enzymes associated to lactic acid bacteria. It has been found that these hydrolytic processes may promote the release of a significant amount of peptides with biological activity.

Among the bioactivities described in the scientific literature, peptides which inhibit the angiotensin converting enzyme (ACE) are highlighted because their potential health benefit for hypertension. ACE is a zinc metallopeptidase which converts a biologically inactive polypeptide, angiotensin I, to a potent vasoconstrictor, angiotensin II. Furthermore, ACE catalyses the degradation of bradykinin, a blood pressure lowering nonapeptide. By these actions, ACE raises blood pressure, and therefore, inhibition of this enzyme results in an antihypertensive effect.

In this chapter, it will be reviewed the presence and bioavailability of ACE-inhibitory peptides in a wide array of cheeses from different world regions, including some well-known types such as Cheddar, Mozzarella, Camembert or Manchego. The analytical techniques for quantification and purification of these peptides will be presented. Moreover, procedures for the determination of the antihypertensive effect will be explained for both in vitro and in vivo methods.

1. INTRODUCTION

Cheese is an important source of nutrients for humans. In general, cheese is rich in fat and casein (constituents of milk which are retained in the curd during manufacture) and it contains relatively small amounts of whey proteins, lactose and water-soluble vitamins.

In the last years, certain components with biological activity have been identified in food-protein (Kitts and Weiler, 2003; Pihlanto and Korhonen, 2003; Hartmann and Meisel, 2007).

These peptides present no biological activity when taking part of the protein structure. They must be released from the native protein to exert their biological effect. Bioactive peptides can be recovered from the protein source by three ways: digestive enzymes (such as pepsin, trypsin and chymotrypsin), fermentation with proteolytic starter cultures or proteolysis by enzymes derived from microorganisms or plants.

Milk proteins are an important source of bioactive peptides (Meisel and Schlimme, 1990; FitzGerald and Meisel, 2000; Clare and Swaisgood, 2000; Shah, 2000) such as antihypertensive, antithrombotic, opioid, immunostimulating, antimicrobial, mineral carrying and cholesterol-lowering peptides

In cheese, these bioactive peptides are generated during the ripening of cheese, when proteins are broken down by proteolytic enzymes into several products, ranging from large peptides to free amino acids. Proteolysis consists in a series of complex and sequential changes caused by proteases from different sources (Upadhyay et al., 2004):

a) The coagulant: depending on the type of coagulant used, the enzymes can be chymosin, pepsin, fungal acid proteases or plant acid proteases. The coagulant retained in cheese curd is a major contributor to proteolysis during ripening.
b) The milk: indigenous proteinases are present in milk, the most important of which is plasmin.
c) Starter lactic acid bacteria (LAB): The starter LAB contains a cell envelope-associated protease (CEE lactocepin, PrtP).
d) Non-starter lactic acid bacteria (NSLAB): Proteases and peptidases from the secondary microflora which grows during ripening.
e) Secondary starter: In many cheese varieties a secondary starter is added deliberately. These microorganisms possess potent enzyme activities.
f) Exogenous proteases and peptidases: mostly used for enzyme modified cheese to accelerate ripening, accentuate flavour or remove bitter compounds

In most of the cheese varieties, proteolysis process starts with casein hydrolysis by coagulant activity and by plasmin or other indigenous proteolytic enzymes. The, the large and intermediate-sized peptides generated in the first stage are hydrolysed by bacterial proteases and peptidases from the starter LAB, NSLAB and perhaps secondary microflora. As a result a large number of peptides of variable chain length are released from the protein (Rank et al., 1985; Upadhyay et al., 2004). The extension of the hydrolysis and the profile of the peptides depend on the cheese variety (Taborda et al., 2003).

The peptides generated during ripening are responsible for the flavour, taste and texture of cheese, but some of them have also some special properties. In some cheese varieties, not only peptides with antihypertensive activity have been reported, but also with antimicrobial or antioxidant activities (Dionysius et al., 2000; Haileselassie et al., 1999; Ong and Shah, 2008a; Gupta et al., 2009). These components provide an added value to cheese because, beyond the nutritional value, the intake of these cheeses with bioactive compounds could have health benefits. For this reason, the potential of distinct dietary peptide sequences to promote human health by reducing the risk of chronic diseases has aroused increasing scientific and commercial interest over the past decade (Hartmann and Meisel, 2007). In this context, this chapter is focused on peptides released from cheese proteins which have shown antihypertensive activity.

1.1. Angiotensin Converting Enzyme and Hypertension

Angiotensin-I-converting enzyme (ACE, also known as peptidyl-dipeptidase A or kininase II)) is a zinc- and chloride-dependent metallopeptidase that acts on a wide range of substrates, displaying both exopeptidase and endopeptidase activity (Sturrock et al., 2004). The primary activity of ACE is to cleave the C-terminal dipeptide of oligopeptide substrates with a wide specificity (Li et al., 2004). It is widely distributed in the body, predominantly as a membrane-bound ectoenzyme in vascular endothelial cells (Sibony et al., 1993).

Angiotensin converting enzyme plays a crucial role in the regulation of blood pressure because it takes part in two important biochemical pathways (Johnston and Franz 1992; Campbell 2003; Li et al., 2004). On the one hand, in the renin-angiotensin system, ACE cleaves the carboxyl terminal His-Leu dipeptide from the inactive decapeptide angiotensin I (Asp-Arg-Val-Tyr-Ile-His-Pro-Phe-His-Leu) transforming it into angiotensin II (Asp-Arg-Val-Tyr-Ile-His-Pro-Phe), an octapeptide with high pressor activity. Angiotensin II not only has vasoconstricting properties but also is involved in the release of a sodium-retaining steroid, aldosterone, from the adrenal cortex, which has a tendency to increase blood pressure. On the other hand, ACE promotes the degradation and inactivation of bradykinin in the the kallikrein-kinin system. Bradykinin is a blood pressure lowering nonapeptide which is transformed into an inactive heptapetide.

Due to these joint actions, inhibition of ACE is considered to be a useful target in the treatment of hypertension. Nowadays, synthetic angiotensin converting enzyme inhibitors like Captopril, Enalaprilat or Lisinopril are widely used to treat cardiovascular problems. Only in the USA, current annual antihypertensive drug costs are approximately $15 billion (Hong et al., 2008). However, the prolonged treatment with these drugs has some adverse side effects. For instance, 5 – 20% of patients exposed to antihypertensive drugs show dry cough. Nevertheless the worst side effect is angioedema (swellings caused by leakage from blood vessels) which affects only from 0.1-0.5% of patients but is life-threatening (Riordan, 2003). The peptides released from food proteins which exhibit ACE inhibitory activity could be an option to reduce the consumption of antihypertensive drugs.

1.2. Inhibition Mechanism and Inhibitory Peptides

Angiotensin converting enzyme has two homologous catalytic domains (N and C domain). The two domains differ in their substrate specificities and physiological functions (Wei et al., 1992). Indeed, in ACE inhibition studies with an ACE-N-selective inhibitor, the inhibition of N domain seems to have no effect on blood pressure regulation (Natesh et al., 2003; Pina and Roque, 2009). This suggests that the C-domain is the dominant angiotensin-converting site and the inhibition of C domain seems to be necessary and sufficient for controlling blood pressure and cardiovascular function (Natesh et al., 2003).

Li et al., (2004) reviewed the binding model proposed by some authors for the interaction between the substrates or competitive inhibitors and the active site of ACE. This model is based on the presumed analogy of ACE to other well characterized enzyme, the zinc metallopeptidase carboxypeptidase A. The model propose that ACE has three subsites (called S1, S1', and S2') that can potentially interact with the three C-terminal amino acids of peptide substrates or inhibitors. The zinc ion of ACE is located between subsites S1 and S1' and participates in the bond cleavage between antepenultimate and penultimate amino acid residues, releasing the C-terminal dipeptide.

Despite the interest on bioactive peptides as an alternative for the control of mild hypertension, the exact mode of interaction with ACE is not fully understood and is mainly supported by information derived from in vitro and in vivo ACE-inhibition studies (Pina and Roque, 2009). The structure-activity relationship of ACE inhibitory peptides from food proteins is not well deciphered. It is known that the binding to ACE is strongly influenced by the C-terminal tripeptide sequence. This tripeptide can interact with the subsites S_1, S_1' and S_2 from the active site of ACE, according to the model proposed before. This is confirmed by the fact that, when elongating the dipeptide with a certain amino acid from the N-terminal, the corresponding tripeptide has more potent inhibitory activity than dipeptide. Nevertheless, further elongation sometimes results in lower activity (Li et al., 2004).

It is possible to find some general characteristic of peptides with high inhibitor activity. According to the reviews by López-Fandiño et al., (2006), Li et al., (2004) and Hong et al., (2008) the main aspects in common are:

a) The relationship between peptide structure and activity indicates that the link to ACE is strongly influenced by the sequence of the C-terminal tripeptide. This sequence may interact with S1, S1 and S2 sites of active site of ACE, as is indicated by the previously proposed model.

b) The enzyme seems to have preference for substrates or inhibitors which have hydrophobic amino acids (aromatics or branched chain) in one of the last three C-terminal positions. Many studies have shown that dipeptides and tripeptides with high inhibitory activity contain tryptophan, phenylalanine, tyrosine and praline residues in their C-terminus as well as a branched aliphatic amino acid in the N-terminal. If a peptide has hydrophilic properties, generally have a low or zero activity, because it can not access to the active site of the enzyme. For example, ACE shows low affinity for substrates or competitive inhibitors with C-terminal dicarboxylic amino acids such as glutamic acid.

c) The ACE inhibitory peptides usually have 2–12 amino acids, although active peptides with up to 27 amino acids have been identified.

d) The structure-activity data suggest that a positive charge, such as lysine (amino-ε group) or arginine (guanidine group) in C-terminus contributes to raise the inhibitory power.

e) When there is a proline amino acid in the C-terminus, the inhibitory capacity is affected by the amino acid adjacent to the proline. To get a good inhibitory activity, it should be a hydrophobic amino acid.

f) ACE also shows high stereospecificity toward radicals of amino acids at the third position of the C-terminus. This radical must have a L configuration. By contrast, ACE shows a lower position stereospecificity in fourth position.

2. ACE-INHIBITORY ACTIVITY IN CHEESES

2.1. Sampling

Sampling is a key step in any analysis. The reliability of the results depends on how representative the sample is. The International Dairy Federation has published the standard procedures for sampling cheeses. Unless the entire cheese is sampled (when it is small enough), it is necessary to take samples from cheese for analysis. The apparatus for sampling most cheese varieties is the cheese trier, although a knife or a cutting wire can be used. According to International Dairy Federation (IDF, 1985), the first step to take the sample is to remove a shallow plug of cheese (15-20 mm deep), this will be the surface sample. Secondly, the trier is inserted in the hole generated previously to take the internal sample. The apparatus which is used in sampling cheese for determine ACE-inhibitory activity must be clean. Cheese samples should be stored at 0 - 4 °C until analysed. The samples must be analysed as soon as possible, preferably no later than 24 hours after sampling.

2.2. Extraction

After sampling, cheese peptides which are in the cheese matrix have to be extracted to analyse them. The extraction process consists of contacting cheese, usually grated, with a solvent in homogenisation equipment like a homogeniser or a stomacher. There are diverse methods to do this extraction using different solvents, contacting times or temperatures. These methods are not specific for ACE-inhibitory peptides extraction, they are used to determine the proteolysis extension and/or to characterise proteolytic products.

One of the most common methods consists in using water to extract the water-soluble fraction (WSE). Several researchers have developed different techniques to obtain water-soluble extracts of cheese using water as solvent (Rank et al., 1985). The optimisation of this process has been carried out by Kuchroo and Fox (1982) using Cheddar cheese. Homogenising grated cheese in water at a ratio of 1:2 (w/v) for 20 min at 20 °C, warming the slurry to 40 °C and holding for 1 h, followed by centrifugation to collect the supernatant liquid seems to be the most convenient and consistent method. This method extracted 70 % of the soluble nitrogen; higher yields could be achieved by repeating the procedure on the precipitate. This procedure and others similar ones have been used in a number of works, including studies about ACE inhibitory peptides from cheese (Smacchi and Gobbetti, 1998; Pritchard et al., 2010; Gómez-Ruiz et al., 2002).

Despite the methods which use water for extraction are similar, there are variations from one author to other. Lignitto et al., (2010) added an organic extraction step to eliminate the cheese fat, Ong et al., (2007) did not warm the slurry. Some authors used a high-powered and fast (short-time) homogenisation step (Ong and Shah, 2008a; Meyer et al., 2009; Saito et al., 2000). Several authors centrifuged the slurry at low temperature (4°C) (Ong and Shah, 2008a; Saito et al 2000) to separate the water-soluble fraction, which is located between the upper layer (fat) and the precipitate (casein).

After the centrifugation the extract is filtered through a filter to obtain a clear water soluble extract. Saito et al (2000) use a dialysis process using seamless cellulose tubing against distilled water for 24 h at 4°C. Tonouchi *et al.*, (2008) used a similar procedure but for 48 h.

After this initial extraction step, it is possible to fractionate the extract according to their molecular weight. The resulting fractions can be analysed separately. The separation can be done by ultrafiltration with different molecular weight cut-off filters (Kuchroo and Fox 1982; Lignitto *et al.*, 2010; Gómez-Ruiz *et al.*, 2006). The chemical fractionation is also possible, using an organic solvent such as ethanol (Haileselassie *et al.*, 1999; Pripp *et al.*, 2006).

Freeze-drying is usually used after the extraction step to increase the shelf life of extracts. They are stored at low temperature (-20 °C). By weighing after freeze-drying it is possible to know the concentration of peptides of the extract (Pritchard *et al.*, 2010).

Water extraction is the most common technique used by researchers for extracting ACE-inhibitory peptides. But using organic solvent is an appropriate technique for extract the more hydrophobic water-soluble components (Rank *et al.*, 1985). As mentioned above, ACE-inhibitors usually contain hydrophobic amino acid. More extraction methods were reviewed by McSweeney and Fox (1997).

2.3. Determination of ACE-Inhibitory Activity: In Vitro Assays

In vitro assays for the assessment of ACE inhibitory activity involve determining angiotensing converting enzyme activity. In these assays, ACE hydrolyses a synthetic tripeptide like hippuryl-L-histidiyl-L-leucyl (HHL) or N-[3-(2-Furyl)acryloyl]- L - phenylalanyl-glycyl-glycine (FAPGG) and the extension of the reaction is determined by spectrophotometric, radioisotopic or fluorometric methods (Vermeirssen *et al.*, 2004).

To express the inhibitor capacity, the half maximal inhibitory concentration (IC_{50}) is used, defined as inhibitor concentration causing a 50 % decrease in the activity of the enzyme. If it is considered that 100 % of enzyme activity corresponds to the activity obtained in the absence of inhibitor, the testing of various inhibitor concentrations can determined the concentration of inhibitor that produces 50% decrease ACE activity. Low IC_{50} values are indicative of a potent ACE inhibitor and a very small concentration of inhibitory substance is needed for decrease the activity of the enzyme. Other way to express inhibition is expressing it as a percentage of inhibition (IACE) of cheese extract. This is very useful when is not possible to reach enough concentration of inhibitor to produce a 50% decrease in the ACE activity.

Some authors consider that expressing bioactivity as inhibitory potential (IP) of cheese is more relevant for consumers than inhibition strength of an extract or a fraction isolated from cheese. According to Pripp *et al.*, (2006) the inhibitory potential (IP) of cheese can be expressed as:

$$IP = IC_{50captopril} \, E / IC_{50E}$$

where $IC_{50captopril}$ and IC_{50E} are the concentrations of captopril and extract from cheese (e.g. mg/mL), respectively, found to inhibit 50% of ACE activity in the assay, and E is the relative amount of extract (mg extract/g cheese).

The spectrophotometric methods present several advantages over other techniques (Holmquist *et al.*, 1979), so they are more widely used. Shalaby *et al.*, (2006) compared two in vitro spectrophotometric assays, using HHL and FAPGG as substrates. FAPGG has better properties than HHL, for instance it has high solubility, high stability and a Michaelis constant value 8 times smaller than that of HHL. Although in both assays the standard deviation for replicate samples was similar, the results of the two assays did not correlate for all samples. The IC_{50} value obtained for a given inhibitor varies according to the source of ACE or with the substrate used in the test (Vermeirssen et al., 2002). Therefore, to get comparable and reproducible results is critical to control the levels of ACE activity in the assay (Murray et al., 2004) as well as using reference substances, such as Captopril, with known blood pressure-lowering effects. Now, both the main assays for determining ACE inhibition and the inhibition values for different cheese varieties are detailed.

2.3.1. Spectrophotometric Assay with HHL

Cushman and Cheung (1971) proposed an in vitro assay for the determination of ACE inhibition using hippuryl-L-histidiyl-L-leucyl (HHL) as substrate. ACE hydrolyses the substrate to yield hippuric acid and histidyl-leucine. The hippuric acid (HA) produced is extracted with ethyl acetate and is quantified by measuring the absorbance of HA at 228 nm. The optimal conditions established using angiotensin-converting enzyme from rabbit lung acetone powder extract were as follows: pH from 8.1 to 8.3, 100mM potassium phosphate buffer with a chloride ion concentration of 300 mM, substrate concentration of 5-10 mM and ACE from 0 to 40 mU/mL. The enzyme is incubated with the substrate for 30 min. at 37 °C and the hydrolysis is stopped with HCl 1N. The hippuric acid produced is extracted with ethyl acetate. After ethyl acetate removal by evaporation, HA is redisolved in water. The amount of hippuric acid was measured at 228 nm against deionised water as blank. According to Cushman and Cheung (1971), the production of HA is linear for at least 30 min whether the concentration of ACE in reaction mixture is up to 12mU per assay. The amount of hippuric acid liberated from HHL under test conditions, but in the absence of an inhibitor, is defined as 100% ACE activity.

The percentage of inhibition (IACE) was calculated using the formula:

Inhibition = (A – B)/ (A - C) x 100

where A is the optical density at 228 nm with ACE but without WSE (Control), B is the optical density in the presence of both ACE and WSE (Inhibitor sample), and C is the optical density without ACE but with WSE (Sample without ACE). Each sample is tested at least in triplicate.

Several authors have done slight variations in this assay. Using 100 mM sodium borate as buffer (Ryhänen et al., 2001; Ong et al., 2007) or changing slightly concentration of enzyme and subtrate. The enzyme source can be either extract from rabbit lung acetone powder or purified ACE from rabbit lung. The powder is cheaper and gives similar results (Vermeirssen et al, 2002), but a previous preparation is required. This method has been used to determine ACE inhibitory activity in numerous of cheese varieties extract.

In Spanish cheeses (Table 1), Gómez-Ruiz et al. (2006) determined the inhibition percentages of WSE and of permeate generated by ultrafiltration of WSE through a membrane of 1000Da.

Table 1. ACE inhibition percentages in Spanish cheeses

Variety	WSE (%)	WSE < 1000 (%)
Idiazábal	87.5 + 2.5	68.6 + 2.4
Roncal	85.8 + 0.5	70.4 + 1.9
Mahón	76.8 + 5.6	56.6 + 4.6
Goat cheese	72.8 + 7.7	59.4 + 4.6
Cabrales	74.7 + 2.1	76.1 + 1.5
Manchego	70.6 + 1.5	65.3 + 2.0

Table 2. ACE inhibition percentages in seven cheese varieties

Variety	WSE (%)
Gouda (8 mo)	75.5
Gouda (24 mo)	78.2
Emmental	48.8
Blue	49.9
Camembert	69.1
Edam	56.2
Harvati	72.7

Several Italian cheeses varieties have been analysed searching for inhibitory peptides. Smacchi and Gobbetti (1998) analysed water-soluble peptides from Mozzarella, Italico, Crescenza, and Gorgonzola. Some fractions of the extracts show high ACE-inhibitory activity. The most active fractions in Mozzarella presented an IACE of 59 %, 82 % in Italico, only 34 % in Crescenda and 80 % in Gorgonzola. Other varieties such as Norvegia, Jarlsberg, Cheddar and Blue, present an inhibition values 75.5, 78.2, 48.8 and 49.9 respectively (Stepaniak et al., 2001).

Bütikofer et al., (2007) determined the inhibition of ACE in vitro of 44 traditional cheeses. The IC_{50} (per mg equivalent cheese per mL) ranged from 2 to 29.5. Subsequently, the water extracts of 7 Swiss cheeses were analysed by Meyer et al., (2009). The semi-hard cheeses Tilsiter, Appenzeller 1/4 fat, Tête de Moine, and Vacherin fribourgeois present an inhibition maximum around 70 % between 200 and 300 days of ripening. The extra-hard and hard cheeses Berner Hobelkäse, Gruyère, and Emmental have lower values (near to 50%). A similar inhibition value was determined for Emmental by Saito et al., (2000). However, in this study, the WSE was pre-treated by hydrophobic chromatography before the ACE assay to determine the inhibitory potential (Table 2).

Also for Gouda, Meisel et al., (1997) found that the highest inhibition activity was 70 % for medium ripening times. Parrot et al., (2003) determined a IC_{50} value of 27.6 ± 8.4 (mg equivalent cheese per mL) for Emmental cheese, which seems to be in agreement with the values reported by Saito et al., (2000), but differs slightly with Bütikofer et al., (2007). The low molecular weight fraction (WSE < 10kDa), presented a higher IC_{50} value (16 ± 8.1 mg equivalent cheese per mL). This can be explained assuming that proteins and/or large peptides do not inhibit ACE.

Okamoto et al., (1995) measured the ACE-inhibitory activity in various fermented foods. Among all investigated foods, the highest activity was obtained in Camembert and Red

Cheddar (0.16mg/mL). However, lower activity was found in Blue (0.27 mg/mL) cheese and none in Cottage cheese.

Apostolidis et al., (2007) studied the inhibitory potential of herb, fruit, and fungal-enriched cheese. It was tested on cheddar, feta, and Roquefort. Inhibition values were between 30 and 74 %. The highest ACE inhibitory activity was observed in plain (74 %) and herb-enriched (73 %) cheddar cheese as well as cranberry-enriched cheese (71 %). In other study, also with cheddar cheese, it was found an IC_{50} value of 0.28 mg/mL after 36 week of ripening (Ong et al., 2007).

With respect to cheeses with probiotics like Festivo cheese (Ryhänen et al., 2001), an IC_{50} of 44 ug/mL was measured in fractions of the water extract. The best IC_{50} value found in probiotic Cheddar cheese was 0.23 mg/mL (Ong et al., 2007) for cheese using *Lb casei* 279 after 24 week of ripening. In later study (Ong and Shah, 2008a) lower IC_{50} values were found in cheese with *Bifidobacterium longum* 1941, B. *animalis subsp. lactis* LAFTI® B94, *Lactobacillus casei* 279, *Lb. casei* LAFTI® L26, *Lb.acidophilus* 4962 and *Lb. acidophilus* LAFTI® L10. The IC_{50} values were between 0.15 and 0.2 mg/mL.

Spectrophotometric methods are used also to evaluate the bioactivity of isolated peptides from cheese. Tonouchi et al., (2008) used the Cushman and Cheung assay to determine the IC_{50} of two peptides from an enzyme modified cheese. LQP and MAP, having IC_{50}: 3.4 mM and 0.8 mM, respectively.

The method has some problems, firstly, it has many steps and a long incubation time is necessary to get a significant amount of product, what means that analysis times will be long. But the mayor drawback is the extraction step, because ethyl acetate can extract also the substrate HHL which absorbs strongly at 228nm (Cushman and Cheung, 1971; Wu et al., 2002) originating interferences.

In order to settle this last problem, some authors have introduced an important variation in the Cushman and Cheung method. The interference caused by HHL is avoided by using chromatography to separate hippuric acid from the reaction media instead of ethyl acetate extraction. Pritchard et al., (2010) analysed ACE inhibitory activity of three commercial Cheddar cheeses. The IC_{50} of cheeses extracts were between 0.05 and 0.15. Low molecular fraction of extract had better IC_{50} than original extract (without fractionating).

2.3.2. Spectrophotometric Assay with FAPGG

The assay for determine ACE activity proposed by Holmquist et al., (1979) is based on the hydrolysis of N-[3-(2-Furyl)acryloyl]- L -phenylalanyl-glycyl-glycine (FAPGG). It was adapted for inhibitory activity measurement (Vermeirssen et al., 2002). In this assay, ACE hydrolyses the substrate producing N-[3-(2-Furyl)acryloyl]-L-phenylalanyl (FAP) and the dipeptide glycyl-clycine (GG), which produce a decrease in absorbance. The use of the furanacryloyl blocking group as chromophoric monitor of substrate hydrolysis provides a simple way to measure ACE activity. The hydrolysis of FA-blocked tripeptides can be monitored in a wide range of substrate concentrations. However, to assess ACE activity with FAPGG as substrate it is needed that the concentration of FAPGG is higher than Michaelis-Menten constant (K_M = 0.3 mM). Under these conditions the reaction has a zero-order kinetic, therefore, the speed of the reaction is independent of substrate concentration and directly proportional to the enzyme concentration. In addition, the hydrolysis of the substrate is linear with the time for at least 15 % of the total reaction time.

Holmquist used a reaction media of 0.05 M buffer Tris-HCl with ion strength of 300 mM and pH 7.5. Later, the assay is standardised for determining ACE activity in serum. The measurement is performed at 37 °C, using wavelength of 340 nm which is the working wavelength (Harjanne, 1984).

The adapted method for determining ACE inhibitory activity (Vermeirssen et al., 2002) is basically the same than Holmquist et al. (1979), with the difference that the inhibitor in study is added to the reaction mixture at different concentrations. In the reaction vessel are introduced both the substrate (FAPGG) and the ACE inhibitor together with the reaction media. The buffer maintains an optimal pH and NaCl ensures the chlorides concentration that maximizes enzyme activity. Subsequently ACE is added and the hydrolysis starts, the reaction takes place at 37 °C.

The assay conditions vary from one author to another, but generally it is established at pH of 7.5-8.3 with Tris-HCl or borate buffer and 0.3 M NaCl(Cushman and Cheung, 1971; Holmquist et al., 1979). As in HHL assay, the enzyme source can be an extract from rabbit lung acetone powder or purified ACE from rabbit lung.

Absorbance is measured at 340 nm, showing a linear decrease with time to higher substrate concentrations 0.3 mM (Holmquist et al., 1979). This absorbance decline is related with the activity of the enzyme. Normally, measuring times do not excess beyond the first 30 min. The percentage of ACE inhibition is calculated from the ratio of the slope in the presence of inhibitor ($pA_{inhibitor}$) to the slope obtained in the absence of inhibitor ($pA_{control}$), according to the formula:

$$\text{Inhibition} = [1-(pA_{inhibitor}/pA_{control})] \times 100$$

Using this method, Pripp et al., (2006) determined the ACE inhibitory activity extracting the ethanol soluble fraction (ESF) of 8 cheeses. Among those studied were the traditional Norwegian cheeses Gamalost and Pultost, both made by heat precipitation of cultured skimmed milk. The other cheeses were Castello (a blue-mould cheese), French Brie, 3 and 9 months ripened Norvegia (a Norwegian Gouda-type cheese), Port Salut and Kesam (a Quarg-type cheese). All of them except Kesam presented IC_{50} ranged between 1.0 and 1.7 mg ESF/mL.

2.4. Factors Affecting ACE Inhibitory Activity

The ACE-inhibitory activity of cheese can be influenced by various factors. Milk pretreatment, cultures, scalding conditions, and ripening time were identified as the key factors influencing the concentration of these 2 naturally occurring bioactive peptides in cheese (Bütikofer et al., 2008). But other factors such milk origin or ripening temperature can be considered.

2.4.1. Time Ripening

Sampling cheese at different ripening times makes possible to follow the changes in ACE inhibitory activity during cheese ripening. ACE activity is determined with one of the methods described above. ACE-inhibitory peptides have usually less than 12 amino acids and to obtain this length an extensively proteolysis is needed. Long ripening times produce high degree of hydrolysis and small peptides which can present ACE-inhibitory activity. Studies on the ACE-inhibitory activity of cheese during ripening show that inhibitory activity increased as proteolysis progressed. In Cheddar cheese both with and without probiotics addition, ACE-inhibitory capacity increases with the time during first 24 weeks, after that it seems to stabilise until 36 weeks (Ong et al., 2007).

However the presence of ACE inhibitory peptides depends on a complex equilibrium between their formation and their degradation by enzymes involved in cheese ripening. It is common that ACE inhibitory activity enhance with the increasing of proteolysis index in ripened cheeses but it decreases when the proteolysis exceeds a certain level. Meisel et al., (1997) determined ACE inhibition of 70% in medium-aged Gouda cheese, whereas lower values were obtained in younger and older Gouda cheeses (51.8 and 34.6%, respectively). This was also observed in Festivo cheese (Ryhämen et al., 2001). ACE inhibition increased from 10% (6 weeks) to 50% after 13 weeks but finally decreased to 30% after 20 weeks. The same trend was found in a study with seven cheese varieties from Switzerland (Meyer et al., 2009). In this study, Tête de Moine, Vacherin fribourgeois, Appenzell, Tilsit, Emmental, Gruyère and Hobelkäse was studied during the period of commercial ripening. The concentration of ACE inhibiting peptides increased during the initial period of cheese ripening but started to decline when proteolysis exceeded a certain level. In this case, the lower inhibition values were associated not only with the ageing but also with the different manufacturing conditions. For Asiago cheese, a semi-hard variety from Italy, the inhibition activity seems descend when ripening time exceeds 6 weeks, but it is not affected by the cheese production system (Lignitto et al., 2010).

Gómez-Ruiz et al. (2002) observed in Manchego cheese that ACE inhibitory activity decreased during first 4 months, reaching the best IC_{50} value in 8-month-old Manchego cheese, the inhibitory activity for longer ripening times (12 months) was worse. In other study with Manchego cheese (Gómez-Ruiz et al., 2004a), it was found that cheese ripening do not follow any common pattern. These results suggest that there was not a linear correlation between ACE inhibitory capacity and the length of ripening. The same trend was described in Swiss cheeses (Bütikofer et al., 2008) since there was no general correlation between the degree of proteolysis and the amount of two powerful antihypertensive peptides (VPP and IPP).

Consequently, cheeses behave as a dynamic system where peptides are being constantly released, some of these peptides are subsequently hydrolyzed and others accumulate over the ripening process (Gómez-Ruiz et al., 2006).

2.4.2. Cheese Making Conditions

The ACE inhibitory activity found in different cheese varieties produced by different technologies is not very different. This seems to point that difference in protein and peptide breakdown due to different cheese technology between varieties may have limited influence on the ACE inhibition capacity of cheeses (Pripp et al., 2006). Lignitto et al., (2010) reached a similar conclusion after analysing the ACE inhibitory effect of WSE of Asiago cheese made with two different production systems. They concluded that the inhibitory peptides must be generated by the same mechanisms present in both cheese production systems.

a) Milk origin

Regarding milk origin, milk proteins from different species (cow, goat and ewe) generated almost similar ACE inhibitory peptides according to their amino acid sequences and the (Gómez- Ruiz et al., 2006). However, Silva et al., (2006) found that caprine cheese systems have higher IC_{50} than ovine cheese systems.

b) Heat treatment

Traditionally, all cheese was made from raw milk, nevertheless, heat treatment of cheese milk became widespread, primarily to ensure the safety of the milk supply and the final product via elimination of adventitious, pathogenic microflora (Hermier and Cerf, 2000). Silva et al., (2006) found that cheeselike systems obtained from raw milk have higher ACE inhibitory activity than those from sterilized milk. This difference is due to heat treatment of milk which causes that the coagulant retained in the curd is the mainly responsible for caseins breakdown. This may account for the differences in the peptide composition, between heat treated and raw milk, in which the microflora, mainly non-starter lactic acid bacteria, also plays an important role, especially in terms of secondary proteolysis. The same was described by Gómez-Ruiz et al., (2002), the highest values of the IC_{50}, and therefore the lowest ACE-inhibitory activity, corresponded to 4-months-aged raw-milk Manchego cheese. Another example is the lower concentration of three ACE-inhibitory peptides (VRYL, LPQNILP and DKIHPF) found in Manchego cheese made pasteurised-milk (Gómez-Ruiz et al., 2004a). In other study (Ong and Shah, 2008a) the concentrations of two potent ACE inhibitors (VPP and IPP) was determined in different cheese varieties. Concentrations of these peptides decreased with increasing heat treatment temperatures.

c) Temperature

The use of elevated ripening temperature has been reported to accelerate ripening by increasing the proteolysis of Cheddar cheese (Folkertsma et al., 1996). The effect of ripening temperature on the ACE inhibitory activity of Cheddar cheeses with probiotics as adjunt culture, had not significant effect in IC_{50} when increasing ripening temperature from 4°C to 8°C (Ong and Shah, 2008a) nor from 4°C to 12°C (Ong and Shah, 2008b).

d) Starter cultures

Gobbetti et al. (2004) suggest that the strain of lactic acid bacteria starter used is one of the main factors that influence the synthesis of hypotensive peptides in dairy products. Some authors have studied the use of probiotics in cheese starters. Probiotics seems to increase the rate of proteolysis. Ong et al. (2007), found that using *Lactobacillus casei* 279 or *Lb. casei* LAFTI® L26 in cheddar cheese the released of ACE inhibitory peptides was higher than the control (without probiotics) only during the first 24 week of ripening at 4°C. However, after this period of time there was not significant difference. In other study (Ong and Shah, 2008a) with using *Lactobacillus casei* 279, *Lb. casei* LAFTI® L26, and *Lb. acidophilus* LAFTI® L10, the same trends was identified. Cheeses made with the addition of *Lb. acidophilus* LAFTI® L10 had the highest ACE-inhibitory activity. The release of VPP and IPP is strongly related to the proteolytic properties of the strains present in the starter culture (Butikofer *et al.*, 2008). The presence of *Lactobacillus helveticus* in the starter culture was associated with elevated concentrations of VPP and IPP, which are potent inhibitory peptides (Meyer *et al.*, 2009). These peptides are more resistant to further degradation than others ACE-inhibitory peptides. However, more research on how different enzymes from starter organisms and process conditions influence on ACE-inhibitory peptides formation is needed (Pripp *et al.*, 2006).

3. PURIFICATION, IDENTIFICATION AND QUANTIFICATION

During ripening, milk proteins are broken down and a vast amount of peptides is generated. Some of them are responsible for ACE inhibitory activity. After certifying the inhibitory activity of the extracts with in vitro assays, it is interesting to know what concrete peptides have this property. To determine this, it is needed to isolate and identify the active peptides. The extract (WSE) from cheese can be fractionated and then separated in individual peptides using high-performance liquid chromatography (HPLC). To identify the bioactive peptides different mass spectrometry (MS) techniques are used in combination with HPLC. However, the number of possible active peptides is huge, so their isolation, identification and quantification are tasks that require considerable time and resources.

The analysis is generally developed by high-pressure liquid chromatography on a reverse-phase (RP-HPLC or RPC). This technique uses a non-polar stationary phase and an aqueous, moderately polar mobile phase. The stationary phase usually is built with compounds having a straight chain alkyl group such as $C_{18}H_{37}$ (C18 columns) or C_8H_{17} (C8 columns). With non polar stationary phases, retention time is longer for molecules which are more non-polar, while polar molecules elute faster. Retention time can be increased by adding more water (or polar solvent) to the mobile phase, thus the affinity of the hydrophobic peptides for the stationary phase will be stronger relative to the now more hydrophilic phase.

The C18 column is the most used stationary phase for analysing peptides in general and, of course, for cheese peptides. The mobile phase is usually formed by two solvent, a mixture water-TCA and a mixture acetonitrile-TCA, TFA can be used instead of TCA (Ryhänen *et al.*, 2001; Ong *et al.*, 2007). A normal flow rate can be 0.5 – 1 mL/min. Each author establishes what are the best operation conditions for his/her study, selecting water/TCA and acetonitrile/TCA ratios and choosing different operating gradients of solvent. For example, Gómez-Ruiz *et al.* (2006) uses firstly a linear gradient of acetonitrile-TCA which increase from 0 to 40% for 60 min, and then from 40 to 70% in 5 min. Instead of RP-HPLC, the reverse-phase fast protein liquid chromatography (RP-FPLC) can be used for the isolation of peptides (Smacchi and Gobbetti, 1998) using similar conditions.

At the outlet of the column there is a detector which monitors the absorbance at 214 nm, although some authors also monitor absorbance at 280 nm (Ryhänen *et al.*, 2001; Gómez-Ruiz *et al.*, 2006). After the column, a fraction collector can recover different peptide fractions on a basis of time either at regular intervals or at specific times to collect specific peaks. The elute fractions can be analysed to know their ACE inhibitory activity (Ong *et al.*, 2007) The fractions with highest inhibition value are usually subjected to further separation and purification by re-injecting them into RP-HPLC. Some times it is necessary to re-inject the fractions more than once (Haileselassie *et al.*, 1999; Smacchi and Gobbetti 1998). In order to obtain pure peptides, it is very important to establish an adequate operation condition (e.g. gradient of the solvents).

The isolated peptides from active WSE fractions have to be identified. They can be sequenced by an automated Edman degradation method, using a protein/peptide sequencer (Ryhänen et al., 2001; Ong et al., 2007). The Edman degradation sequentially removes one residue at a time from the amino end of a peptide. The peptide to be sequenced is adsorbed onto a solid surface. The Edman reagent, phenylisothiocyanate (PTC), is added together with a mildly basic buffer solution (e.g. 12% trimethylamine). PTC reacts with the uncharged terminal amino group of the peptide to form a phenylthiocarbamoyl derivative. Then, under mildly acidic conditions, a cyclic derivative of the terminal amino acid (thiazolinone derivative) is liberated, which leaves an intact peptide shortened by one amino acid. Once the amino acids are removed from the sample, they must be analyzed to determine their identity. Since the cleaved amino acid derivative is not generally suitable for analysis, it is converted to a more stable phenylthiohydantoin (PTH)-amino acid by extracting thiazolinone amino acid into organic solvent and treating it with acid. The PTH-amino acid derivative can be identified by chromatographic procedures. The Edman procedure can then be repeated on the shortened peptide, yielding another PTH-amino acid, which can again be identified by chromatography. This method is adequate for identifying peptides shorter than 50 amino acids due to the cyclical derivatization not always going to completion.

The molecular weight is always determined by mass spectrophotometry (MS). The main differences between one authors and others are in the ion source, in the mass analyzer and in the ion collection/detection system. On the one hand, some authors use this technique together with peptide sequencing. Ong et al. (2007) and Ong and Shah (2008a) use a matrix-assisted laser desorption/ionization time-of-flight mass spectrophotometry (MALDI-TOF-MS). Also, it is very usual to use system which combines chromatography and mass spectrophotometry. Tonouchi et al. (2008) use liquid chromatography in conjunction with MS. The column is connected to the MS which is equipped with quadrupole mass spectrometer using electrospray ion source with positive ion polarity mode. On the other hand, there are authors considering that identification of peptide components in complex protein hydrolysates in which the sequence of the precursor proteins are known, requires more information than just the masses of the peptides, but does not require complete sequencing of the peptide components (Gómez-Ruiz et al., 2004a). So the separation step (RP-HPLC) is usually combined with a tandem mass spectrometer (MS^n) in order to determine the molecular masses and the amino acid sequences of peptides.

Haileselassie et al. (1999) analysed the fractions collected after RP-HPLC. The fractions were dissolved and introduced into Atmospheric Pressure Ionization Mass Spectrometry (API-MS). Mass spectra were obtained in the positive mode on a triple stage mass spectrometer. Simple algorithms were used to correlate the charges produced by these compounds to their molecular masses. A similar LC-MS system was used by Lignitto et al. (2010). The mass spectrometer consisted of electrospray ionization in positive ion mode and single quadrupole analyzer. The most abundant peptides were identified according to their molecular weights and their significant fragment ions. The identified peptides were semiquantified by comparison with an internal standard (Phe–Phe). A HPLC-MS/MS technique was used by Gómez-Ruiz et al. (2006) to identify Manchego peptides. But the result for some peptides was not totally satisfactory, so they used of-line MS/MS to more accurate peptide identification. Bütikofer et al. (2007) and then Meyer et al. (2009) use a triple mass spectrometry (LC-MS^3) after the liquid chromatography to quantify VPP and IPP content. The application of this method allows the recording of specific fragments of these two peptides that can be used for quantification in case of limited chromatographic resolution of complex peptide mixtures. Oshawa *et al.* (2008), also quantify these peptides using liquid chromatography ion trap time of flight mass spectrometry (LCMS-IT-TOF), equipped with a RP-aqueous column. Finally, the origin of each peptide was determined from protein sequence analysis with a protein-data base.

Table 3. ACE inhibitory peptides identified in cheese

Peptide	Origin	Cheese
FP	Various fragments	Manchego[1], Idiazábal[1]
PP	Various fragments	Manchego[1], Roncal[1], Goat cheese[1], Cabrales[1]
QP	Various fragments	Manchego[1], Roncal[1], Goat cheese[1], Idiazábal[1]
IPP	β-CN (f 74–76)	Swiss cheeses[2]
LQP	β-CN f (88-90)	Enzyme modified cheese[3]
MAP	β-CN f (102-104)	Enzyme modified cheese[3]
PFP	Various fragments	Manchego[1]
RPK	αs_1-CN f(1-3)	Cheeselike system of goat milk[4]
VPP	β-CN (f84–86))	Swiss cheeses[2]
ERYL	αs_1-CN f(89-92)	Manchego (8month)[5]
PKHP	αs_1-CN f(4-7)	Roncal[1]
VPQL	αs_1-CN f(106-109)	Manchego (8month)[5]
VRGP	β-CN f(201-204)	Goat cheese[1]
VRYL	αs_2-CN f(205-208)	Manchego (8month)[5]
YQEP	β-CN f(191-119)	Cheeselike system of ovine milk[4], Cheeselike system of goat milk[4]
DKIHP	β-CN f(47-51)	Manchego[1], Roncal[1], Goat cheese[1], Cabrales[1], Idiazábal[1]
VPKVK	β-CN f(95-99)	Cheeselike system of ovine milk[4], Cheeselike system of goat milk[4]
DKIHPF	β-CN f(47-52)	Manchego[1], Manchego (8month)[5] Roncal[1], Goat cheese[1], Cabrales[1], Idiazábal[1], Cheddar (with Lb. Casei LAFTI 26)[6]
RPKHPI	αs_1-CN f(1-6)	Festivo[7], Cheddar (with Lb. Casei LAFTI 26)[6], Cheddar (with Lb. Casei LAFTI 10)[8]
ARHPHPH	κ-CN (f96-102)	Cheddar (with Lb. Casei LAFTI 10)[8]
KHPIKHQ	αs_1-CN f(3-9)	Manchego (8month)[5]
LPQNILP	β-CN f(70-76)	Manchego (8month)[5]
RPKHPIK	αs_1-CN f(1-7)	Festivo[7], Cheddar (with Lb. Casei LAFTI 26)[6], Cheddar (with Lb. Casei LAFTI 10)[8]
VPSERYL	αs_1-CN f(86-92)	Manchego (8month)[5]
YQKFPQY	αs_2-CN f(90-96)	Cheeselike system of goat milk[4]
DVPSERYL	αs_1-CN f(85-92)	Manchego (8month)[5]

Table 3. (continued)

Peptide	Origin	Cheese
KHPIKHQG	αs_1-CN f(3-10)	Manchego (8month)[5]
KKYNVPQL	αs_1-CN f(102-109)	Manchego (8month)[5]
RPKHPIKH	αs_1-CN f(1-8)	Cheeselike system of goat milk[4]
YQEPVLGP	β-CN f(191-198)	Cheeselike system of ovine milk[4], Cheeselike system of goat milk[4]
EDVPSERYL	αs_1-CN f(84-92)	Manchego (8month)[5]
FVAPFPEVF	αs_1-CN f(24-32)	Cheddar (with Lb. Casei LAFTI 26)[6], Cheddar (with Lb. Casei LAFTI 10)[8]
KKYKVPQLE	αs_1-CN f(102-110)	Cheddar (with Lb. Casei LAFTI 26)[6]
RPKHPIKHQ	αs_1-CN f(1-9)	Festivo[7], Cheddar (with Lb. Casei LAFTI 26)[6], Cheddar (with Lb. Casei LAFTI 10)[8], Gouda (8 month)[9]
YPFPGPIPN	β-CN f(60–68)	Gouda (8 month)[9], Manchego (8month)[5]
KEDVPSERYL	αs_1-CN f(83-92)	Manchego (8month)[5]
RPKHPIKHQG	αs_1-CN f(1-10)	Manchego (8month)[5]
MPFPKYPVQPF	β-CN f(114-119)	Gouda (8 month)[9]
RPKHPIKHQGLPQ	αs_1-CN (f 1-13)	Gouda (8 month)[9]
LVYPFPGPIHNSLPQ	β-CN f(58-72)	Crescenza[10]
YQEPVLGPVRGPFPIIV	β-CN f(193-209)	Cheddar (with Lb. Casei LAFTI 26)[6]
YQEPVLGPVRGPFPIIV	β-CN f(193-209)	Cheddar (with Lb. Casei LAFTI 10)[8]

[1] Gómez-Ruiz et al. (2006); [2] Butikofer et al. (2008); [3] Tonouchi et al. (2008); [4] Silva et al. (2006); [5] Gómez-Ruiz et al.(2004a); [6] Ong et al. (2007); [7] Rÿhanen et al. (2003); [8] Ong and Shah (2008a); [9] Saito et al. (2000); [10] Smacchi and Gobbetti (1998)

After all purification steps, final fractions often still contain multiple compounds that can cause a discrepancy between the activity found in the purified fractions and the activity of the individual chemically synthesised peptides (Gómez-Ruiz et al., 2002). To determine the IC_{50} values in ACE inhibitory activity and antihypertensive effects in vivo, the peptides must be chemically synthesized according to information obtained from structural analyses.

A number of peptides with ACE-inhibitory activity have been identified in cheeses (Gómez-Ruiz et al., 2004a). In Table 3, only peptides with an IC_{50} lower than 300 uM are shown.

4. BIOAVAILABILITY

The ACE inhibitory potential of these peptides is not always related to its antihypertensive effect. Some peptides, known to exhibit a great in vitro ACE inhibitory activity do not possess any activity after oral or intravenous administration. For instance, αs_1-casein f(23-27), a potent ACE inhibitor in vitro, was shown to have no hypotensive effect in vivo (Maruyama et al., 1987)

Physiological effects of bioactive peptides depend on their ability to maintain their activity until reaching their targets, which can be modified during the digestive hydrolysis and their absorption through the intestinal epithelium until entering the blood stream. There are three stages able to alter the bioavailability of ACE inhibitory peptides: the gastrointestinal digestion, intestinal absorption and blood enzymes (Vermeirssen et al., 2004).

Research on gastrointestinal digestion of milk proteins or polypeptides, as well as the resistance against digestion of some sequences of known inhibitory activity has been performed by several in vitro tests. In theses assays, the gastrointestinal digestion has been simulated by two consecutive hydrolysis stages employing pepsine and pancreatic enzymes (tripsine, quimotripsine, carboxi and aminopeptidase), respectively. These studies conclude that gastrointestinal digestion is a key factor determining the ACE inhibitory activity of these molecules (López-Fandiño et al., 2006), since some active peptides lost their inhibitory activity after the protein hydrolysis and others which initially were inactive developed ACE inhibitory activity after the digestion. To this regard, it was reported that inhibitory peptides where Proline is placed at C-terminal position, are normally more resistant to enzyme degradation. Tripeptides containing the Proline-Proline sequence at C-terminal position are reported to be resistant to Proline specific peptidases (FitzGerald and Meisel, 2000). Therefore, there is evidence that orally supplied di- and tri-peptides containing Proline, which originally exhibited in vitro antihypertensive activity, remained stable after digestion and thus conserved their original activity after intestinal absorption. This assumption has been proved by several in vivo tests where the oral administration of these peptides, especially di- and tri-peptides, even at low doses, resulted in hipotensive effects (Li et al., 2004).

During digestion, peptides will be hydrolysed not only by gastrointestinal enzymes but also by the brush-border peptidases on intestinal epithelial cells. The human colonic carcinoma cell line Caco-2 has the ability to differentiate into enterocyte-like cells that express several characteristic features of mature small intestinal cells (Hidalgo et al., 1989). Caco-2 cells form monolayers with tight junctions and express brush-border enzymes including peptidases. These cells provide a good in vitro model for the digestion of peptides. (Howell et al., 1992). Another factor limiting the bio-availability of peptides is their stability in the blood stream. Peptides must be resistant to the enzymes present in blood, including the ACE itself, which could hydrolyse the inhibitory peptides (Vermeirssen et al., 2004).

According to the modification of the inhibitory capacity by gastrointestinal enzymes or ACE and other enzymes contained in the blood stream, inhibitory peptides fall into three groups (Fujita et al., 2000):

a) Inhibitor type peptides: those whose inhibitory capacity remains unchanged after gastrointestinal digestion or blood transport.
b) Substrate type peptides: those which are hydrolysed by ACE or gastrointestinal enzymes, giving rise to peptides with lower inhibitory power.
c) Proinhibitor type: those which acquire ACE inhibitory activity after hydrolysis by ACE or gastrointestinal enzymes.

Bioavailability studies on cheese involve submitting cheese extracts to assays which recreate the hydrolysis reaction that occur during digestion. If a peptide from the cheese has been previously isolated and identified, it can be synthesized and used for the assays instead of cheese extract.

Parrot et al., (2003), proposed a in vitro enzymatic digestion protocol for peptides from dairy products. The method involves the hydrolysis of water soluble extract (WSE) with gastrointestinal enzymes. The Ace-inhibitory activity is measured before and after the hydrolysis. In the study found that IC_{50} value of Emmental WSE decrease round 32-33 % after digestion by pepsin and trypsin or by pepsin and pancreatin. The same result was found when the proteins and large peptides are release by ultrafiltration from the WSE (<10kDa). Gastrointestinal digestion causes an increase from 16 to 25 (mg equivalent cheese per mL). This decrease in inhibitory activity is due to the hydrolysis of substrate type peptides.

In a study with Manchego cheese, several ACE-inhibitory peptides were identified (Gómez-Ruiz et al., 2004a). Subsequently, eleven of these peptides were synthesized and subjected to a simulated digestion with pepsine, trypsin and chymotrypsin (Gómez-Ruiz et al., 2004b). ACE inhibition was measured before and after digestion, the fragments released during the process were identified. As a result of the reactions, some of the peptides were hydrolysed loosing inhibitory power, however, others such a TQPKTNAIPY increased its ACE-inhibitory activity. Its IC_{50} changed from 4.22 to 0.66 (mg/mL), some of the peptides generated from TQPKTNAIPY were TNAIPY (IC_{50}= 2.52 mg/mL) and TNAIP which contains proline as the C-terminal amino acid, It is known that the presence of proline makes amino acid sequences less susceptible to proteolytic enzymes. Four peptides remained intact after simulated digestion, the short peptides FP and IPY, but also two peptides of 6 amino acid residues (VRGPGP and LEIVPK). Interestingly, all of them contain proline either at the last C-terminal position or at the penultimate position.

In Lignitto et al., (2010), it was found that the low molecular weight (<3kD) compounds found in Asiago d'allevo cheese do not modify their inhibition activity after simulated gastrointestinal digestion, moreover, the digestion of bigger compounds (<10kD) seems to enhance their inhibitory capacity. A true inhibitor was found in an enzyme modified cheese (Tonouchi et al., 2008). The IC_{50} value of MET-ALA-PRO was affected neither by digestive enzymes nor by pre-incubation with ACE. The antihypertensive peptides, VPP and IPP, have been identified in several cheeses (Butikofer et al., 2008). These peptides are highly resistant to the hydrolysis of gastrointestinal enzymes and as well as bush-border enzymes (including ACE) (Ohsawa et al., 2008).

5. IN VIVO ASSAYS FOR THE ANTIHYPERTENSIVE EFFECT

As commented above, a peptide possessing a high in vitro ACE inhibitory potential does not necessarily conserve its antihypertensive properties after an in vivo essay, owing to the physiological transformations which this peptide may undertake during its digestion and intestinal absorption (Vermeirssen *et al.*, 2004). Only a reduced number among all the peptides known to exhibit in vitro ACE inhibitory activity has been tested on animal or human subjects (Saito, 2008; FitzGerald *et al.*, 2004).

In vivo inhibitory activity of peptides is usually tested in spontaneously hypertensive rats (SHR), which are considered as a good model of human hypertension. In many cases, the results of these tests highlight the differences between the in vitro activity of a given peptide and its corresponding in vivo effects (FitzGerald *et al.*, 2004). In vivo tests permit to differentiate the ACE inhibitors from antihypertensive peptides (Saito, 2008). Tests on human subjects are the last step to validate the antihypertensive activity of a given peptide. Studies on rats are conducted under controlled conditions of temperature, moisture and feeding. The sample can be a cheese extract or an isolated peptide, which is normally, administrated dissolved into matrix, which may consist in a saline solution. Three types of rats are considered for the tests:

a) Positive control group, whose individuals are supplied with a drug known to cause an antihypertensive effect, such as captopril.
b) Negative control group, which is supplied with the matrix deprived of the antihypertensive compounds.
c) Study group, exposed to the peptide or peptic fraction of interest.

The effect of antihypertensive peptides can be tested on Wistar-Kyoto rats (WKY), which are rats with normal values for the arterial tension. In this case, only two groups are considered: a negative control group and a study group. These studies are carried out to know how antihypertensive peptides affect to population without hypertension. Regarding the time trends and prevalence of the effects, some studies may be focused on the short term effects, where the rats are fed with a desired peptide and dose, and the arterial pressure is measured before administration and after 2, 4, 6 and 8 hours. When the antihypertensive effects are studied in a long term, the rats are fed with the inhibitory peptide during several days, normally at a fixed hour, and the arterial pressure is registered throughout the considered period. In some occasions, the animal has to be sacrificed after the intake of the desired peptide. This permits to determine the level of antihypertensive peptides and the activity of ACE converting enzyme in different organs, such as the aorta, lungs, kidneys, heart and brain (Masuda *et al.*, 1996).

In cheeses, Saito *et al.*, (2000) studied the antihypertensive effect of Gouda cheese in SHR. The sample was a solution of 1 mg/mL of distilled water using a dosage of 6.1 to 7.5 mg/kg of body weight. The systolic blood pressure (SBP) was measured before and after 6 hour of oral administration (by gastric intubation). They found that Gouda (8 months), Blue, Edam and Havarti originated a significant decrease in SBP (mmHg). The strongest antihypertensive effect was observed in Gouda (8 months) which reduce 24.7 ± 0.3 mm Hg the blood pressure.

In an enzyme modified cheese, a tripeptide (MAP) with ACE-inhibitory activity was identified. After being synthesized, its antihypertensive activity in vivo was studied (Tonouchi *et al.*, 2008). The dosage applied was 3 mg peptide/kg and SBP was measured before and 4 and 8 hour after oral administration. The decrease in blood pressure was significant at 8h, the peptide reduced SBP in 17 mm Hg.

Studies with dogs were carried out by Isea and Villalobos (1999). They studied the antihypertensive effect of the water extract of Manchego cheese on the arterial blood pressure of five dogs. The dogs were kept under known food administration for twenty days, previous to the experiment. The extracts at different doses were administrated through the femoral vein and blood pressure was measured with a manometer. The result pointed to a significant blood pressure diminution after cheese extract administration.

Regarding human test, many tests conducted on human subjects have shown a decrease in the blood pressure after the intake of some milk protein hydrolysates or lacto-fermented products. A complete review covering the main in vivo antihypertensive tests on human subjects is given by Korhonen (2009).

Two peptides, VPP and IPP, first isolated from *Lactobacillus helveticus* fermented milk (Nakamura *et al.*, 1995a) have been identified in several Swiss cheeses (Bütikofer *et al.*, 2008, 2007). The concentration of these peptides is similar to those found in fermented milk products with blood pressure lowering properties. The antihypertensive effect in vivo of VPP and IPP has been proved in this fermented milk product using spontaneously hypertensive rats (Nakamura *et al.*, 1995b; Masuda *et al.*, 1996). But also in human studies, where a dose dependent blood pressure lowering effect of the two tripeptides IPP and VPP has been proven (Hata *et al.*, 1996; Seppo *et al.*, 2003). These tests consist in placebo-controlled studies intended to observe the effect of supplementation of antihypertensive peptides on hypertensive individuals. One group was fed with a lacto-fermented product supplemented with the peptides of interest, while the other group was supplied with a similar product deprived of the active compounds. The blood pressure is monitored during several weeks, as well as the appearance of possible side effects. This study can also be conducted on healthy individuals, with the aim to study the effects of these peptides on their diet.

REFERENCES

Apostolidis, E., Y.-I. Kwon and K. Shetty (2007). Inhibitory potential of herb, fruit, and fungal-enriched cheese against key enzymes linked to type 2 diabetes and hypertension. *Innovative Food Science and Emerging Technologies* 8, 46–54.

Bütikofer, U., J. Meyer, R. Sieber and D. Wechsler (2007). Quantification of the angiotensin-converting enzyme-inhibiting tripeptides Val-Pro-Pro and Ile-Pro-Pro in hard, semi-hard and soft cheeses. *International Dairy Journal* 17, 968–975.

Bütikofer, U., J. Meyer, R. Sieber, B. Walther and D. Wechsler (2008). Occurrence of the Angiotensin-Converting Enzyme–Inhibiting Tripeptides Val-Pro-Pro and Ile-Pro-Pro in Different Cheese Varieties of Swiss Origin. *Journal of Dairy Science* 91, 29–38.

Campbell, D.J. (2003). The renin-angiotensin and the kallikrein-kinin systems. *The International Journal of Biochemistry and Cell Biology* 35, 784-791.

Clare, D.A. and H.E. Swaisgood (2000). Bioactive milk peptides: A prospectus. *Journal of Dairy Science*, 83, 1187-1195.

Cushman, D.W. and H.S. Cheung (1971). Spectrophotometric assay and properties of the angiotensin-converting enzyme of rabbit lung. *Biochemical Pharmacology* 20, 1637-1648.

Dionysius, D.A., R.J. Marschke, A.J. Wood, J. Milne, T.R. Beattie, H. Jiang, T. Treloar, P.F. Alewood and P.A. Grieve (2000). Identification of physiologically functional peptides in dairy products. *The Australian Journal of Dairy Technology* 55, 103.

FitzGerald, R.J. and H. Meisel (2000). Milk protein-derived peptide inhibitors of angiotensin-I-converting enzyme. *British Journal of Nutrition* 84, S33-S37.

FitzGerald, R.J., B.A. Murray and D.J. Walsh (2004). Hypotensive peptides from milk proteins. *Journal of Nutrition* 134, 980S-988S.

Folkertsma, B., P.F. Fox and P.L.H. McSweeney (1996). Accelerated ripening of Cheddar cheese at elevated temperatures. *International Dairy Journal* 6, 1117-1134.

Fujita, H., K. Yokohama and M. Yoshikawa (2000). Classification and Antihypertensive Activity of Angiotensin I-Converting Enzyme Inhibitory Peptides Derived from Food Proteins. *Journal of Food Science* 65, 564-569.

Gobbetti, M., F. Minervini and C.G. Rizzello (2004). Angiotensin I-converting-enzyme-inhibitory and antimicrobial bioactive peptides. *International Journal of Dairy Technology* 57, 173-188.

Gómez-Ruiz, J.A., M. Ramos and I. Recio (2002). Angiotensin-converting enzyme-inhibitory peptides in Manchego cheeses manufactured with different starter cultures. *International Dairy Journal* 12, 697–706.

Gómez-Ruiz, J.A., M. Ramos and I. Recio (2004a). Identification and formation of angiotensin-converting enzyme-inhibitory peptides in Manchego cheese by high-performance liquid chromatography–tandem mass spectrometry. *Journal of Chromatography A* 1054, 269–277.

Gómez-Ruiz, J., M. Ramos and I. Recio (2004b). Angiotensin converting enzyme-inhibitory activity of peptides isolated from Manchego cheese. Stability under simulated gastrointestinal digestion. *International Dairy Journal* 14, 1075–1080.

Gómez-Ruiz, J.A., G. Taborda, L. Amigo, I. Recio and M. Ramos (2006). Identification of ACE-inhibitory peptides in different Spanish cheeses by tandem mass spectrometry. *European Food Research and Technology* 223, 595–601.

Gupta, A., B. Mann, R. Kumar and R.B. Sangwan (2009). Antioxidant activity of Cheddar cheeses at different stages of ripening. *International Journal of Dairy Technology* 63, 339–347.

Haileselassie, S. S., B. H. Lee and B. F. Gibbs (1999). Purification and Identification of Potentially Bioactive Peptides from Enzyme-Modified Cheese. *Journal of Dairy Science* 82, 1612–1617.

Harjanne, A. (1984). Automated kinetic determination of angiotensin-converting enzyme in serum. *Clinical Chemistry* 30, 901-902.

Hartmann, R. and H. Meisel (2007). Food-derived peptides with biological activity: From research to food applications. *Current Opinion in Biotechnology* 18, 1–7.

Hata, Y., M. Yamamoto, M. Ohni, K. Nakajima, Y. Nakamura and T. Takano (1996). A placebo-controlled study of the effect of sour milk on blood pressure in hypertensive subjects. *American Journal of Clinical Nutrition* 64, 767-771.

Hermier, J. and O. Cerf (2000). Heat treatments. Pages 239–254 in *Cheesemaking—From Science to Quality Assurance*. A. Eck and J.C. Gillis, ed. Lavoisier, Paris, France.

Hidalgo, I.J., T.J. Raub and R.T. Borchardt (1989). Characterization of the human colon carcinoma cell line (Caco-2) as a model system for intestinal epithelial permeability. *Gastroenterology* 96, 736–749.

Holmquist, B., P. Bünning and J.F. Riordan (1979). A continuous spectrophotometric assay for angiotensin converting enzyme. *Analytical Biochemistry* 95, 540-548.

Hong, F., L. Ming, S. Yi, L. Zhanxia, W. Yongquan and L. Chi (2008). The antihypertensive effect of peptides: A novel alternative to drugs? *Peptides* 29, 1062-1071.

Howell, S., A.J. Kenny and A.J. Turner (1992). A survey of membrane peptidases in two human colonic cell lines, Caco-2 and HT-29. *Biochemical Journal* 284, 595–601.

International Dairy federation (1985). Milk and milk products. *Methods of sampling* (Standard 50B).

Isea, G. and J. Villalobos (1999). *Effect of the Aqueos Extract of Manchego Cheese on the Dog Arterial Blood Pressure*. Revista Cientifica de la Facultad de Ciencias Veterinarias de la Universidad del Zulia 9, 231-234.

Johnston, J.I. and V.L. Franz (1992). Renin-angiotensin system: a dual tissue and hormonal system for cardiovascular control. *J Hypertens* 10, 13–26.

Kitts, D.D. and K. Weiler (2003). Bioactive proteins and peptides from food sources. Applications of bioprocesses used in isolation and recovery. *Current Pharmaceutical Design* 9, 1309–1323.

Korhonen, H.J. (2009). Bioactive milk proteins and peptides: From science to functional applications, *The Australian Journal of Dairy Technology* 64, 16–25.

Kuchroo, C. N. and P. F. Fox (1982). Soluble nitrogen in Cheddar cheese. *Comparison of extraction procedures*. Milchwissenschaft 37:331.

Li, G.-H., G-W Le, Y-H Shi and S. Shresthaa (2004). Angiotensin I converting enzyme inhibitory peptides derived from food proteins and their physiological and pharmacological effects. *Nutrition Research* 24, 469-486.

Lignitto, L., V. Cavatorta, S. Balzan, G. Gabai, G. Galaverna, E. Novelli, S. Sforza and S. Segato (2010). Angiotensin-converting enzyme inhibitory activity of water-soluble extracts of Asiago d'allevo cheese. *International Dairy Journal* 20, 11–17.

López-Fandiño, R., J. Otte and J. van Camp (2006). Physiological, chemical and technological aspects of milk-protein-derived peptides with antihypertensive and ACE-inhibitory activity. *International Dairy Journal* 16, 1277-1293.

Maruyama, S., H. Mitachi, J. Awaya, M. Kurono, N. Tomizika and H. Suzuki (1987). Angiotensin I converting enzyme inhibitory activity of the C-terminal hexapeptide of α_s s1-casein. *Agricultural Biological Chemistry* 51, 2557-2561.

Masuda, O., Y. Nakamura and T. Takano (1996). Antihypertensive peptides are present in aorta after oral administration of sour milk containing these peptides to spontaneously hypertensive rats. *Journal of Nutrition* 126, 3063-3068.

McSweeney, P.L.H. and P.F. Fox (1997). Chemical methods for the characterization of proteolysis in cheese during ripening. *Lait* 77, 41-76.

Meisel, H. and E. Schlimme (1990). Milk proteins: precursors of bioactive peptides. *Trends in Food Science and Technology* 1, 41- 43.

Meisel, H., A. Goepfert and S. Günther (1997). *ACE-inhibitory activities in milk products.* Milchwissenschaft 52, 307-311.

Meyer, J., U. Bütikofer, B. Walther, D. Wechsler and R. Sieber (2009). Changes in angiotensin-converting enzyme inhibition and concentrations of the tripeptides Val-Pro-Pro and Ile-Pro-Pro during ripening of different Swiss cheese varieties. *Journal of Dairy Science* 92, 826–836.

Murray, B.A., D.J. Walsh and R.J. FitzGerald (2004). Modification of the furanacryloyl-Lphenylalanylglycylglycine assay for determination of angiotensin-I-converting enzyme inhibitory activity. *Journal of Biochemical and Biophysical Methods* 59, 127-137.

Nakamura, Y., N. Yamamoto, K. Sakai, A. Okubo, S. Yamazaki and T. Takano (1995a). Purification and characterization of angiotensina I-converting enzyme inhibitors from sour milk. *Journal of Dairy Science* 78, 777-783.

Nakamura, Y., N. Yamamoto, K. Sakai and T. Takano. (1995b). Antihypertensive effect of sour milk and peptides isolated from it that are inhibitors to angiotensin I-converting enzyme. *Journal of Dairy Science* 78, 1253-1257.

Natesh, R., S.L.U. Schwager, ED. Sturrock and K.R. Acharya (2003). Crystal structure of the human angiotensin-converting enzyme–lisinopril complex. *Nature* 421, 551-554.

Ohsawa, K., H. Satsu, K. Ohki, M. Enjoh, T. Takano and M. Shimizu (2008). Producibility and Digestibility of Antihypertensive ☐-Casein Tripeptides, Val-Pro-Pro and Ile-Pro-Pro, in the Gastrointestinal Tract: Analyses Using an in Vitro Model of Mammalian Gastrointestinal Digestion. *Journal of Agricultural and Food Chemistry* 56, 854–858.

Okamoto, A., H. Hanagata, E. Matsumoto, Y. Kawamura, Y. Koizumi and F. Yanagida (1995). Angiotensin-converting enzyme inhibitory activities of various fermented foods, *Bioscience, Biotechnology, and Biochemistry* 59, 1147–1149.

Ong, L., A. Henriksson and N.P.Shah (2007). Angiotensin converting enzyme-inhibitory activity in Cheddar cheeses made with the addition of probiotic Lactobacillus casei sp. *Dairy Science and Technology* (Lait) 87,149–165.

Ong, L. and N.P. Shah (2008a).Release and identification of angiotensin-converting enzyme-inhibitory peptides as influenced by ripening temperatures and probiotic adjuncts in Cheddar cheeses. *Food Science and Technology* 41, 1555-1566.

Ong, L. and N.P. Shah (2008b). Influence of Probiotic Lactobacillus acidophilus and L. helveticus on Proteolysis, Organic Acid Profiles, and ACE-Inhibitory Activity of cheddar Cheeses Ripened at 4, 8, and 12 °C. *Journal of Food Science* 73, 111-120.

Parrot, S., P. Degraeve, C. Curia and A. Martial-Gros (2003). In vitro study on digestion of peptides in Emmental cheese: Analytical evaluation and influence on angiotensin I converting enzyme inhibitory peptides. *Nahrung/Food* 47, 87 – 94.

Pihlanto, A. and H. Korhonen (2003). Bioactive peptides and proteins. *Advances in Food and Nutrition Research* 47, 175–276.

Pina, A.S. and A.C.A. Roque (2009). Studies on the molecular recognition between bioactive peptides and angiotensinconverting enzyme. *Journal of Molecular Recognition* 22, 162-168.

Pripp, A.H., R. Sørensen, L. Stepaniak and T. Sørhaug (2006). Relationship between proteolysis and angiotensin-I-converting enzyme inhibition in different cheeses. *Food Science and Technology* 39, 677–683.

Pritchard, S.R., M. Phillips and K. Kailasapathy (2010). Identification of bioactive peptides in commercial Cheddar cheese. *Food Research International* 43, 1545–1548

Rank, T.C., R. Grappin and N.F. Olson (1985). Secondary proteolysis of cheese during ripening. A review, *Journal of Dairy Science* 68, 801– 805.

Riordan, J.F. (2003). Angiotensin-I-converting enzyme and its relatives. *Genome Biology* 4, 225.

Ryhänen, E.L., A. Pihlanto-Leppälä and E. Pahkala (2001). A new type of ripened, low-fat cheese with bioactive properties. *International Dairy Journal* 11, 441–447.

Saito, T. (2008). Antihypertensive Peptides Derived from Bovine Casein and Whey Proteins. *Advances in Experimental Medicine and Biology* 606, 295-317.

Saito, T., T. Nakamura, H. Kitazawa, Y. Kawai and T. Itoh (2000). Isolation and Structural Analysis of Antihypertensive Peptides That Exist Naturally in Gouda Cheese. *Journal of Dairy Science* 83, 1434-1440.

Seppo, L., T. Jauhiainen, T. Poussa and R. Korpela (2003). A fermented milk high in bioactive peptides has a blood pressure-lowering effect in hypertensive subjects. *American Journal of Clinical Nutrition* 77, 326-330.

Shah, N.P. (2000). Effects of milk-derived bioactives: an overview. *British Journal of Nutrition* 84, S3– S10.

Shalaby, S.M., M. Zakora and J. Otte (2006). Performance of two commonly used angiotensinconverting enzyme inhibition assays using FA-PGG and HHL as substrates. *Journal of Dairy Research* 73, 178-186.

Sibony, M., JM. Gasc, F. Soubrier, F. Alhenc-Gelas and P. Corvol (1993). Gene expression and tissue localization of the two isoforms of ACE. *Hypertension* 21:827–35.

Silva, S. V., A. Pihlanto and F. X. Malcata (2006). Bioactive Peptides in Ovine and Caprine Cheeselike Systems Prepared with Proteases from Cynara cardunculus. *Journal of Dairy Science* 89, 3336–3344.

Smacchi, E. and M. Gobbetti (1998). Peptides from several Italian cheeses inhibitory to proteolytic enzymes of lactic acid bacteria, Pseudomonas fluorescens ATCC 948 and to the angiotensin I-converting enzyme. *Enzyme and Microbial Technology* 22, 687–694.

Stepaniak, L., L. Jedrychowski, B. Wróblewska and T. Sørhaug. (2001). Immunoreactivity and inhibition of angiotensin-I converting enzyme and lactococcal oligopeptidase by peptides fromcheese. *Italian Journal of Food Science* 13, 373– 381.

Sturrock, E.D., R. Natesh, J.M. Van Rooyen and K.R. Acharya (2004). Structure of angiotensin I-converting enzyme. *Cellular and Molecular Life Sciences* 61, 2677-2686 .

Taborda, G., E. Molina, I. Martínez-Castro, M. Ramos and L. Amigo (2003). Composition of the water-soluble fraction of different cheeses. *Journal of Agricultural and Food Chemistry* 51, 270-276.

Tonouchi, H., M. Suzuki, M. Uchida and M. Oda (2008). Antihypertensive effect of an angiotensin converting enzymeinhibitory peptide from enzyme modified cheese. *Journal of Dairy Research* 75, 284–290.

Upadhyay, V.K., P.L.H McSweeney, A.A.A. Magboul and P.F. Fox (2004). Proteolysis in Cheese during Ripening. Pages 391-434 in *Cheese: Chemistry, Physics and Microbiology,* Third edition - Volume 1: General Aspects. Elsevier Ltd

Vermeirssen, V., J. Van Camp and W. Verstraete (2002). Optimisation and validation of an angiotensin-converting enzyme inhibition assay for the screening of bioactive peptides. *Journal of Biochemical and Biophysical Methods* 51, 75-87.

Vermeirssen, V., J. Van Camp and W. Verstraete (2004). Bioavailability of angiotensin I converting enzyme inhibitory peptides. *British Journal of Nutrition* 92, 357–366.

Wei, L., E. Clauser, F. Alhenc-Gelas and P. Corvol (1992). The two homologous domains of human angiotensin I-converting enzyme interact differently with competitive inhibitors. *Journal of Biological Chemistry* 267, 1398-13405.

Wu, J., R.E. Aluko and A.D. Muir (2002). Improved method for direct high-performance liquid chromatography assay of angiotensin-converting enzyme-catalyzed reactions. *Journal of Chromatography* 950, 25 - 130.

In: Cheese: Types, Nutrition and Consumption
Editors: Richard D. Foster, pp. 247-266

ISBN 978-1-61209-828-9
©2011 Nova Science Publishers, Inc.

Chapter 13

NEW APPROACHMENT ON CHOLESTEROL REMOVAL IN CHEESE

Hae-Soo Kwak
Department of Food Science and Technology,
Sejong University, Seoul, Korea

ABSTRACT

Cheese is a nutritious food with various balanced nutrients, such as proteins, peptides, amino acids, fats, fatty acids, vitamins and minerals. However, the amounts of cholesterol is very high, e.g. 102mg/100g Cheddar cheese. Most of consumers are not prefer the cholesterol. Dairy scientists have been tried for lowering the cholesterol in cheeses for a long time. The method found initially is reducing fat in cheese that is poor in taste. Recently, we have been studied about removing specifically cholesterol during cheese making without changing anything from cheese including nutrients, flavor, taste and texture. The method developed is entrapping cholesterol by crosslinked β-cyclodextrin (β-CD). Cholesterol can be removed from milk for soft cheeses and from cream for semi hard and hard cheeses. In cholesterol-removed Cheddar cheese ripening, ripening time could be shortened about 50%. Crosslinked β-CD is lower solubility than β-CD, and particle size is bigger. So entrapment and separation from cream are possible and the β-CD is recycable about 10times. We developed various cholesterol-removed cheeses, such as Cheddar cheese, Mozzarella cheese, Camembert cheese, blue cheese, Gouda cheese, Feta cheese and process cheese. Cholesterol-removed cheeses will be commercialized in near future. I will describe the developed technique in detail in this chapter.

1. INTRODUCTION

Even though cheese is a nutritious food with various balanced nutrients the amounts of cholesterol are highly quantitated in cheese, such as 102mg/100g Cheddar cheese [1], 122mg/100g process cheese [2,3], 95mg/100g Cream cheese [4]. Most of consumers are not prefer such as cholesterol. Therefore, dairy related scientists have been tried to lower the cholesterol in cheese and other dairy products for a long time. The method found so far is just the reduction of milk fat from the products which are poor in taste and texture. During last decade, the scientists have developed specifically cholesterol-reducing technology from mostly milk and dairy products by different methods, such as biological, chemical and physical process. We also have been extensively studied about removing cholesterol from various cheeses (Cheddar, Process, Mozzarella, Camembert, blue, Feta, Cream) and other animal originated foods (egg, mayonnaise, lard, fish oil) as one of physical processes by β-cyclodextrin (β–CD). It was found that cholesterol-removed cheeses did not change nutrients, flavor, texture and taste during cheese making and ripening. We developed cholesterol removal rate ranged from 90 to 93% in most of cheeses and other products.

However, we faced certain limitation to industrialize this technology due to high cost of β–CD and environmental problem. To solve those points, it was necessary that β–CD should be recyclable. Recently, we developed crosslinking technique with β–CD and adipic acid [5,6]. This crosslinked β–CD was developed to be satisfied for cholesterol removal rate over 90%, about 10 times of recycling and low solubility of water from 16 to 11%. Cholesterol can be removed for soft cheeses from milk and for semi hard and hard cheese by cream when β–CD is used. Also during ripening of Cheddar cheese, acceleration of the ripening was found to be shortened about half time. We developed various cholesterol-removed cheeses, such as Cheddar cheese, Mozzarella Cheese, Camembert cheese, Blue cheese, Cream cheese, Feta cheese and Process cheese. I describe the developed technique about cholesterol-removal cheese and other food products in this chapter.

2. CHOLESTEROL REMOVAL FROM FOODS

A strong positive correlation exists between increased serum cholesterol concentration and risk of coronary heart disease. Animal and human experiments showed that plasma cholesterol as shown chemical structure in Fig. 1 is raised by an increased intake of cholesterol and saturated fat [7]. Therefore, consumers are increasingly concerned about the cholesterol level in their diets and there have been dramatic increase in no-, low- and removed cholesterol products in the market [8].

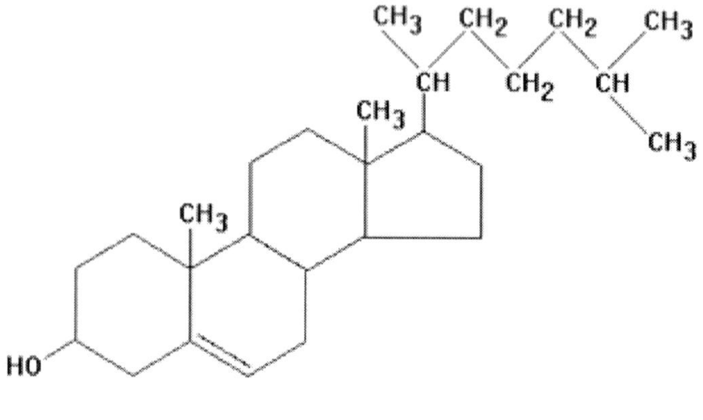

Figure 1. Chemical structure of cholesterol.

The removal of cholesterol in milk fat can be accomplished by many different means, including biological (microorganisms, enzymes); chemical (solid-liquid extraction, extraction with organic solvents, complex formation) or physical processes (distillation, crystallization, supercritical fluid extraction). Among the methods, cholesterol removal from microorganism [9] showed that Kefir-added milk reduced 41-84% cholesterol by *Streptococcus thermophilus, Lactobacillus delbrueckii* subsp. *buigaricus, Bifidobacterium bifidum* and *lactobacillus acidophilus*. However, this method reduces limited ranges of cholesterol, needs long time (24 hours) and cannot keep quality of milk. Also during adding the microorganisms, pathogenic or toxic bacteria could be contaminated and lower the quality of products.

The method of extraction with organic solvents was reported [7] that cholesterol was removed over 95% from butter fat and fish oil. But extraction with distillation takes out flavor from the fat, and the fat could be hydrolyzed or polymerized by heating. These reactions may lead to low quality products. Melting crystallization is the method that fat is concentrated by vacuum, cooled down to the crystallized and separated out the cholesterol from milk fat. Shukla et al. developed cholesterol-removed butter [10], but the butter was poor in texture and had high melting point. This abnormal product did not favor to most consumers.

Supercritical fluid extraction is relatively advanced technology [7, 10, 11]. This method is to extract the target material by carbon dioxide with high density and low viscosity under the condition of over critical temperature and pressure. This method has been applied into oil extraction from oil seeds, removal of bitterness from hops, removal of caffein from coffee and cholesterol removal from animal originated foods. This technology has advantages over other technology, such as inexpensive energy, high productivity and using safe solvent to prevent explosion or toxin. Shukla et al. reported [10] that they fractionated milk fat to make butter with low cholesterol. However, developed butter is not similar to market butter due to using fractionated fatty acids. This butter is limited to certain consumers and specific food ingredient. Therefore, this method is still under experimental stage. As mentioned above, most of cholesterol removal technologies developed by physical, chemical and biological means remove cholesterol as well as nutrients and flavors. Some other methods have additional disadvantage, such as high cost.

Absorption methods for cholesterol removal from milk fat are possible to treat at low temperature (5°C), thereby minimize to lower quality and flavor loss and economical. Additionally, cholesterol removal can be selective [12]. Treatment with saponin for cholesterol removal is the formation of insoluble complexed cholesterol using saponin. Chang et al. reported [13] that they determined the optimum conditions for cholesterol removal from homogenized milk by treatment with saponin. The result of the experiment showed that 73.7% of the removal under the conditioned factors. In conclusion, saponin is strongly selective in cholesterol, so final product does not change the quality. But cholesterol removal rate is limited and saponin is costly to apply into foods. Therefore, currently β-cyclodextrin (β–CD) is focused on cholesterol removal in foods due to the most effective method in cheese and other dairy products.

The unique method to make up the disadvantages of developed other methods for cholesterol removal is the absorption method by β–CD. β–CD is a cyclic oligosaccharide composed of seven glucose units linked by α-(1-4) bonds as shown in A of Fig. 2. It has a cavity at the centre of molecule which allows the complex formation with cholesterol. β–CD is non toxic, edible, non hydroscopic, chemically stable and easy to separate from the complex. Thus, β–CD provides advantages when used for removal of cholesterol from various foods. Cholesterol in milk is contained in milk fat globule membrane over 80% and rest of cholesterol is in milk plasma. In our preliminary study, only 25 to 30 % of cholesterol was removed from raw milk. This result is due to large fat globules in unhomogenized milk, which cannot interact with β–CD. Therefore, homogenization is necessary to remove cholesterol in milk. β–CD has various advantages, such as direct cholesterol removal from milk fat, treatment under low temperature (5°C), minimizing the change of quality by microbial contamination and loss of flavors, low expenses of treatment and selective removal of cholesterol. And also β–CD is recognized as food additives worldwide.

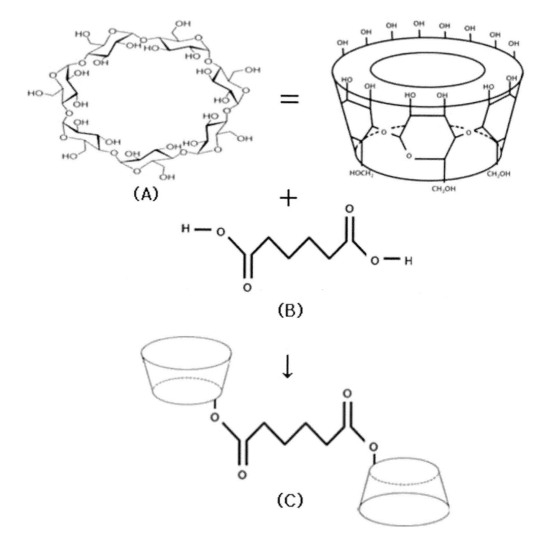

Figure 2. Chemical structure of crosslinked β-cyclodextrin reacted by adipic acid (A): β-cyclodextrin, (B): adipic acid (C): crosslinked β-cyclodextrin.

2. CHOLESTEROL REMOVAL FROM β–CYCLODEXTRIN

Recently beta cyclodextrin (β–CD) was proved to remove more than 90% of the cholesterol in milk fat. However, individual food products need to be optimized to remove cholesterol as much as possible. Effective removal of cholesterol was extensively studied in milk, cheese and other dairy products. In homogenized milk (3.6%) fat by application of β–CD, β–CD at 0.5 to 1.5% removed 92.2 to 95.8% of cholesterol, respectively, when stirred at 10° C at 166 x g for 10 min [14]. Alonso et al. confirmed [15] that cholesterol removal in milk by β–CD in laboratory, semi-industrial and industrial scale. In my lab, cream (36% in milk fat) was treated with β–CD to remove cholesterol with various factors using response surface methodology [2]. In our result, cholesterol could be removed maximum 97.8% under the conditions of 15% β–CD, 40°C stirring temperature, 20 min stirring time and 1,200 rpm stirring speed. After regular cream study to remove cholesterol, whipping cream was also treated by β–CD to examine the changes in functional properties of cholesterol-removed whipping cream [16]. Before processing whipping stirring cream, cream (36% milk fat) was treated to remove cholesterol optimizing with 10% β–CD, 20 min time and 800 rpm stirring speed for more than 90% removal. Higher stirring time and speed increase the apparent viscosity of whipped cream treated with β–CD. The overrun increased to 150% and foam instability was 2.5 ml defoamed cream with 10 min stirring time and 100 rpm speed. In the results, cholesterol-removed whipping cream could be produced without adverse effect. After whipping cream study, we had been continued examining compound whipping cream by palm oil to reduce cholesterol. When the ratio of cream to palm oil was 1:1, positive results was found in cholesterol removal and product quality [17].

We had been consecutively studied the cholesterol-removed butter and lowering blood cholesterol added by gamma linolenic acid (GLA). Cholesterol removal rate reached 93.2% by β–CD in butter before GLA addition. As expected, TBA value increased with GLA addition in cholesterol-reduced butter. During storage, the production of short-chain free fatty acid (SCFFA), which is influenced flavor and taste of butter, increased significantly in GLA-added butter. Color and overall acceptability among several sensory characteristics were also significantly different from the sample butter. We observed blood cholesterol in rat. Total blood cholesterol increased slowly and triglyceride level decreased significantly in the sample butter fed rat. Actually this study was the first trial to reduce total blood cholesterol level in butter and provided such a functional butter with keeping quality [18].

As mentioned above about cholesterol removal in dairy products, β–CD has the advantage of removing cholesterol from dairy products at efficiency over 90%, however, it suffers from various disadvantages due to environmental pollution and more consumption of β–CD due to its ineffective recovery. Also β–CD could be recovered to at some level, but it is difficult to remove in cream. Therefore, to overcome the problems, the recovery and recycling of β–CD are required.

4. RECYCLING OF β – CYCLODEXTRIN

Several methods have been developed for the dissociation of cholesterol from cholesterol–β–CD complex to recycle, such as using hydrogen bond inhibitor, resin, heating, sodium chloride and organic solvents. Firstly, using hydrogen bond inhibitor is the method that hydrogen inhibitor is added into cholesterol–β–CD complex to prevent sedimentation of non–β–CD materials to precipitate β–CD only and then crystallize it to recycle. The advantage of this method is inexpensive, simple and short time. However, it is easy to be mixed non–β–CD materials and pure β–CD after precipitation. This mixture forms haze which is not suitable for some products needed clearance. Secondly, using resin is the method that resin absorbs cholesterol and passes β–CD resin.

Finally, the organic solvents can be utilized to separate out β–CD from cholesterol–β–CD complex by selected organic solvent with variables, such as temperature, time, speed et al. The method has advantages including simple, economical and industry applicable. However, most of organic solvents are remained with β–CD even though they are trace level. To solve the problem, we can use the organic solvents recognized as food additives, such as acetic acid, isopropanol, ethanol et al.

We had examined organic solvents to find possibility of β–CD recycling for cholesterol removal in cream. To optimize conditions four different factors, such as ratio of solvent to cholesterol–β–CD complex, mixing speed, temperature and time for cholesterol dissociation in cream (milk fat 36%). Used solvents were acetic acid and isopropanol (3:1). Using the ratio of 6:1 (solvent to the complex) showed 82.5% cholesterol dissociation when mixed at 100 rpm at 56° C for 1 hour. In a continued study, using recycled β–CD only removed at best 75% cholesterol in cream. So we tried to mix unused β–CD with the ratio of 6 to 4 and found to increase more than 90% cholesterol removal [19]. However, to recycle β–CD by organic solvents, centrifugation is needed, but cholesterol–β–CD complex could not be clearly separated out of cream. Also it is necessary to mix used and unused β–CD to improve cholesterol removal.

To solve the problem on recovery and recycling with organic solvents, another trial was employed to study the possibility of solid support β–CD immobilization. We had prepared the β–CD immobilized glass bead of different conditions, such as mixing time, mixing temperature, tube size of silanization and β–CD immobilization reactions [20]. In the results, the glass beads (diameter 1mm) at 20 mM 3-isocyanatopropyl triethoxysilane, 30 mM β–CD and 16 h of mixing time in 7 mm diameter tube at 10 ° C were selected as optimized conditions. Under the condition we found that the cholesterol removal rate was only 41%. In recycling study, cholesterol removal was the same rate as the first result, but recycling efficiency was close to 100%. Even though the recycling was effectively positive, cholesterol removal was futher behind yet than needed. Therefore, we had searched for effective method in cholesterol removal and recycling, and finally found crosslinking of β–CD as the most remarkable way.

5. CROSSLINKING OF Β–CD

Recently, using β–CD powder allows over 90% of cholesterol removal in milk and dairy products. However, large amount of β–CD is consumed for the process due to ineffective recovery and no recycling. To overcome these problems, we attempted to study the immobilization of β–CD on solid support. But as mentioned above, the removal of cholesterol was limited to only around 40%. So we postulated that the crosslinking of β–CD might be possible to increase the cholesterol removal and to recover the used β–CD for recycling.

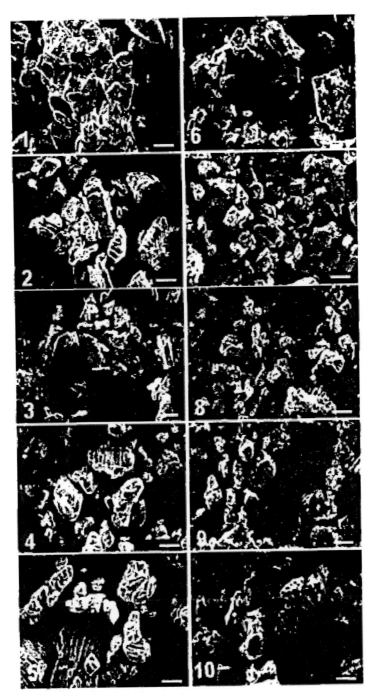

Figure 3. Scanning electron micrographs of crosslinked β-cyclodextrin after recycling process [6]. The gradual reductions in size and associated morphological changes after recycling process were revealed by SEM observations. 1. After one time reuse, 2. After two time reuse, 3. After three time reuse, 4. After four time reuse, 5. After five time reuse, 6. After six time reuse, 7. After seven time reuse, 8. After 8 time reuse, 9. After 9 time reuse, and 10. After ten time reuse. Scale bars = 20 μm.

Functionality of starch is commonly modified by the crosslinking. Various crosslinking agents, such as phosphorous, oxychloride, sodium trimetaphosphate, adipic acid, formaldehyde, epichlorohydrin et al. have been extensively used to produce crosslinked starches, which inter- or intramolecular mono- and diethers are formed with hydroxyl group of starch. This chemically modified changes in starch increase or decrease in viscosity. So, crosslinked starches are used mainly as thickening agents and stabilizers in sauces and dressings for pizzas. Highly crosslinked starch are more stable at various pHs, which are indispensable for manufacturers of food. Among crosslinking agents, epichlorohydrin has been well known as a most effective agent.

Therefore, we tried to develop crosslinked β–CD with epichlorohydrin and determined the optimum conditions with 10 min mixing time, 5°C mixing temperature and 400 rpm mixing speed [21]. After producing the crosslinked β–CD, it was applied into milk to reduce cholesterol resulting in 83.3% of maximum reduction cholesterol with 1% crosslinked β–CD addition. In recycling test, the crosslinked β–CD resulted in almost 100% efficiency. Even though recycling rate reached to almost 100%, the crosslinked β–CD with epichlorohydrin revealed lower level in cholesterol removal than powdered β–CD. Also epichlorohydrin was found to be not allowed to use in food processing due to its toxicity. To solve the problems of the crosslinking agent, adipic acid was considered to produce crosslinked β–CD, because adipic acid is recognized as a food additive, which is used for beverage and confectionary as acidulant and preservatives. We prepared crosslinked β–CD with adipic acid as shown in Figure 2 and also conditions are optimized for over 90% cholesterol removal. Additionally, effective recycling was also observed. Conclusively, we found the first evidence of possibility for applying crosslinked β–CD by adipic acid in food industry [5].

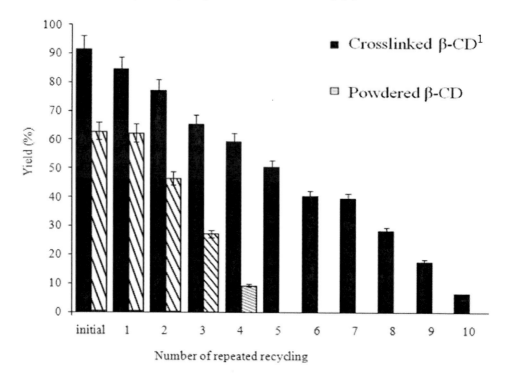

Figure 4. Recycable yield of crosslinked β-cyclodextrin to remove cholesterol in milk [5]. [1]Milk was treated with 2% adipic acid reacted crosslinked β-CD.

Table 1. Cholesterol removal using crosslinked β-CD with repeated times of recycling in milk.

Number of repeated recycling	Cholesterol removal[1] (%) Powdered[2]	Crosslinked[3]
Initial	92.41^a	92.39^a
1st	89.37^a	92.51^a
2nd	84.98^b	92.32^{ab}
3rd	79.34^c	92.13^{ab}
4th	72.26^d	92.21^{ab}
5th	-	92.42^{ab}
6th	-	91.83^{ab}
7th	-	90.58^b
8th	-	89.51^b
9th	-	84.02^c
10th	-	81.42^d

[1] Means within column by the same letter are not significantly different (P<0.05).
[2] Milk was treated with powdered β-CD.
[3] Milk was treated with 2% adipic acid reacted crosslinked β-CD.

After confirming crosslinked β–CD with adipic acid on effective cholesterol removal and recycling rates in milk, we had studied about the structural changes during recycling on SEM as shown in Fig. 3. The size reduction and morphological changes were found during the recycling process and propound changes were observed at 8th time reuse. Also we compared the recyclable yield of crosslinked β–CD between 2% adipic acid reacted crosslinked β–CD and powdered β–CD in milk. The crosslinked β–CD showed possibility of the recycling as shown in Fig. 4. After removing cholesterol from milk, the used crosslinked β–CD was washed by organic solvents for cholesterol dissociation and reuse. In recycling study, the cholesterol removal rate kept continually over 90% till 8th time reuse in milk as shown in Table 1 and cream [6]. In this results, we concluded that crosslinked β–CD is effective, economical and industry applicable in milk, cheese, other dairy products and other animal resourced foods for cholesterol removal.

6. ENTRAPMENT OF NUTRIENT

Even though the crosslinked β–CD was proved to be effective and advantageous in cholesterol removal, we were curious about whether the β–CD entraps only cholesterol or additionally other nutrients. So we measured the amount of possibly entrapped nutrient, such as lactose, short-chain free fatty acid (SCFFA), free amino acid, water-soluble vitamin and the quantities of residual β–CD after cholesterol removal from milk and cream by crosslinked β–CD [22, 23]. For this study, we added the amounts of crosslinked β–CD from 0.4 to 1.2% into milk and from 4 to 12% into cream. Lactose was not entrapped from 4.86% in milk and entrapped only 0.03% from 2.74% in cream. The total amounts of SCFFA were exhibited 11.70 and 16.63 ppm from milk and cream and entrapped 0.00 to 0.03 and 0.06 ppm, respectively. Entrapped free amino acids for milk and cream were 0.39 to 0.48 µmol/ml and 0.28 to 0.91 µmol/ml, respectively. Some amount of water-soluble vitamins are entrapped and it is in the range of 0.00 to 0.06 ppm for thiamine, 0.01 to 0.06 ppm for niacin, 0.02 to 0.05 ppm for L-ascorbic acid and 0.01 to 0.06 ppm for riboflavin, respectively, in milk. The amount of the vitamins in cream also showed similar trend to these in milk. In the results of this study, we observed that the concentrations of added crosslinked β–CD into the milk and cream did not affect the amounts of the entrapped nutrients.

We had been studied the amounts of residual β–CD after treating β–CD in milk and cream. The amounts of residual β–CD in milk were proportionally increased from 1.22 to 3.00 ppm with increase the concentration of crosslinked β–CD from 0.4 to 1.2%, respectively. An increase in the concentrations of β–CD from 4 to 12% for cream also caused a proportional increase in the amounts of residual β–CD from 1.86 to 6.11 ppm, respectively. Based on the data obtained from this study, we could conclude that the amounts of entrapped nutrients are negligible and the residual β–CD was trace amount in milk and cream during cholesterol removal by crosslinked β–CD [22,23].

7. CHOLESTEROL REMOVAL IN CHEESE

On the basis of health aspects, cheese consumers are not ready to sacrifice the taste and other aspects. This implies that cheese industry faces the challenge to produce fat-reduced cheeses which have similar properties to normally fat containing products. However, serious problem in low fat cheese is that fat reduction has profound negative effects on the final flavor and texture, such as lack of flavor and defects of fullness of texture. Thus, extensive research has been concentrated on the optimization of the flavor, sensory and texture quality of fat-reduced cheeses. However, most of consumers may not prefer such a low fat cheese due to unpleasant flavor, taste and texture.

To solve this serious problem of cheese, we have been studying for a long period of time about cholesterol removal without reducing fat in cheese. From now on, I would like to describe about cholesterol removal on various cheeses.

7.1. Cheddar Cheese

Generally, milk is not homogenized in cheese making, but to remove cholesterol, milk must be homogenized prior to cheese making due to low rate of cholesterol removal (about 30%) from unhomogenized milk. Since Cheddar cheese consumption dominates in USA and other countries, we had started cholesterol removal of cheese study from Cheddar cheese [24]. The cheeses were made by 2 different treatments, such as control (no homogenization, no β–CD) and sample (1,000 psi milk homogenization, 1% β–CD). The cholesterol removal of the sample cheese was 79.3% which was much lower than that of expected (over 90%). The production of short-chain free fatty acids (SCFFA) which is influenced in flavor and taste increased with ripening time in both control and sample. However, the releasing quantity of SCFFA was higher in milk–treated cheese than control between 5 and 9 month ripening which indicated accelerated ripening. Neutral volatile compounds were not much different between control and sample. In bitter-tasted amino acids which may be a serious problem, milk-treated cheese produced much higher than control. In sensory study, texture score is highly effected due to the decrease in texture with increasing ripening time of cholesterol-reduced cheese [24]. In this study, we observed that the cheese made by β–CD–treated milk at low pressure homogenization reduced cholesterol with non-effective level of intensive bitter taste, rapid cheese ripening and no capture of flavor compounds by β–CD. Even though homogenized milk can reduce cholesterol over 90% in Cheddar cheese after several trials, homogenization in cheese making leads to various disadvantages like a slow drainage, a reduced tension and a decreased elasticity of the cheese curd. To solve the problems, we tried to separate cream from the milk as next step study.

In the second study, we separated cream from milk, treated cream by 10% β–CD and blended with skim milk at 1,000 psi homogenization. The cholesterol removal of the cheese was improved to 92.1%, however, the production of SCFFA, neutral volatile compounds, bitter amino acid, texture and accelerated ripening time were still almost identical to the first study [1].

Even though some of the defects appeared in the second study, cholesterol-removed functional Cheddar cheese may be possible to develop, therefore, we attempted to promote the cheese to reduce blood cholesterol by adding functional material, such as phytosterol, which has the blood cholesterol lowering property. Phytosterol ester at the range of 2 to 8% was added during mixing the β–CD–treated skim milk and cream also showed cholesterol reduction over 90%. And the concentrations of SCFFA and free amino acids increased proportionally with the increasing phytosterol ester. In sensory study, intensity of rancid, bitterness and off-flavor increased significantly, while texture decreased during ripening in the sample cheese. As a main study of this experiment, total blood cholesterol level was lowered by 18% when rats were fed with 8% phytosterol-added and cholesterol-reduced cheese. Even though the quality of the cheese was needed to be improved more, the possibility of blood cholesterol lowering Cheddar cheese was appeared in the first trial [25]. As the second trial, evening primrose oil (EPO) was applied into Cheddar cheese to lower blood cholesterol. Experimental cheese was ripened at 7° C for 8 weeks while control 32 weeks. TBA value as an oxidation indicator was higher in all cholesterol-reduced Cheddar cheese than in control. In blood cholesterol analysis, total cholesterol and high–density lipoprotein were not significantly different but triglyceride decreased significantly in samples [26]. In this study, we found that functional materials are needed more to select by research.

During developing cholesterol-removed Cheddar cheese, we developed simultaneously crosslinked β-CD to recover the cholesterol-entrapped β-CD complex and recycle the used β-CD. So, we tried to apply the β-CD in cheeses. Crosslinked β-CD also was proved effective cholesterol removal in cheese and other dairy products, and accelerated ripening effects in Cheddar cheese. However, this Cheddar cheese has some defects which has strong bitterness and crumble texture. To improve these defects, we made experimental cheese treated by several main factors, such as salt concentration, cooking time and cooking temperature [27]. When we added 3% salt, total SCFFA increased to 53 ppm in 9 week ripening period. On the other hand, when added 1% salt, it increased to 126 ppm in the same time. In bitterness study, 3% salt-added sample cheese increased to 55 μmol/g in the bitter amino acids in 9 week ripening period. However, 1% salt-added sample increased 100 μmol/g in the same time. In the result of sensory test, we observed that the lower the salt concentration the stronger the bitterness. In the texture study, hardness of 3% salt-added cheese was just half of that in 1% salt-added sample in 9 week ripening period.

In the change of the cooking time and cooking temperature, there was no significant difference (p<0.05). In a subsequent study, we found ripening of acceleration by the crosslinked β-CD based on the SCFFA and free amino acids. In texture, the sample cheese was significantly greater at 5 week ripening than those in the control cheese at 4 month ripening. Even though the cholesterol-removed cheese was showed some variations such as bitterness, rancidity and off-flavor at the early stage of ripening than those in control, the sample cheese changed to similar or lower scores than control with ripening. Therefore, this study showed that crosslinked β-CD-treated Cheddar cheese was accelerated effective ripening as well as removed cholesterol. I expect that Cheddar cheese manufacturers may be very interest with these benefits and apply this technique in near future.

7.2. Process Cheese

Natural cheese such as Cheddar is the important ingredient in process cheese and it also produced by mixing different ages and degrees of maturity of natural cheese along with salt, butter and other ingredients to obtain a uniform product [28]. The popularity of the process cheese contributes to its numerous applications and it is one of the leading cheese varieties in the world followed by Cheddar cheese and Mozzarella cheese.

Since process cheese is mainly produced by Cheddar cheese with different ripening, accelerated ripened and the cholesterol-reduced process cheese is effectively economical and health beneficial. As the first trial of cholesterol-removed process cheese by crosslinked β-CD, we made block-type process cheese [29]. For cholesterol-removed process cheese making, it was formulated with 72% of cholesterol-removed Cheddar cheese (50% 3 week, 2% 6 week and 30% 9 week ripened), 10% of cholesterol-removed butter, 3% emulsifying salt, 5% skim milk powder and 10% water. The composition of block-type process cheese was close to the control cheese. The cholesterol removal rate was over 90% from the cholesterol content of control process cheese of 122.0 mg/100g. Total amount of SCFFA did not differ between the sample and control cheese, but the production of free amino acids and bitter amino acids was higher in cholesterol-removed process cheese in all storage times compared with those in the control. In sensory study, acidic, salty and bitterness were high, but elasticity was low. Finally, we concluded that cholesterol removed block-type process cheese is possible to apply into industry scale.

As a continued study, we examined the cholesterol-removed process cheese spread as a major variety of process cheese with the cholesterol-removed block-type process cheese. Cholesterol removal of the cheese spread was also over 90%. SCFFA of the cheese spread was almost identical to the control, but free amino acids were higher in the spread than in the control during storage for 6 months. Rheological properties such as hardness, adhesiveness, elasticity, were relatively similar to each other cheeses but gumminess and brittleness were higher in the spread. Overall acceptability in sensory analysis showed no significant difference between experimental spread and control during storage. Therefore, we may suggest that functional and economical efficient process variety may be developed by crosslinked β-CD as a newly approached science and technology.

7.3. Mozzarella Cheese

Last decade, Mozzarella cheese as a traditional Italian cheese has been rapidly increased consumption in all over the world due to the expanding popularity of Pizza. However, most consumers are concerned about the excessive intake of cholesterol. Therefore, we were interested to study about cholesterol removal from Mozzarella cheese after developing cholesterol removal over 90% by β-CD [3]. To reduce cholesterol from Mozzarella cheese, homogenization is necessary in milk. However, homogenized milk adversely affects protein structure and causes casein micelles and their subunits to be incorporated into the fat globule membrane. These fat and casein interaction leads to a weaker cheese curd, curd shattering and improper curd matting [30]. Therefore, in Mozzarella cheese making, homogenization results milk solids loss and fat leakage in pizza making.

Since homogenization is important to reduce cholesterol and is negatively effect to quality of Mozzarella cheese, we tried to optimize conditions for homogenization of the cheese milk. In the result, the homogenization pressure influenced seriously on the cholesterol reduction in milk. The highest cholesterol reduction was 75.6% when the pressure increased up to 70.0 Kg/cm^2 with 1.0% β-CD and 70°C. In the quality of the sample cheese, the meltabilty of the cheese decreased with higher pressure. The stretchability decreased to 40% of the control cheese and oiling-off also dropped down sharply from homogenization pressure. Compared with other cheeses, cholesterol-reduced Mozzarella cheese decreased cholesterol reduction, stretchability and texture. In this study, we experienced that Mozzarella cheese could be reduced cholesterol with some adversed effects by β-CD.

7.4. Camembert Cheese

Camembert cheese is characterized by the growth of the white mold *Penicillium camemberti* on the surface during ripening. Lactic acid produced by starter culture is metabolized by the mold increasing the pH above 7.0 on the surface toward the end of ripening. The ripening of the Camembert is relatively quick due to its high moisture and the rapid growth mold. During ripening, Camembert softens extensively, leading actually to be an almost liquid-like consistency.

We had experiment for cholesterol removal in Camembert cheese from separation of cream from the raw milk. The 10% crosslinked β-CD and bulk pasteurized cream (36% milk fat) was stirred in a blender at 800 rpm for 30 min. The cream was blended with skim milk and then homogenized with 500 psi at 50°C and cooled to 32°C to produce Camembert cheese. In the results of this study, we found that the composition of the cholesterol-removed Camembert cheese was similar to the control cheese and the cholesterol removal reached over 90% as expected. SCFFA productions between the sample and control cheese were not different during ripening periods. Mostly contributed SCFFA released were butyric and capryic acid in both groups. The rheological characteristics except springiness were increased till 2 week ripening and decreased thereafter. Moldy characteristics were increased sharply through the ripening period in both sample and control cheeses. We found out the results that cholesterol-removed Camembert cheese and the regular cheese do not differ in most physicochemical and sensory properties [31, 32]. Therefore, cholesterol-removed Camembert cheese using crosslinked β-CD could be developed.

7.5. Blue Cheese

Blue cheese is characterized by the growth of *Penicillium* in tissues throughout the cheese matrix and produced by mold spore of *P. roqueforti* or *P. glaucum* into milk or cheese curds. These molds are rich in protease and lipase which undergo extensive proteolysis and lipolysis in blue-type cheeses resulting in odor, flavor, appearance and texture development. Proteolysis leads to gradual softening of cheese body and production of the water-soluble nitrogenous-compounds which form cheese flavor.

We had developed cholesterol-removed blue cheese by crosslinked β-CD. The preparation of cholesterol removal was almost identical to Camembert cheese making, but cholesterol-removed cream was standardized with skim milk to a fat content of 12%, homogenized with 500 psi and then repeated with 1,000 psi at 50°C. It was mixed with skim milk again to a fat content of 3.4% and cooled to 30°C to incubate. After that procedure, we followed the regular blue cheese making [33]. The experimental blue cheese was vacuum-packaged and ripened at 10°C for 8 weeks to examine [34].

We observed that the composition of cholesterol-removed blue cheese was similar to the control cheese and the cholesterol removal was over 90% as shown in Camembert cheese. Amounts of SCFFA and free amino acids between sample cheese and control were not different at every storage period. Butyric and capric acid mostly dominated over other SCFFA in both cheeses. In rheological properties, hardness was continuously increased during 8 week ripening, however, cohesiveness, gumminess and brittleness were increased till 6 week and stopped thereafter. We found out that the most significant change during ripening was moldy property in appearance, flavor and taste as expected. Overall acceptability of the sensory score was not significantly developed during 8 week ripening in both groups. Since we could not find profound difference in most physicochemical and sensory properties between cholesterol-removed Blue cheese and the control, we may say that the cholesterol-removed blue cheese can be developed using crosslinked β-CD.

7.6. Feta Cheese

For many centuries, Feta cheese was well known only in Balkan region, however, migration from the area to the other countries of the world made new markets for the Feta cheese and trade was established internation-wide. Feta is a soft white cheese and it is ripened in brine and is salty, slightly acidic and pleasant in sensory property with a world-wide acceptance. The body texture is creamy, smooth and firm, which makes the cheese sliceable. Even though gas holes are not allowable, irregular small mechanical openings are commonly desirable. Traditionally, Feta cheese has been made with sheep's milk, but mixtures of sheep's and goat's milk impart specific flavor. We had been also studied about cholesterol removal in Feta cheese and compared the physicochemical and sensory properties of the sample cheese and control during 12 week ripening [35]. The composition of cholesterol-removed Feta cheese by crosslinked β-CD was similar to the control cheese. As we expected, cholesterol was removed over 90%. SCFFA and free amino acids were produced almost same amounts between the sample cheese and control during ripening periods. Most rheological properties of both cheeses were continuously decreased throughout the ripening period. In sensory characteristics, we could not find out any difference or defects and the overall acceptability of the sample was slightly better than control cheese. Therefore, we can also expect the possibility of cholesterol-removed Feta cheese by crosslinked β-CD.

7.7. Cream Cheese

Cream cheese is manufactured in many forms ranged from plain to flavored in Europe and some countries of North America. Imitation type cheese also found in USA made from whole milk component with lower concentrations of fat than prescribed by federal standards of identity. As a reflection of the fat, conscious age, Cream cheese production and consumption might be declined, but obviously this is not the case. Maybe the excellent subtle flavors originated from the lactic acid fermentation or the rich pool of quality nutrients, or many old and new culinary uses associated with cheese tell why it keeps the popularity. Sometimes it is used as a replacement for high fat spreads. The consumption of Cream cheese and Neufchatel cheese combined has been gradually increased in USA since 1995.

There is a wide variety of Cream cheese with different dry matter and fat content. The Food and Drug Administration in USA stated in as early as 1952 that Cream cheese should not have less than 33% fat content and not more than 55% moisture. Cream cheese in Canadian standards are the same except the minimum requirement of 30% fat. However, France required fat in dry matter not less than 75% in Triple creme.

For the study of cholesterol-removed Cream cheese, we had been experimented in various ways, such as cholesterol removal, sensory evaluation, texture and using whole milk powder during storage periods. To manufacture cholesterol-removed cream cheese, cholesterol-removed cream (36% milk fat) was standardized with skim milk to a fat content of 11%, pasteurized, homogenized and cooled down to 30°C to incubate for making Cream cheese. After making the cheese, it was stored at 4°C for 8 weeks.

The composition of cholesterol-removed Cream cheese was significantly similar to the control and over 90% of cholesterol reduction was observed in the sample cheese. Total amounts of SCFFA and free amino acids were significantly lower in the cholesterol-removed cheese than in the control throughout the storage. Most rheological attributes decreased sharply in the control compared with the sample cheese. In sensory study, spreadability and wateryness in the sample cheese were significantly higher than in the control cheese. Sensory score for sourness increased significantly in the control cheese from 4 to 8 week storage, but those in the cholesterol-removed cheese by crosslinked β-CD increased slowly during all the storage periods [4]. After physicochemical and sensory study, we observed neutral volatile compounds in cholesterol-removed Cream cheese compared to the control during 4 week storage. Tentatively identified volatile compounds were detected 12 acids, 2 ketones, 1 amine, 1 alcohol, 1 ketone and 1 alkene. The identified compounds from the sample cheese were same as those from regular control cheese [36].

We attempted to substitute whole milk powder and fresh cream (36% milk fat) to make Cream cheese and cholesterol-removed Cream cheese, and identified volatile flavor compounds, texture and sensory properties in both cheeses. Tentatively identified flavor compounds were detected 11 acids, 2 ketones, 1 imide, 1 amine, 1 alcohol, 2 lactone, 2 alkene and 1 alkane. Identified flavor compounds from cholesterol-removed Cream cheese made from whole milk powder were same as those from control. The rheological and sensory properties were not significantly different from both cheeses. On the basis of our results, even though Cream cheese made from whole milk powder is slightly different from that of the whole milk in identified flavor, cholesterol-removed Cream cheese made from the whole milk powder showed no adverse changes in flavor, texture and sensory analysis [37].

In conclusion, crosslinked β-CD plays very important role to remove specifically cholesterol over 90% in variety of cheeses. We found out that physicochemical, textural and sensory properties in cholesterol-removed cheeses were not different from controls during ripening and storage. Therefore, consumers may prefer cholesterol-removed cheeses in near future.

8. OTHER PRODUCTS

During the study of cholesterol-removed cheese and dairy products, we found some other animal based products need to remove cholesterol. So we have been researched out the optimization of cholesterol-removal from the products, such as egg, mayonnaise, lard and fish oils, each egg contains about 200 to 250 mg cholesterol when hen lays egg. To utilize the egg to other foods, cholesterol removal is required to develop functional food, such as mayonnaise. Also to make cholesterol-reduced sausage, lard should be cholesterol free. Fish liver oils also contain high amounts of cholesterol to be removed. We have been studied various other products along with the cheese and dairy products which I would like to introduce.

8.1. Egg

Even though egg is a nutritious with various balanced nutrients, one egg contains about 272mg of cholesterol, and National Research Council in USA recommends total intake of less than 300 mg/day. Therefore, there have been increase in no-, low-, and reduced-cholesterol products in the market place. We had optimized cholesterol removal in egg yolk by crosslinked β–CD [38]. The optimum conditions were based on the ratio of egg-yolk-to-water, the concentration of crosslinked β–CD, mixing temperature, time and speed by the addition of crosslinked β–CD-complex. Egg yolk-water mixture increased cholesterol removal with the increasing level of the β–CD (10-25%). The optimum conditions of cholesterol removal about 95% in egg yolk were 25% of crosslinked β–CD at the ratio of egg yolk-to-water and 800 rpm mixing at 45°C for 30 min and 2,890xg centrifugal speed. In recycling study, the removal rates were measured using 10 times recycled crosslinked β–CD in egg yolk. The average rate of cholesterol removal during 8 time recycling was 85%. This study indicated that water-mixed egg yolk could apply into functional mayonnaise.

8.2. Mayonnaise

Mayonnaise is one of the most widely used condiments or sauces in the world. It constitutes plant oil, egg yolk, vinegar et al. as main ingredients. Among them egg yolk plays a important role in mayonnaise making as an emulsifying agent. Since egg yolk contains high amounts of cholesterol, mayonnaise also composes 50~70mg/100g cholesterol. Recently, consumers have increasingly demanded the cholesterol-reduced mayonnaise, so egg yolk-replaced products by egg white has been developed and shown in market places. However, this substituted product has disadvantages with sensory defects. Various methods were tried to reduce cholesterol, but most of methods are non-selective, and reduce flavor and nutrients.

We had been carried out to develop cholesterol-removed mayonnaise with crosslinked β–CD and blood cholesterol lowering effect by adding phytosterol and study it's physicochemical and sensory properties during 10 months at 9°C [39]. The compositions of mayonnaise treated with crosslinked β–CD and added phytosterol were similar to the control. The range of cholesterol removal was from 90.7 to 92.5%. The TBA absorbance of the sample showed that the more phytosterol contained, the lower the TBA values which suggested that phytosterol may prevent developing oxidation. The viscosity of the mayonnaise decreased with higher amounts of phytosterol during storage. In color measurement, lightness and yellowness decreased and redness increased. In sensory properties, most characterstics were similar to the control mayonnaise without phytosterol. In conclusion, cholesterol-removed mayonnaise is very similar to control.

8.3. Lard

Edible commercial lard, used for hardening agents, shortening cocoa butter substitutes, cooking oil sausage and restructured ham contain a high level of cholesterol with about 50-100 mg/100g. We determine the optimum conditions of different factors, such as ratio of lard to water, β–CD concentration etc on the reduction of cholesterol from lard by using crosslinked β–CD. The cholesterol removal was ranged from 91.2 to 93.0% with 5% crosslinked β–CD. In recycling study, the rate of cholesterol removal was 92.1% in the first trial similar to the new crosslinked β–CD (92.3%). Up to 8 time use, the cholesterol removal was not significantly different. The optimum conditions of cholesterol removal by crosslinked β–CD were 1:3 ratio of lard to water, 5% crosslinked β–CD concentration, 40°C mixing temperature, 1 hr mixing time and 150 rpm mixing speed [40]. So the cholesterol-removed lard could be used for making sausage, restructured ham and other foods.

8.4. Fish Oils

Squid liver oil produced from squids is a products containing high amounts of docosahexaenoic acid (DHA) and eicosapentaenoic (EPA), and high unsaturated ω-3 fatty acids, which are essential for health benefits. However, squid liver oil contains also higher content of cholesterol (1,640 mg/100g). Therefore, removing cholesterol from the oil can be a good way to develop neutraceutical food products.

To remove the cholesterol from squid liver oil, we had studied optimum conditions. Different factors were crosslinked β–CD concentration, mixing temperature, ratio of the oil to water, mixing time and speed. It was found that cholesterol removal from the oil was significantly affected by all factors mentioned such as follows; the conditions were 1:3 ratio of squid liver oil to water, 25% diluted and crosslinked β–CD concentration, 20 min mixing time, 800 rpm mixing speed and 55°C mixing temperature for about 89% cholesterol removal. In recycling study, the first recycling trial was 81.05% and over 70% of cholesterol removal was observed [41].

Another fish oil studied was cod liver oil consisting of ω-3 fatty acid, comprising high levels of DHA and EPA, triacylglycerols, mono-, di- acylglycerols, free fatty acid and vitamins A, D and E. The oil has been used as nutritional supplement in the world. However, cod liver oil contains higher amounts of cholesterol with 554mg/100g. We studied to find the optimum conditions for crosslinked β–CD to remove cholesterol from the oil [42]. The ratio of the oil to water was 1:2, the β–CD concentration 25%, and mixing time 20min, mixing speed 400 rpm and mixing temperature 60°C with about 89% cholesterol removal. In recycling study, the first recycling was 85% and 82% cholesterol removal was observed up to 3 time trials.

CONCLUSIONS

Even though β–CD could be entrapped cholesterol over 90% from animal originated food products, such as cheese and other dairy products, crosslinking of the β–CD is important to apply into making commercial food products. We experimented positively various cheeses to remove cholesterol without changing taste and texture. Therefore, it is concluded that functional cheeses could be developed with advanced technology by crosslinking β–CD.

REFERENCES

[1] Kwak, H. S., Chung, C. S., Shim, S. Y., and Ahn. J. (2002). Removal of cholesterol from Cheddar cheese by β-cyclodextrin. *J. Agric. and Food Chem, 50,* 7293-7298.

[2] Kim, S. Y., Hong, E. K., Ahn, J., and Kwak, H. S. (2009). Chemical and sensory properties of cholesterol-reduced processed cheese spread. *Int. J. Dairy. Technol, 62(3),* 348-353.

[3] Kwak, H. S., Nam, C. G., and Ahn, J. (2001). Low cholesterol Mozzarella cheese obtained from homogenized β-cyclodextrin-treated milk. *Asian-Aust. J. Anim. Sci, 14(2),* 268-275.

[4] Han, E. M., Kim, S. H., Ahn J., and Kwak, H. S. (2008). Comparison of cholesterol-reduced cream cheese manufactured using crosslinked β-cyclodextrin to regular cream cheese. *Asian-Aust. J. Anim. Sci, 21(1),* 131-137.

[5] Han, E. M., Kim, S. H., Ahn, J., and Kwak, H. S. (2005). Cholesterol removal from homogenized milk with crosslinked β-cyclodextrin by adipic acid. *Asian-Aust. J. Anim. Sci, 18(12),* 1794-1799.

[6] Han, E. M., Kim, S. H., Kim, K. W., and Kwak, H. S. (2007). Morphological change of crosslinked β-cyclodextrin after recycling. *Kor. J. Dairy Sci and Technol, 25(1),* 9-13

[7] Sieber, R. (1993). Cholesterol removal from animal food can it be justified. *Fed. Dairy. Res. Int, 45,* 1243-1247

[8] Ahn, J., and Kwak, H. S. (1999). Optimizing cholesterol removal in cream using β-cyclodextrin and response surface methodology. *J. Food Sci, 64(4),* 629-632.

[9] Hedges, A., Shieh W., and Ameral, R. (1993). Process for removal of residue of cyclodextrin. Austrailia Patent, WO 93/24022.

[10] Shukla, A., Bhaskar, A. R., Rizvi, S. H., and Mulvaney, S. J. (1994). Physicochemical and rheological properties of butter made from supercritically milk fat. *J. Dairy Sci,* 77. 45-54

[11] Lim, S. B., Jwa, M. K., and Kwak, H. S. (1998). Cholesterol removal from milk fat by supercritical carbon dioxide extraction in coupled with adsorption. *Kor. J. Food Sci. Tech,* 30(3), 574-580.

[12] Okenfull, D. G., Sidhu, G. S., and Rooney, M. L. (1991). Cholesterol reduction. Austraila Patent, WO 91/11114.

[13] Chang, E. J., Oh, H. I., and Kwak, H. S. (2001). Optimization of cholesterol removal conditions from homogenized milk by treatment with saponin. *Asian-Aust. J. Anim. Sci,* 14(6), 844-849. Lee, D. K., Ahn, J., and Kwak, H. S. (1999). Cholesterol removal from homogenized milk with β-cyclodextrin. *J. Dairy Sci,* 82, 2327-2330. Alonso, L., Cuesta, P., Fontecha, J., Juarez, M., and Gilliland, S. E. (2009). Use of β-cyclodextrin to decrease the level of cholesterol in milk fat. *J. Dairy Sci,* 92(3), 863-869

[14] Shim, S. Y., Ahn, J., and Kwak, H. S. (2003). Functional properties of cholesterol-removed whipping cream treated by β-cyclodextrin. *J. Dairy Sci,* 86, 2767-2772.

[15] Shim, S. Y., Ahn, J., and Kwak, H. S. (2004). Functional properties of cholesterol removed compound whipping cream by palm oil. *Asian-Aust. J. Anim. Sci,* 17(6), 857-862.

[16] Jung, T. H, Kim, J. J. Ahn, J., and Kwak, H. S. (2005). Properties of cholesterol reduced butter and effect of gamma linolenic acid added butter on blood cholesterol. *Asian-Aust. J. Anim. Sci,* 18(11), 1646-1654.

[17] Kwak, H. S., Suh, H. M., Ahn, J., and Kwon, H. J. (2001). Optimization of β-cyclodextrin recycling process for cholesterol removal in cream. *Asian-Aust. J. Anim. Sci,* 14(4), 548-552.

[18] Kwak, H. S., Kim, S. H., Choi, H. J., and Kang, J. (2004). Immobilized β-cyclodextrin as a simple and recyclable method for cholesterol removal in milk. *Arch. Pharm. Res,* 27(8), 873-877.

[19] Kim, S. H. Ahn, J. and Kwak, H. S. (2004). Crosslinking of β-cyclodextrin on cholesterol removal from milk. *Arch Pharm. Res,* 27(11), 1183-1187.

[20] Ha, H. J., Jeon, S. S., Chang, Y. H. and Kwak. H. S. (2009). Entrapment of milk nutrients during cholesterol removal from milk by crosslinked β-cyclodextrin. *Kor. J. Food Sci. Anim. Resour,* 29(1), 566-572. Ha, H. J., Lee, J. E., Chang, Y. H., and Kwak, H. S. (2010). Entrapment of nutrients during cholesterol removal from cream by crosslinked β-cyclodextrin. *Int. J. Dairy Technol,* 63(1), 119~126.

[21] Kwak, H. S. Chung, C. S. Seok, J. S. Seok., and Ahn. J. (2003). Cholesterol removal and flavor development in Cheddar cheese. *Asian-Aust. J. Anim. Sci.* 16(3), 409-416.

[22] Kwak, H. S., Ahn, H. J., and Ahn, J. (2005). Development of phytosterol ester-added Cheddar cheese for lowering blood cholesterol. *Asian-Aust. J. Anim. Sci,* 18(2), 267-276.

[23] Kim, J. J., Yu, S. H., Jeon, W. M., and Kwak, H. S. (2006). The effect of evening primrose oil on chemical and blood cholesterol lowering properties of Cheddar cheese. *Asian-Aust. J. Anim. Sci,* 19(3), 450-458.

[24] Seon, K. H., Ahn, J., and Kwak, H. S. (2009). The accelerated ripening of cholesterol-reduced Cheddar cheese by crosslinked β-cyclodextrin during ripening. *J. Dairy Sci,* 92(1), 49-57.

[25] Guinee, T. P., Caric, M., and Kalab, M. (2004). Pasteurized processed cheese and substitutes/imitation cheese products. In: Fox, P.F. (ed), *In Cheese: Chemistry and Microbiology.* (2), (pp. 349-394) Elsevier applied Science, London, UK.

[26] Kim, S. Y., Park, S.Y., Ahn. J., and Kwak, H. S. (2008). Properties of cholesterol-reduced block-type process cheese made by crosslinked β-cyclodextrin. *Kor. J. Food Sci. Anim. Resour,* 28(4), 463-469.

[27] Metzger, E. L., and Mistry, V. V. (1993). Effect of homogenization on quality of reduced-fat Cheddar cheese. 2. Rheology and microstructure. J. Dairy Sci. 76. Suppl.1. D163, 145.

[28] Bae, H. Y., Kim, S. Y., Kim, H. Y., and Kwak, H. S. (2008). Properties of cholesterol-reduced Camembert cheese made by crosslinked β-cyclodextrin. *Int. J. Dairy. Technol,* 61(4), 364-371.

[29] Bae, H. Y., Kim, S. Y., and Kwak, H. S.. (2008). Comparison of cholesterol-reduced Camembert cheese using crosslinked β-cyclodextrin to regular Camembert cheese during storage. *Milchwissenschaft,* 63(2), 153-156.

[30] Kosikowski, F. V., and Mistry, V. V. (1997). Cheese and fermented milk foods. (pp. 277-280). F. V. Kosikowski, L.L.C. 1 Peters Lane Westport, CT 06880.

[31] Kim, H. Y., Bae, H. Y., and Kwak, H. S. (2008). Development of cholesterol-reduced blue cheese made by crosslinked β-cyclodextrin. *Milchwissenschaft,* 63(1), 53-56.

[32] Bae, H. Y., Kim, S. Y., Ahn, J., and Kwak, H. S. (2009). Properties of cholesterol-reduced Feta cheese made by crosslinked β-cyclodextrin. *Milchwissenschaft,* 64(2), 165-168.

[33] Jeon, S. S., Chung, C. H., and Kwak, H. S. (2010). Comparison of identified flavor compounds, texture and sensory properties in regular cream cheese and cream cheese made from whole milk powder. *J. Dairy Sci,* 93. E-Suppl. 1. T74.

[34] Jeon, S. S., Lee, S. J., and Kwak, H. S. (2010). Comparison of identified flavor compounds, texture and sensory properties in cream cheese and cholesterol-removed cream cheese made from whole milk powder. Annual Meeting of Kor. Soc. for Food Sci. Anim. Resour. International Convention Center. Jeju, Kor. Abs#209.

[35] Kim, S. H., Han, E. M., Ahn, J., and Kwak, H. S. (2005). Effect of crosslinked β-cyclodextrin on quality of cholesterol-reduced cream cheese. *Asian-Aust. J. Anim. Sci.* 18(4), 584-589.

[36] Jung, T. H., Ha, H. J., Ahn, J. and Kwak, H. S. (2008). Development of cholesterol-reduced mayonnaise with crosslinked β-cyclodextrin and added phytosterol. *Kor. J. Food Sci. Anim. Resour,* 28(2), 211-217.

[37] Kim, S. H., Kim, H. Y., and Kwak, H. S. (2007). Cholesterol removal from lard with crosslinked β-cyclodextrin. *Asian-Aust. J. Anim. Sci,* 20(9): 1468-1472.

[38] Lee, J. E., Seo, M. H., Chang, Y. H., and Kwak, H. S. (2010). Cholesterol removal from squid liver oil by crosslinked β-cyclodextrin. *J. Am. Oil Chem. Soc,* 87, 233-238.

[39] Chang, Y. H., Lee, J. E., and Kwak, H. S. (2010). Optimization of the conditions for removing cholesterol from cod liver oil by β-cyclodextrin crosslinked with adipic. *J. Am. Oil Chem. Soc,* 87, 803-808.

In: Cheese: Types, Nutrition and Consumption
Editors: Richard D. Foster, pp. 267-287

ISBN 978-1-61209-828-9
©2011 Nova Science Publishers, Inc.

Chapter 14

NUTRITIONAL BENEFITS IN CHEESE

Hae-Soo Kwak[1], Palanivel Ganesan[1] and Youn-Ho Hong[2]

[1]Department of Food Science and Technology, Sejong University, Seoul, Korea
[2]Department of Food and Nutrition, Chonnam National University, Gwangju, Korea

ABSTRACT

Cheese serves as a one of the good sources for essential nutrients, such as proteins, lipids, minerals and vitamins. It can enhance health benefits by the production of certain peptides and free amino acids which has various bioactive properties, such as anti-microbial, anti-carcinogenic, anti-thrombotic and so on. Certain biologically active lipids, such as conjugated fatty acid (CLA) and milk fat globule membrane (MFGM), present in cheeses are also found to be health beneficial. Thus, it plays a very important role in the diet of human; however, it suffers from adverse nutritional image due to the presence of saturated fatty acid, cholesterol and salt content. It can be overcome by the production of cheese with low fat or cholesterol removal and by the addition of certain functional living materials, such as probiotic bacteria. The non-starter lactic acid bacteria (NSLAB) used in the cheeses found to be bioactive, such as inactivation of antigenotoxins and production of gamma-aminobutyric acid generation of bioactive peptides. This chapter describes the nutritional significant of cheese components, and their role in enhancing the health benefits.

1. INTRODUCTION

Nutritious rich food, cheese is made mostly from the milk of cows, buffaloes, sheeps or goats, and it is an important food component in the healthy diet of American, Asian and European [1]. It provides a rich source of proteins, peptides, amino acids, short-, medium- and long- chain fatty acids, vitamins, and essential minerals including calcium. A large variety of cheeses has been produced in the world to meet the requirements of taste and health need of individuals. But their consumption varies with individual, race, ethnicity of people and type of milk in cheese preparation. Among the varieties, Cheddar was found to be more popular variety in UK and Mozeralla in USA. In recent years, cheese found to be health beneficial due to the presence of health promoting factors, such as essential amino acids, free fatty acids and so on.

Numerous factors which include type of milk, lactation period, ripening process, type of starter used can vary the nutritional components of the cheese. The fully ripened cheese contains highly water soluble components than its source, milk [2]. It also contains several peptides which has various bioactive roles in humans. These peptides can be generated not only during the ripening process of cheese but also can generate during the digestion process in human tract. Bioactive peptides generated during the ripening as well as during digestion are found to be health beneficial, such as ACE-inhibitory activity [3]. The peptides derived from the casein and whey proteins are also serving as prominent source for the nutraceutical functional foods. Cheese also generates certain free amino acids by the actions of enzymes produced by the starter culture and rennet. However, the amount of free amino acids present in cheese varies with the source of milk and rennet used. The amount of sulfur containing amino acids is relatively low in cheese peptides when compared to the source milk proteins. In general, the amino acid index varies between 91 and 97 if the total amino acid of milk protein were considered to be 100. Biogenic amine formed during decarboxylation of free amino acids by the action of microorganisms which are added during the preparation process or by contaminant also lowers the amino acid index in cheese. The enhanced digestibility of cheese can be produced by the breakdown of casein during ripening of cheese.

The potential and the nutrient significant of cheese are of wide range due to the presence of potentially significant amount of both saturated and unsaturated fat. However, different type of fats has different health effects and not all saturated fats elevated the plasma cholesterol. Certain fats in cheese are found to be health beneficial, such as conjugated linoleic acid (CLA) which shows various biological activity include anticancer, antithrombotic, antidiabetic and antiatherosclerosis. The average content of CLA in cheese is found to be 0.5 to1.7g/100 g of free fatty acids. These contents found to be unaffected during various processes and storage of cheese. In order to reduce the cholesterol level in cheese certain processes has been used, such as the use of cholesterol-reduced milk fat made by adsorption on to beta cyclodextrin.

Cheese also acts as good source minerals, vitamins, and probiotic bacteria which have various health enhancing effects. Cheese contains concentrated source of calcium and it helps in the prevention of osteoporosis of future. Among the various vitamins in cheese, water soluble vitamins are extensively lost during the cheese preparation. But some water soluble vitamins are retained, such as niacin, folate and vitamin B_{12}. Folic acid is important for the reduction of homocysteine in blood. Fat soluble vitamins, such as Vitamin A, are essential in immune system which also found high in cheese. Lactic acid bacteria (LAB) also play an important role in the enhancement of nutritional components of cheese by the production of certain exopolysaccharides. It enhances the flavor of cheese during ripening by the action of its enzymes. It also produces certain peptides and amino acids which increase the bioactivities of cheese. This chapter discusses the current knowledge on beneficial effects of cheese-derived peptides, amino acids, fatty acids, minerals, vitamins, probiotics, and other substances on human health.

2. Proteins

Proteins are of unique macronutrients since it cannot be stored as nonfunctional form in our body, as such other macro nutrients. The other macronutrients such as fat can stored in adipocytes whereas carbohydrate can stored as glycogen. The major milk proteins include caseins, β-lactoglobulin, lactoferrin, serum albumin and immunoglobulins which exerts various biological activities as a whole protein or peptides. Among the milk proteins, caseins are the main protein in cheese; which exist in the form of aggregates after combination with colloidal calcium phosphate known as casein micelles [4]. Caseins in cheese are of nutritionally rich due to the high supply of essential amino acids, phosphate and calcium. They also act as a good source of energy in the human diet.

The nutrition value of cheese protein was slightly lower than the milk protein due to the loss of sulfur containing protein in whey during cheese making process. However, use of certain techniques in cheese preparation, such as ultra filtration for concentration of milk and addition of whey proteins in milk, prevent the loss of biologically active protein. The digestibility of cheese protein was higher than the source milk and this greatly increased during the curing process of cheese. Predigestion step was commonly referred to the curing process of cheese and this process enhances the conversion of proteins to smaller peptides and amino acids. The water-insoluble casein in cheese is mostly converted to water-soluble nitrogenous compounds during the curing process. These smaller peptides are readily absorbed by the intestine and some amino acids formed during curing process helps in increased secretion of gastric juice, such as aspartic and glutamic acids. Thus, cheeses provide a good source of peptides and amino acids from casein and thereby prevent the dismantling of vital proteins in our body.

2.1. Lactoferrin

Lactoferrin is the multifunctional glycoprotein existed in the cheese at the range of 672 µg g−1 (soft cheese) to 1218 µg g−1 (semi-hard cheese) [5]. These proteins have various physiological roles which include host defense against variety of microorganisms, iron homeostasis, anticancer, antiviral and antiinflammatory activity [6]. It possesses two metal binding sites which can able to bind iron and thereby has an antimicrobial effect against wide range of microorganism including yeast [7]. The enzymes, such as pepsin, chymosin, cathepsin and other natural milk enzymes have a potential proteolytic effect on lactoferrin in cheese. It also leads to generation of peptides, such as lactoferricin and lactoferrampin, which also exhibit antimicrobial activity. The main peptide lactoferricin contains 25 aminoacids from the N terminus of lactoferrin molecule which exhibit antiviral against hepatitis C and also anticancer effects. The lactoferrin undergoes extensive denaturation in sterilized milk and yogurt; however, cheese contains detectable range which may be the alternative nutrient source for biologically active lactoferrin.

2.2. Peptides

Cheese flavor and texture are mostly contributed by the proteolysis of cheese protein which leads to generation of various biologically and nutritionally rich peptides and amino acids. The proteolysis actions are mostly catalyzed by the enzymes, such as proteases, and peptidases, and the extent of proteases are depend upon many factors, such as type of lactic starter [8], coagulant used, the condition in which cheese is matured such as time, temperature and humidity and so on. In general, β-casein is degraded less extensively in Parmesan, Emmental and Tilsit, than $α_{s1}$-casein, with higher retaining of $γ_1$-casein and $γ_2$-casein. However, in Roquefort cheese, β-casein is almost degraded. The plasmin action in cheese can be determined by the presence of less $γ_1$-casein and more $γ_2$-casein. These peptides are of great interest beyond the nutritional and sensory value due to the production of biologically active peptides (BPs). Some of the bioactive peptides are listed in Table 1.

Table 1. Bioactive peptides in various cheeses

Cheese type	Bioactive peptides	Bioactivity	References
Parmigiano–Reggiano	β-cn f(8–16), f(58–77), αs2-cn f(83–33)	Phosphopeptides, precursor of β-casomorphin	[77]
Cheddar	αs1- and β-casein fragments	Several phosphopeptides	[78]
Italian varieties: Mozzarella, Crescenza, Italico, Gorgonzola	β-cn f(58–72)	ACE inhibitory	[3]
Gouda	αs1-cn f(1–9), β-cn f(60–68)	ACE inhibitory	[79]
Festivo	αs1-cn f(1–9), f(1–7), f(1–6)	ACE inhibitory	[12]
Emmental	αs1- and β-casein fragments	Immunostimulatory, several phosphopeptides, antimicrobial	[16]
Manchego	Ovine αs1-, αs2- and β-casein fragments	ACE inhibitory	[10]
Emmental	Active peptides not identified	ACE inhibitory	[9]

2.3. Bioactive Peptides (BPs)

Cheese can produce BPs not only during the ripening process but also during the digestion of cheese in the gastro intestinal tract on *in vitro* conditions [9]. These BPs have a positive impact on the health of human, and their activity is based on their amino acid composition and their ability to reach the target site. Bps from cheese show hypotensive and or angiotensin- I converting enzyme inhibition (ACE) [10], anti-hypertension activity, antithrombosis activity, anticarcinogenic activity, opioid activities, stimulation of immunity and so on [11]. However, BPs should be bioavailable to survive digestion and to reach the target site. BPs which contains amino acids, such as proline and hydroxyl proline, are found to be resistant to the digestive enzymes. The BPs also exhibit various physiological effects in our body during transport such as modulation of gut secretion, blood pressure lowering and antioxidant. So the transport of the BPs is regulated on the size, charge molecular weight and bonding of the peptide. The predominant size of peptide varies between 2-50 AAs. Further individual BPs such as β-casein, has been shown multiple functions, such as opiod and ACE-enzyme inhibition. Some of the bioactive peptides from cheese are discussed below.

2.3.1. Antihypertensive Peptides

Among the biologically active peptides in cheese ACE- inhibiting peptides make up the major contribution. These peptides are of particularly important because it enhances the level of vasodialatory peptide (bradykinin) and corresponding decrease in the vasoconstrictory peptide (angiotensin-II) which ultimately results in the reduction of risk of cardio vascular disease (CVD). The starter culture used in the preparation of the cheese also contributes the synthesis of these peptides and it varies with the type of starter used in the cheese. In *Festivo* cheese made with starter cultures, such as *L. acidophilus* and bifidobacteria has multifactorial health benefits, such as antihypertensive peptides, probiotics and bioavailability of calcium[12]. In Manchengo cheese made with various starter cultures shows the maximum antihypertensive activity at 8 months. Further addition of probiotic culture enhances the release of ACE-Inhibitory peptides in Cheddar cheese during ripening.

The ACE-inhibitory activity of cheese can also be determined by the degree of proteolysis and low level of proteolysis exhibits low ACE-Inhibitory activity [13]. The peptides obtained after 8 month storage of cheese are normally found to be high ACE-inhibitory activity. However, higher degree of proteolysis also causes sufficient loss in ACE-Inhibitory activity of certain cheese. In case of Parmesan cheese, the ACE-Inhibitory peptide obtained from $α_{s1}$-casein seen in 6 months was degraded after 15 months storage. But extend of degradation varies with the type and storage of cheese, Gouda cheese show highest activity during 2 year old storage [14]. The inhibition strengths of these peptides are also varies among the cheese, Smacchi and Gobbetti [3] reported inhibition strengths of various Italian cheese in brackets, Gorgonzola (80% Inhibition), Mozarella (59% Inhibition) and Italico (82% inhibition) are found to lower the risk of CVD.

Apart from the long chain peptides some new oligopeptides also show the biological activity. Some of the oligopeptides from Grano padono cheese shows various biological activities. Some researchers also reported that various Swiss origin hard (44 samples), semi hard and soft cheese contains two tri peptides. These tripeptides (Valyl-prolyl-proline and isoleucyl-prolyl-proline) concentration varies in the cheese based on the pasteurization of milk and ripening time of cheese. Higher concentration of these tripeptides obtained from raw milk and long ripened cheese such as Emmental than soft cheese obtained from pasteurized milk. However, some sheep cheese obtained from the 15-day-old storage shows higher ACE-inhibitory activity [10].The ACE-inhibitory activity of peptides obtained from the cheese are not as potent as drugs used for the treatment. However, they show as a moderate bioactivity which can be used as functional food in our daily diet.

2.2.2. Immunopeptides

Casein peptides from milk obtained after the hydrolysis shows various immune functions. [15]. However, the role of immunopeptides of cheese against human body defense are quite complex. Gagnaire *et al.* reported that Emmental cheese contains 28 peptides which show immune-stimulatory as well as antimicrobial activity in vitro. Initially, Jolles *et al.* reported that trypsin hydrolyzed human milk possess immunostimulatory activity. Some of the bioactive sequence of casein and lyophilized extract of Gouda cheese also shows also modulating activity inhuman cells. The exact mechanism and activity of cheese derived peptides which exert the immunomodulatory are still questionable.

2.2.3. Antimicrobial Peptides

Antimicrobial peptides have been identified in various cheeses which makes the microbial resistance impropable. Among the agents used for the generation of antimicrobial peptides chymosin makes the major which generate similar sequence of peptides from various cheeses of different sources which includes cow, sheep, and goat. Some researchers reported that nine varieties of Italian cheese show the antimicrobial activities. The ripening time generate the greater sequence of this antimicrobial peptide, however increasing the ripening time also leads to the hydrolysis of peptides and loss of the bioactivity in various cheese. Some researchers also reported that 91 peptides in Emmental cheese among them 21 shows mixed bioactive which includes mineral carrying, antimicrobial and so on. The peptides which act against microorganism are in broad range from bacteria to fungi.

2.2.4. Antioxidant Peptides

Ripening of cheese generates various peptides with antioxidant activities. These peptides are obtained from the milk protein domains which show antioxidant activity. Songiseep *et al.* [19] reported that the antioxidant activity of cheese increase with increasing stage of ripening of cheese and addition of adjunct culture in cheese cause to increase the formation of peptides. Some other research also reported that Cheddar cheese enriched with fruit extract showed the antioxidant activity [20] and their extend of bioactivity depends upon the ripening stage. Recently, Pritchard et al., 2010 identified peptides with MW greater that 10 kDa has higher inhibition of DPPH in various commercial and organic cheese produced in Australia [21, 22].

2.3. Free Amino Acids (FAA)

Cheese making involves various biochemical processes among them proteolysis gains more importance in the generation of FAA and flavor of cheese. It generates both essential FAA and nonessential FAA in higher levels. Table 2 shows FAAs contents of Cheddar cheese assayed by USDA (2008). The pattern of proteolysis and generation of FAA can be summarized as follows: initially the caseins are hydrolyzed by residual coagulant activity retained in the curd, by plasmin, and also by other proteolytic enzymes to a range of intermediate-sized peptides, which are hydrolyzed by proteinases and peptidases from the starter lactic acid bacteria, non-starter lactic acid bacteria (NS-LAB) and secondary microflora to shorter peptides and amino acids.

Table 2. Essential and nonessential amino acid content of Cheddar cheese [80]

Amino acids	Amount (g/100g cheese)
Essential amino acids	
Histidine	0.87
Isoleucine	1.545
Leucine	2.39
Lysine	2.07
Methionine	0.65
Phenylalanine	1.31
Threonine	0.89
Tryptophan	0.32
Valine	1.66
Nonessential amino acids	
Alanine	0.70
Arginine	0.94
Cystine	0.13
Tyrosine	1.20

The characteristic free amino acid (FAA) pattern varies with cheese type based on enzymatic degradation of peptides and amino acid interconversion [23]. The concentrations of the different amino acids in a cheese are related to the manufacturing technology (type of curd, addition of starters, ripening conditions), duration of ripening, and the extent and type of proteolysis. FAA shows different bioactive properties in various cheeses. Sulphur AAs, such as cysteine, methionine and γ-glutamylcysteine are known as strong xenobiotic deactivating and anti-neoplastic agent. The tryptophan, was found to relieve stress and induce sleep. The branched-chain FAA (Leu, Ile, Val), along with aromatic FAA (Phe, Tyr, Trp) and Met, are present in all cheese types which are the main precursors of key aroma compounds. Certain FAA are extremely important in taste and flavor development, e.g. Arg is related to bitterness, while Pro, Ser and Asn are related to sweetness. Hence the increase in the Ser and Asp concentrations may help to mask any bitter flavors that may be developed as a result of the possible formation of bitter peptides in the cheese. Most of the goat cheeses contains amino acids such as glutamic acid, lysine and leucine, but in some cheese like soft rennet fresh goat milk Cacioricotta cheeses researchers found a notable amount of taurine [24]. Mostly these amino acid is lost in whey and they recovered in cheese most likely due to the high heat treatment of milk leads to denatured whey protein entrapment in curd. Some of the whey protein entrapment in curd also leads to the increase of essential free amino acids such as cysteine, isoleucine, leucine, lysine, threonine and tryptophan.

2.3. Γ-Amino Butyric Acid (GABA, 4-Amino Butanoic Acid, $C_4H_9NO_2$)

GABA is non protein amino acid and it is well known for various beneficial effects such as antihypertensive, calming effects, diuretics and various neuronal effects [25]. GABA is generated during ripening stage of cheese predominantly by the action of various LAB species used in the starter culture. Types of LAB also influence the rate of production of GABA. The production of GABA leads to increase in the carbon dioxide formation which ultimately results in the formation of eyes and cracks in Gouda cheese. GABA also found to reduce the blood pressure in the experimental animals through intravenous administration [26].

Glutamate decarboxylase activity of LAB lead to synthesis of GABA from L-glutamate and it leads to screening of various LAB species to the development of functional cheese. Among the various strains screened in 22 Italian cheeses, some of them were identified as GABA producing strains such as *Lactobacilli brevis, Lactobacilli paracasei* and *Lactobacilli plantarum* [27]. Recently, few researchers produced Cheddar cheese with *Lactobacilli. casei* Zhang which shows high biological activity of peptides includes ACE-inhibitory activity and non protein amino acid such as GABA. LAB has a capacity to produce GABA from L-glutamate, however some researcher reported that *Lactobacilli paracasei* PF6 and *Lactobacilli plantarum* C48 can synthesize GABA in the absence of L-glutamate as precursor in the stimulated gastro intestinal conditions [27].

3. FAT

Fat content is essential in cheese and it is varies based on the milk content and the process involved in the production of cheese. The fats contribute flavor and texture to the cheese and the types of fats involved in cheese are of triglycerides, saturated fatty acids and unsaturated fatty acids including mono and poly unsaturated fatty acids. The fatty acids contents of milk vary with the species of animals. For example milk fat from sheep and goat are rich in medium chain triacylglycerols (MCT) and FAs C6-10. The fatty acids C6:0, C8:0 and C10:0 are found to vary in goats, sheep, and cows and found advantages to consumer health [29]. Some fatty acids are originated in the mammary gland of cow through de novo biosynthesis [30]. Among the fatty acids *De novo* biosynthesis contributes 45% of the fatty acids produces short and medium chain fatty acids and remaining through the diet of cow which contributes longer-chain length fatty acids. The dietary lipids are modified by the rumen bacteria leads to mixture of fatty acids including the conjugated linoleic acid (CLA). Milk fat are therefore cheese fat except in the case of Mold cheese [31].

Fat in cheese consumption believed that associated with CVD because lipoproteins deposit fat around the body [32]. However, balance of the fatty acids in the diet may alter the level of deposition. The main nutritional concern of the cheese is of saturated fat which may raise plasma atherogenic LDL. Among the cheese Cheddar contains high total fat, of which 62% of the fatty acids are SFA, 27% are MUFA and 3% are PUFA. Even though the link of high fat in cheese concern with CVD [33] they cannot prove casualty, due to various other factors such as life style, smoking, obesity and other foods consumed in diet. However, all fats do not have plasma cholesterol raising effects and it varies with the chain length of SFAs. The longer chain length fatty acid such as stearic acid found to be lower than medium chain (lauric, myristic and palmitic) and shorter chain length fatty acids. Some fatty acid such as stearic acid are converted to MUFA oleic acid in cheddar cheese which is considered to be the healthier source of fat in diet since it does not associated with CVD. From the point, all fats in Cheddar cheese are not raise the plasma cholesterol levels as a marker for CVD.

Guidelines regarding the dietary of fat often neglect the individual SFAs for the beneficiary activities. Some of the beneficiary activities includes anti cancer, antiviral, anti bacterial and anti carier properties. Lauric acid play an important role in anti viral, anti bacterial properties [34] and also act as an anti- carier properties [35]. The fatty acid such as butyric acid also plays an important role in expression of genes and prevention of growth of cancer [36]. Some other lipids such as trans fatty acids in cheese also shows various beneficial role in health.

3.1. Conjugated Linoleic Acid (CLA)

CLA are trans fatty acids which are double bonded unsaturated and exist in two steroisomeric forms; the cis and trans configuration. Only small amount of trans fatty acids are found in cheese and are found to be health beneficial. The main dietary source of CLA are milk, other ruminant fats and also by rumen bacteria [37]. The trans fatty acid which from other source such as hydrogenated vegetable oils shows the risk of CVD [38] by increasing the level of the small dense elevated LDL cholesterol level. In contradictory the ruminant source of CLA found to be beneficial to health.

The various beneficial role of CLA includes body fat reduction, inhibition of tumour, anti atherosclerosis and anti obesity [39]. The mechanism of CLAs involve in the reduction of body fat are rather complex and multi functional such as by increasing the expenditure of energy, modulating cytokines and increasing the rate of β-oxidation. Among the CLA in cheese 75% or more of CLA in cheese is *cis*9, *trans*11 CLA isomer, while trace levels of *trans*10, *cis*12 CLA isomer are also present [40], and are shown in Fig 1. It was reported that the amount of CLA were different according to the types of cheese. The CLA content of cheese shows in Table 3. Prandini *et al.* [41] compared various Italian and French cheese, and reported that sheep cheeses had the highest levels of CLA (9.86 mg/g fat), α-linolenic acid (0.75%) and trans-vaccenic acid (1.63%), and the lowest contents of linoleic acid (1.80%) and oleic acid (16.83%). The comparison of cheeses obtained from milk of the same ruminant species but through different production technologies reported statistically significant differences in the fatty acid profiles that could be due to a different degree of lipolysis in the cheeses compared. Judging from the data of animal trial, it is recommended about 500 mg of CLA per day for human consumption can be effective in preventing cancer.

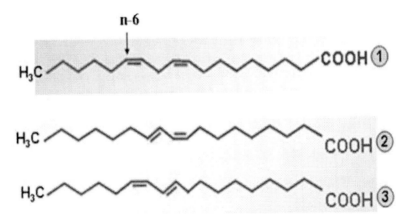

Figure 1. Structure of linoleic acid and its major CLA derivatives. [93] 1. Linoleic acid (typical n-6 PUFA); 2. *cis*-9,*trans*-11-octadecadienoic acid (9-CLA, in fact an n-7 fatty acid); 3. *trans*-10, *cis*-12-octadecadienoic acid (10-CLA).

Table 3. CLA content of various cheeses [41, 81]

Cheese type	Lipid basis amount (mg of CLA/g of lipid)
Alpine	4.79 ± 1.07
Blue 1	4.87 ± 0.10
Blue 2	7.96 ± 0.12
Brie	4.75 ± 0.28
Cheddar- medium	4.02 ± 0.29
Cheddar-sharp	4.59 ± 0.30
Cheddar-gold	3.72 ± 0.17
Cream	4.3 ± 0.42
Cottage	4.8 ± 0.30
Edam	5.38 ± 0.90
Emmantal	7.66 ± 1.42
Fontiona Valdostana	8.11 ± 1.53
Goat	4.29 ± 1.78
Grana/parmigiano	3.85 ± 0.51
Montery jack	4.8 ± 0.38
Mozzarella	4.31 ± 0.21
Parmeasan	4.0 ± 0.53
Pecorino	7.77 ± 2.25
Swiss	5.45 ± 0.59
Viking	3.59 ± 0.01
Processed American	3.64 ± 0.15

Values are means standard error.

3.2. Milk Fat Globule Membrane (MFGM)

MFGM is found in significant quantities in various cheese which is rich in proteins, glycoproteins, fats such as sphingolipids, glycerophopholipids, ezymes and other found and other minor components [42] are shown in Fig 2. The pressing of cheese causes various changes in MFGM and it includes (i) breaking of outer double layer from fat globules and be expelled with the serum during pressing and (ii) the monolayer of membrane material (mainly proteins and phospholipids) may remain around the fat inclusions [43]. Thus, breaking of the MFGM and coalescence of the fat globules may result in the liberation of the double layer of surface-active and hydrophilic components, consisting mainly of phospholipids, lipoproteins and proteins which have some functional and nutritional properties [43].

Phospholipids from the MFGM may also interact with proteins, i.e. caseins and whey proteins. Some of the fragments of MFGM are present either in fat or at the serum pockets. Polar lipids such as phospholipids are spontaneously associate with water and various liquid phases. [44]. Some of the MFGM lipids are varies in shape based on the composition such as cubic, lamellar or hexagonal crystalline [44]. In excess of water, the membrane lipids in the lamellar form can be dispersed in vesicular form. The phospholipid of MFGM has potential physiological effects on brain health, against colon cancer, gastrointestinal pathogens, cholesterol binding *in vivo* [45] and inhibition of tumour growth. It also enhances the texture [43] and water holding capacity of certain cheese. MFGM act as carbon source for lactic acid bacteria during ripening and increase the flavor in cheese by providing enzymes [43]. Intense flavor in cheeses was obtained from the proteolysis and lipolysis of MFGM enzymes. MFGM also helps in prevention of excessive lipolysis and act as a barrier which results in the reduction of rancid flavor in cheese [46].

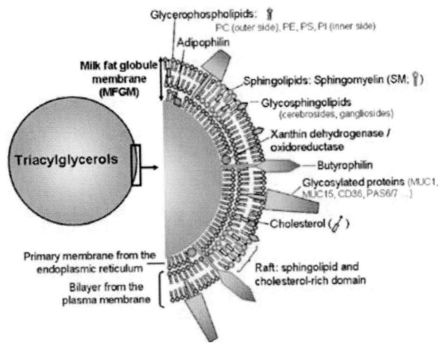

Figure 2. Schematic representation of the structure of milk fat globule membrane [94].

3.2.1. Bioactive MFGM Lipids

Among the various lipids some polar and complex lipids of MFGM found to be health enhancing functions [47]. The phospholipids of MFGM shows anticancer activity. The other lipids of MFGM are also associated in reduction of age-related diseases, and apoptosis [48, 49]. The inhibition of intestinal absorption of cholesterol and suppression of colon tumors are most effectively done by sphingomyelin [45]. Some steriodal vitamins such as Vitamin K has protective actions against hepatocarcinoma and atherosclerosis. The toctirenols also possess various health beneficial properties such as nueroprotective, anticancer and antioxidant activities [50].

3.2.2. Bioactive MFGM Proteins

Most of the proteins in MFGM shows bioactive functions, some of them involved in cell signaling, fat transport and/or metabolism, protein synthesis and so on. Beyond the functions they also show various bioactive role in humans. The Mucin 1 protein shows preventive role in the attachment of fimbriated microorganisms. Some other protein like fatty acid binding protein also shows the anti cancer activity. Some of the proteins in MFGM has unknown activity, however few report suggested that some MFGM proteins have negative effects, but it should be confirmed with the animal models before it should be exploited [51].

4. MINERALS

Mineral concentration in cheese varies with the type of cheese, manufacturing procedure, coagulation method and the amount of salt added in cheese [52]. The mineral migration in cheese causes also some changes in concentration of minerals during cheese ripening. The pH gradient effect causes such changes that lead to the movement of minerals from centre to the external layer of cheese block or vice versa [53]. Recently, Gonzalez-Martin [54] developed mineral measurement in various cheeses using near infrared spectroscopy with a fibre optic probe and found that potassium and sodium concentrations were higher. Thus cheese is a rich source of major and minor minerals which include calcium, phosphorous, sodium, chloride, potassium and zinc which are required by our diet. Some of the mineral composition in cheese is summarized in Table.4.

Table 4. Minerals of various cheeses

Name	Ca^a	P^a	Na^a	Mg^a	K^a	Zn^b	Cu^b	Mn^b	Fe^b	References
Sainte Maure (days)	21		12.7		4.01					[82]
Rocamadour	2.53	5.07		0.37	3.69	13.1				[83, 84]
Babia Laciana	1.99	4.19	3.45	0.22	2.99	14.7	2.05	2.42	3.47	[85]
Bastelicaccia	6.55									[86]
Vadeteja	6.43	4.4	12.1	0.26	2.61	26.3	1.7	1.02	3.55	[85]
Armada	8.67	6.47	8.34	0.32	2.21	36.1	1.72	0.89	3.79	[85]
Fresh cheese	14.1	8.12	10	0.63	2.54	34.6	1.68	0.4	4.01	[87]
Washed curd	12.4	7.1	7.8	0.55	1.71	36.6	1.34	0.43	4.59	[87]
Majorero	13.7	8.18	9.8	0.62	1.62	45.1	2.05	0.37	3.88	[87]
Serra da Estrela	10	8		1	1.7	94.3	2.3	1.25		[88]
Pecorino	14	9		0.8						[89]
Los Pedroches	11	7		0.9	1.8	38	1.4			[90]
Canestrato Pugliese	21	10		0.8						[91]
Roquefort	11	7		0.5	2.1	64	1.4	0.4	7	[92]

[a] g/kg total solids.
[b] mg/kg total solids.

4.1. Calcium

Calcium is an important macro mineral for our body and it is present abundance in cheese. The level of calcium in cheeses is vary with the type and found to be higher in hard cheese m (8.1 g/kg) which are 4 times higher in cheeses made with mold and in milk. The availability of calcium in milk is in different forms either casein–bound, ionic or in colloidal form as calcium phosphate. The coagulation process of cheese curd will be affected if the calcium in milk is not in equilibrium form, for example during cold storage ionic form depletion lead to the detriment. In order to overcome these difficulties certain amount of calcium chloride is added in the cheese making process and it enhances the level of calcium in various cheeses and it is very beneficial to health concern. It also enhances the cheese making process by reducing the coagulation time and the gel firmness [55].

Cheese calcium is highly bioavailable due to the complex form between the cheese peptides and calcium, this prevents the calcium against precipitation and aid in absorbtion of the intestine [56]. The cheese consumption helps to prevent the tooth caries by enhancing remineralization and reducing demineralization process [57]. It also acts as a good source of calcium for the lactose intolerant individuals, where most of the lactose is metabolized and largely removed in whey [58]. The consumption of calcium is necessary since the body will demineralize the bone calcium when blood calcium level is inadequate. Therefore, it is necessary to consume a sufficient amount of calcium for maintaining a good skeleton.

Cheese calcium consumption helps not only maintain healthy bones but also plays an important role in reducing blood pressure, helps in losing weight when consumed with low energy diets. The exact mechanisms by which consumption of calcium and reduction of body weight are unclear. It may be pre assumed that complex formation of fatty acid and calcium prevents the absorbtion. Further, dietary calcium stimulate lipolysis and decreases the lipid accumulation by suppressing the calciterol.

4.2. Phosphorus

Cheese also act as good source of phosphorous which exist in various forms such as soluble phosphate exist in the serum phase and bound phosphate exist in the paracasein part of cheese curd. The bound phosphate also in two forms one as bound organic phosphate and another is bound inorganic phosphate which is classified based on the covalent attachment of phosphate with casein [59]. The average concentration of phosphorous in cheese is varies with the type of cheese and the milk used for cheese preparation. Some study show that phosphorous content in cow and goat cheese are found to be lower than cheese obtained from the ewes. The average concentrations of phosphate in cow cheese are about 3.73g/kg, reported by Gonzalez [54] through near infra red spectroscopy study with fibre optic probe.

The phosphate helps in maintaining pH and also enhances the gel strength of cheese by cross linking within or between the casein. However, the level of different phosphate varies in Cheeses, For example in Cheddar cheese the organic phosphate level decreases with increasing ripening time most likely due to the dephosphorylation of casein and phospho peptides. The dephosphorylation was due to the several acid phosphatases which derived from the milk and other cheese bacteria. These enzymes also aids in the production of some bioactive peptides with phosphate which has also various health enhancing effects. Even though phosphorous is essential nutrients and over consumption of phosphorous with low calcium diet leads to various deteriorating effects including osteoporosis. The optimum molar ratio of calcium to phosphorous is 1:1 and in the well balanced diet can overcome this deficiency.

4.3. Salt

Salt plays a very important role in the cheese making process. It has various roles such as preservatives in cheese by preventing the growth of spoilage bacteria [60] and also enhances the activity of both lipolytic and proteolytic enzymes, which promote the flavor of cheese. It also accelerates the whey expulsion and affects the rheolgy [61]. The addition of salt varies with types of cheese such as Cheddar- the salt added in curd, Edam-cheese immersed in brine and Blue cheese-salt rubbed outside [62]. Salt are very essential for life and it involves in various biochemical process for the normal function of our body. Some of the biological roles of salt include nutrient absorption and transport, nerve impulse transmissions for muscle and cardiac function [63]. The minimal requirement of salt for body is about 0.5g/day [64].

Among the main functions of salt in diet the maintenance of blood volume and blood pressure makes up more. The excess consumption of the salt may also leads the hypertension and CVD. In order to reduce the salt content, the sodium level in the cheese alternative attempt has taken by using KCl. This practice is dropped off due to the off flavors of KCl contribute to the cheese when they used in excess. The most negative impact of the salt is can increase pressure. However, individual health is also important than the salt that causes the pressure. Even though salt can increase blood pressure the cheese acts as a balanced diet with the supply of calcium and bioactive peptides which can modulate the increase pressure.

5. VITAMINS

The vitamin content is variable between types and variety of cheese. It also depends on the milk vitamins, microbial cultures and also the conditions in which cheese is matured [65]. Milk vitamins, such as vitamin A and D, are retained mostly in the cheese curd together with other fat-soluble vitamins as shown in Table 5 [67]. In most cheese, some water-soluble vitamins, such as folate, niacin, B_{12} and riboflavin, are noted in sufficient quantities to have a significant effect on human nutrition [1]. The water soluble vitamins are heat sensitive than fat soluble vitamins and sufficient amount of vitamins are lossed in pasteurization of milk and also in whey. The loss of water soluble vitamins in goat cheese is of about: 10–20% for ascorbic acid, <1% for riboflavin, 5–7% for pyridoxin, folates and cobalamin, around 10% for thiamin, 0% for niacin, pantothenic acid and biotin. However, sufficient amount of water soluble vitamins are produced by the LAB culture used. Folate content was noted high in the soft lactic goat milk chesses [67]. Folate and vitamin B_{12} can help reducing high levels of homocysteine in blood, an amino acid that has been linked with cardiovascular disease [68], while niacin and riboflavin are important for the metabolism of carbohydrates, fats, and proteins [69].

Table 5. Vitamin content of Cheddar cheese

Vitamin	Unit	Content per 100g
Vitamin A	RE (µg)	388
Vitamin D	µg	0.6
Folate	µg	30
Niacin	NE (mg)	7
Vitamin B_{12}	µg	2.4
Riboflavin	mg	0.4

6. PROBIOTICS

Probiotics is the term used for the administration of living microorganisms in food which exert certain health enhancing function in our body. The various health enhacing function of the probiotic bacteria includes enhancing immune system, reduce the bold cholesterol, anticarcinogenic and so on. Some LAB such as *Pediococcus, Lactobacillus* inhibits the growth of toxigenic mould by production of certain anti metabolites such as hydroxyl fatty acids, hydrogen peroxide [70]. Cheese act as a good source for the deliver of probiotic organisms since it act as a buffer and create high acidic environment which is favorable for the survival of probiotic through out GIT [71].

Consumption of cheese with probiotic bacteria has various health enhancing effects such as increasing the saliva secretion rate and thereby enhancing the oral health with reducing the hyposalivation and the mouth dryness [72]. The consumption of cheese with *L. rhamnosus* HN001 and *L. acidophilus* are found to increase the immune response of healthy elderly people. Some of the age related deteriotion of the immune system can also be reduced by the consumption of cheese. Cheese with certain LAB species can also able to reduce the growth of certain toxigenic microbes by the production of certain metabolites. Some of the cheese LAB species shows antigenotoxic properties and antimutagenic properties [73], thereby it may reduces the risk of cancer [74]. Among the LAB species Lactobacilli casei isolated from traditional Italian ewe cheeses show microbial antigenotoxic–antimutagenic properties [75, 76]. Thus, cheese also serve as an alternative functional with the implement of certain beneficial bacteria, and further research also should focused to enhance the value of these functional cheese based on the disease specific.

CONCLUSIONS

The most nutritionally completed food in the diet of world represented by cheese. It is a good source of proteins, peptides, amino acids, lipids, free fatty acids, minerals such as calcium, phosphate and vitamins. They can serve as an enhancer of the health of world population. Certain fats such as CLAs in cheese proved to be cardio protective. Though some saturated lipids and salts can increase the risk of CVD, but it can be balanced by a concomitant increase in anti-atherogenic HDL-cholesterol levels. In addition generation of bioactive components, such as GABA and antigenotoxins by certain LAB species are found to increase the health potential value of the cheese. Further cheese can enhance the well being of the diet of groups consuming inadequate source of calcium.

From the chapter, it is clear that there is a lack of certain information such as certain vitamins, minerals and carbohydrates produced from the bacteria and source milk. Further, study should be focused on the cheese based on the various type of milk, beneficial bacteria role and their metabolites function in cheese. Those studies might enhance the nutritional role of cheese.

REFERENCES

[1] Ash, A., and Wilbey, A. (2010). The *nutritional significance of cheese in the UK diet. Int. J. Dairy Tech, 63,* 305-319.

[2] Kosikowski, F. V., and Mistry, V.V. (1997). Cheese and Fermented Milk Foods Volume 1: Origins and Principles. (pp.539). F V Kosikowski. Westport, CT:

[3] Smacchi, E., and Gobbetti, M. (1998). Peptides from several Italian cheeses inhibitory to proteolytic enzymes of lactic acid bacteria: Pseudomonas fluorescens ATCC 948 and to the angiotensin I-converting enzyme. *Enz. Microbiol. Technol, 22,* 687-694.

[4] Farrell, H. M., Jimenez-Flores, R., Bleck, G. T., Brown, E. M., Butler, J, E., Creamer, L. K., Hicks, C. L., Hollar, C. M., Ng-Kwai-Hang, K. F., and Swaisgood, H. E. (2004). Nomenclature of the proteins of cows' milk—sixth revision. *J. Dairy Sci, 87,* 1641-1674.

[5] Dupont, D., Arnould, C., Rolet-Repecaud, O., Duboz, G., Faurie, F., Martin, B., and Beuvier, E. (2006). Determination of bovine lactoferrin concentrations in cheese with specific monoclonal antibodies. *Int. Dairy J, 16,* 1081-1087.

[6] Elbarbary, H. A., Abdou, A. M., Park, E. Y., Nakamura, Y., and Mohamed, H. A. (2010). Novel antibacterial lactoferrin peptides generated by rennet digestion and autofocusing technique. *Int. Dairy J, 20,* 646-651.

[7] Steijns, J. M., and van Hooijdonk, A. C. M. (2000). Occurrence, structure, biochemical properties and technological characteristics of lactoferrin. *Br. J. Nutr, 84,* S11-S17.

[8] Kunji, E. R. S., Mierau, I., Hagting, A., Poolman, B., and Konings, N. (1996). The proteolytic system of lactic acid bacteria. *Antonie van Leeuwenhoek, 70,* 187-221.

[9] Parrot, S., Degraeve, P., Curia, C., and Martial-Gros, A. (2003). In vitro study on digestion of peptides in Emmental cheese: analytical evaluation and influence on angiotensin I converting enzyme inhibitory peptides. *Nahrung, 47,* 87-94.

[10] Gomez-Ruiz, J. A., Ramos, M., and Recio, I. (2002). Angiotensin converting enzyme-inhibitory peptides in Manchego cheeses manufactured with different starter cultures. *Int. Dairy J, 12,* 697-706.

[11] Butikofer, U., Meyer, J., Sieber, R., and Wechsler, D. (2007). Quantification of the angiotensin-converting enzymeinhibiting tripeptides Val-Pro-Pro and Ile-Pro-Pro in hard, semi-hard and soft cheeses. *Int. Dairy J, 17,* 968-975.

[12] Ryhanen, E., Pihlanto-Leppala, A., and Pahkala, E. (2001). A new type of ripened, low-fat cheese with bioactive properties. *Int. Dairy J,* 11 441-447.

[13] Meisel, H., Goepfert, A., and Gunther, S. (1997). ACE-inhibitory activities in milk products. *Milchwissenschaft, 52,* 307-311.

[14] Saito, T., Nakamura, T., Kitazawa, H., Kawai, Y., and Itoh, T. (2000). Isolation and structural analysis of antihypertensive peptides that exist naturally in Gouda cheese. *J. Dairy Sci, 83,* 1434-1440.

[15] Gill, H. S., Doull, F., Rutherfurd, K. J., and Cross, M. L. (2000). Immunoregulatory peptides in bovine milk. *Br. J. Nutr,* 84, S111-S117.

[16] Gagnaire, V., Molle, D., Herrouin, M., and Leonil, J. (2001). Peptides identified during Emmental cheese ripening: Origin and proteolytic systems involved. *J. Agric. Food Chem, 49,* 4402-4413.

[17] Jollès, P., Parker, F., Floch, F., Migliore, D., Alliel, P., Zerial, A., and Werner, G.H. (1981). Immunostimulating substances from human casein. *J. Immun, 3,* 363-369.

[18] Rizzello, C. G., Losito, I., Gobbetti, M., Carbonara, T., De Bari, M. D., and Zambonin, P. G. (2005). Antibacterial activities of peptides from the water-soluble extracts of Italian cheese varieties. *J. Dairy Sci, 88,* 2348-2360.

[19] Songisepp, E., Kullisaar, T., Hutt, P., Elias, P., Brilene, T., Zilmer, M., and Mikelsaar, M. (2004). A new probiotic cheese with antioxidative and antimicrobial activity. *J. Dairy Sci,* 87, 2017-2023.

[20] Apostolidis, E., Kwon, Y. I., and Shetty, K. (2007). Inhibitory potential of herb, fruit, and fungal-enriched cheese against key enzymes linked to type 2 diabetes and hypertension. *Innovat. Food Sci. Emerg. Tech, 8,* 46-54.

[21] Pritchard, S.R., Phillips, M., and Kailasapathy, K. (2010). Identification of bioactive peptides in commercial Cheddar cheese. *Food Res. Int, 43 (5).* 1545-1548.

[22] Pritchard, S.R., Phillips, M., and Kailasapathy, K. 2010. Identification of bioactive peptides in commercial Australian organic cheddar cheeses. *Aust. J. Dairy Tech. 65 (3),* 170-173.

[23] Polo, C., Ramos, M., and Sanchez, R. (1985). Free amino acids by high performance liquid chromatography and peptides by gel electrophoresis in Mahon cheese during ripening. *Food Chem, 16,* 85-96.

[24] Caponio, F., Gomes, T., Allogio, V., and Pasqualone, A. (2000). An effort to improve the organoleptic properties of a soft cheese from rustic goat milk. *Eur. Food Res. Technol, 211,* 305-309.

[25] Lacroix, N., St-Gelais, D., Champagne, C. P., Fortin, J., and Vuillemard, J. C. (2010) Characterization of aromatic properties of old-style cheese starters. *J. Dairy Sci,* 93, 3427-3441.

[26] Lacerda, J. E., Campos, R. R., Araujo, C. G., Andreatta-Van Leyen, S., Lopes, O. U. and Guertzenstein, P. G. (2003). Cardiovascular responses to microinjections of GABA or anesthetics into the rostral ventrolateral medulla of conscious and anesthetized rats. *Braz. J. Med. Biol. Res,* 36, 1269-1277.

[27] Siragusa, S., De Angelis, M., Di Cagno, R.Rizzello, C,G., Coda, R., and Gobbetti, M. (2007). Synthesis of γ-aminobutyric acid by lactic acid bacteria isolated from a variety of Italian cheeses. *Appl. Environ. Microbiol. 22,* 7283-7290.

[28] Wang, H. K., Dong, C., Chen, Y. F., Cui, L.M., and Zhang, H. P. A new probiotic Cheddar cheese with high ACE-inhibitory activity and gamma-aminobutyric acid content produced with Koumiss-derived Lactobacillus casei Zhang. *Food Technol. Biotechnol, 48,* 62-70.

[29] Sanz sampelayo, M. R., Chilliard, Y., Schmidely, P., and Boza, J. (2007). Influence of type of diet on the fat constituents of goat and sheep milk. *Small. Rumen. Res. 68,* 42-63.

[30] Palmquist, D. L. (2006). Milk fat: origin of fatty acids and influence of nutritional factors thereon. In: P. F. Fox., and P. L. H. McSweeney (Eds) *Advanced Dairy Chemistry Lipids,* (pp. 43-92) Springer: New York.

[31] Walther, B., Schmid, A., Sieber, R., and Wehrmuller, K. (2008). Cheese in nutrition and health. *Dairy Sci. Technol,* 88, 389-405.

[32] Ballantyne, C. M. and Hoogeveen, R. C. (2003). Role of lipid and lipoprotein profiles in risk assessment and therapy. *Am. Heart J,* 146, 227-233.

[33] Kromhout, D., Menotti, A., Bloemberg, B., Aravanis, C., Blackburn, H., Buzina, R., Dontas, A. S., Fidanza, F., Giampaoli, S., Jansen, A., et al. (1995). Dietary saturated and trans fatty acids and cholesterol and 25-year mortality from coronary heart disease: the Seven Countries Study. *Prev. Med, 24,* 308-315.

[34] Thormar, H., and Hilmarsson, H. (2007). The role of microbicidal lipids in host defense against pathogens and their potential as therapeutic agents. *Chem. Phys. Lipids, 150,* 1-11.

[35] Schuster, G. S., Dirksen, T. R., Ciarlonw, A. E., Burnett, G. W., Reynolds, M. T., and Lankford, M. T. (1980). Anticaries and antiplaque potential of free fatty acids in vitro and in vivo. *Pharmacol. Therapeut. Dent, 5,* 25-33.

[36] German, J. B. (1999). Butyric acid: a role in cancer prevention. *Nutr. Bull, 24,* 293-299.

[37] Kuhlsen, N., Pfeuffer, M., Soustre, Y., MacGibbon, A., Lindmark-Mansson, H., and Schrezenmeir, J. (2005). Trans fatty acids: scientific progress and labelling. *Bulletin Int. Dairy Fed, 393,* 1-20.

[38] Mensink, R. P., Zock, P. L., Kester, A. D. M., and Katan, M. B. (1998). Effects of dietary fatty acids and carbohydrates on the ratio of serum total to HDL cholesterol and on serum lipids and apolipoproteins: a meta-analysis of 60 controlled trials. *Am. J. Clin. Nutr, 77,* 1146–1155.

[39] Park, Y., and Pariza, M. W. (2007). Mechanisms of body fat modulation by conjugated linoleic acid (CLA). *Food Res. Int, 40,* 311-323.

[40] Yurawecz, M.P., Roach, J. A. G., Sehat, N., Mossoba, M.M., Kramer, J.K.G., Fritsche, J., Steinhart, H., and Ku, Y. (1998). A new conjugated linoleic acid isomer, 7 trans, 9 cis-octadecadienoic acid, in cow milk, cheese, beef and human milk and adipose tissue. *Lipid, 33,* 803-809.

[41] Prandini, A., Sigoloa, S., and Piva, G. (2010). A comparative study of fatty acid composition and CLA concentration in commercial cheeses. J. Food Compos. Anal, (*In press*).

[42] Lopez, C. (2010). Lipid domains in the milk fat globule membrane: Specific role of sphingomyelin. *Lipid Technol, 22,* 175-178.

[43] Lopez, C., Camier, B., and Gassi, J.-Y. (2007). Development of the milk fat microstructure during the manufacture and ripening of Emmental cheese observed by confocal laser scanning microscopy. *Int. Dairy J. 17,* 235-247.

[44] Larsson (1994) In: K. Larsson, Editor, Lipids—Molecular Organization, Physical Functions and Technical Applications, The Oily Press, Dundee, Scotland (1994).

[45] Noh, S. K., and Koo, S. L. (2004). Milk sphingomyelin is more effective than egg sphingomyelin in inhibiting intestinal absorption of cholesterol and fat in rats. *J. Nutr. 134,* 2611-2616.

[46] Vanderghem, C., Bodson, P., Danthine, S., Paquot, M., and Blecker, C. (2010). Milk fat globule membrane and buttermilks: from composition to valorization. *Biotechnol. Agron. Soc. Environ. 14,* 485-500.

[47] Bourlieu, C., Bouhallab, S., and Lopez, C. (2009). Biocatalyzed modifications of milk lipids: applications and potentialities. *Trends Food Sci Technol, 20,* 458-469.

[48] Parodi, P.W. (2001). Cow's milk components with anti-cancer potential. *Aust. J. Dairy Technol,. 56,* 65-73.

[49] Spitsberg, V. L. (2005). Invited review: bovine milk fat globule membrane as a potential nutraceutical. *J.Dairy Sci, 88,* 2289-2294.

[50] Sen, C. K., Khanna, S., and Roy, S. (2006). Tocotrienols: Vitamin E beyond tocopherols. *Life Sci. 78,* 2088-2098.

[51] Riccio, P. (2004). The proteins of the milk fat globule membrane in the balance. *Trends Food Sci. Technol, 15,* 458-61.

[52] Lucey, J. A., and Fox, P. F. (1993). Importance of calcium and phosphate in cheese manufacture: a review. *J. Dairy Sci, 76,* 1714-1724.

[53] Moreno-Rojas, R., Pozo-Lora, R., Zurera-Cosano, G., and Amaro- Lopez, M. (1994). Calcium, magnesium, manganese, sodium and potassium variations in Manchego-type cheese during ripening. *Food Chem, 50,* 373-37

[54] Gonzalez-Martín, I., Hernandez-Hierro, J. M., Revilla, I., Vivar-Quintana, A., and Lobos Orteg, I. (2011). The mineral composition (Ca, P, Mg, K, Na) in cheeses (Cow's Ewe's and Goat's) with different ripening times using near infrared spectroscopy with a fibre-optic probe. *Food chem.* (In press).

[55] Kruif, C. G., and Holt, C. (2006). Casein micelle structure, functions and interactions. In: P. F. Fox., and P. L. H. McSweeney (Eds) Advanced Dairy Chemistry-Proteins (pp. 262-265). New York: Kluwer Academic/Plenum Publishers.

[56] Ebringer, L., Ferencik, M., and Krajcovic, J. (2008). Beneficial health effects of milk and fermented dairy products – review. *Folia Microbiol, 53,* 378-394.

[57] Kashket, S., and DePaola, D. P. (2002). Cheese consumption and the development and progression of dental caries. *Nut. Rev, 60,* 97-103.

[58] Walther, B., Schmid, A., Sieber, R., and Wehrmuller, K. (2008). Cheese in nutrition and health. *Dairy Sci. Technol, 88,* 389-405.

[59] Upretia, P., and Metzge, L. E. (2007). Influence of calcium and phosphorus, lactose, and salt-to-moisture ratio on Cheddar cheese quality: pH changes during ripening. *J. Dairy Sci, 90(1),* 1-12.

[60] Adams, M. R., and Moss, M. O. (2008). Food Microbiology. (pp. 112-115). The Royal Society of Chemistry, Cambridge.

[61] Fox, P. F., Guinee, T. P., Cogan, T. M., McSweeney, P. L. H. (2004). Cheese: Chemistry, Physics and Microbiology – Volume1: General Aspects. (pp. 207-249). Elsevier Academic Press, London.

[62] Robinson, R. K., and Wilbey, R. A. (1998). Cheese making Practice. (pp. 98) Aspen publishers, Maryland.

[63] Morris, M. J., Na, E. S., and Johnson, A. K. (2008). Review: salt craving: the psychobiology of pathogenic sodium intake. *Physiol. Behav, 94,*709-721.

[64] Simpson, F. O. (1988). Sodium intake, body sodium and sodium excretion. *The Lancet, 332,* 25-29.

[65] Oste, R., Jagerstad, M., and Andersson, I. (1997). Vitamins in milk and milk products. In Advanced Dairy Chemistry – Volume 3: Lactose, Water, Salts and Vitamins, 2nd edn. pp. 347–388. Fox P F and McSweeney P L H, eds. New York: Kluwer Academic/Plenum Publishers.

[66] Parodi, P. W. (2004). Milk fat in human nutrition. *Aust. J. Dairy Tech, 59,* 3-59.

[67] Favier, J. C., and Dorsainvil, E. (1987). Composition des fromages de chèvre, *Cah. Nutr. Diet,* 17-123.

[68] Quinlivan, E. P., McPartlin, J., McNulty, H., Ward, M., Strain, J. J., Weir, D. G., and Scott, J. M. (2002). Importance of both folic acid and vitamin B12 in reduction of risk of vascular disease. Lancet 359 227-228.

[69] Powers, H. J. (1999). Current knowledge concerning optimum nutritional status of riboflavin, niacin and pyridoxine. *Proc. Nutr. Soc, 58,* 435-440.

[70] Dalie, D. K. D., Deschamps, A. M., and Richard-Forget, F. (2010). Lactic acid bacteria – Potential for control of mould growth and mycotoxins: A review. *Food Control, 21,* 370-380.

[71] Cruz, A. G., Buriti, de Souza, C. H. B. Faria, J. Saad, S.M. I. (2009). Probiotic cheese: health benefits, technological and stability aspects. *Trends Food Sci. Tech, 20,* 344-354.

[72] Hatakka, K., Ahola, A. J., Yli-Knuuttila, H., Richardson, M., Mossau, T., and Meurman, J. H. (2007). Probiotic reduce the prevalence of oral *Candida* in the elderly – a randomized controlled trial. *J. Dent. Res, 86,* 125-130.

[73] Hsieh, M. L. and Chou, C. C. (2006). Mutagenicity and antimutagenic effect of soymilk fermented with lactic acid bacteria and bifidobacteria. *Int. J. Food Microbiol, 111,* 43-47.

[74] Massi, M., Vitali, B., Federici, F., Matteuzzi, D., and Brigidi, P. (2004). Identification method based on PCR combined with automated ribotyping for tracking probiotic Lactobacillus strains colonizing the human gut and vagina. *J. Appl. Microbiol, 96,* 777-786.

[75] Caldini, G., Trotta, F., Corsetti, A., and Cenci, G. (2008). Evidence for in vitro antigenotoxicity of cheese non starter lactobacilli. *Antonie Van Leeuwenhoek, 93,* 51-59.

[76] Corsetti, A., Caldini, G., Mastrangelo, M., Trotta, F., Valmorri, S., and Cenci, G. (2008). Raw milk traditional Italian ewe cheeses as a source of Lactobacillus casei strains with acid-bile resistance and antigenotoxic properties. *Int. J. Food Microbiol, 125,* 330-335.

[77] Addeo, F., Chianes, L., Salzano, A., Sacchi, R., Cappuccio, V., Ferranti, P., and Malorni, A. (1992). Characterization of the 12% trichloroacetic acid-insoluble oligopeptides of Parmigiano–Reggiano cheese. *J. Dairy Res, 59,* 401-411.

[78] Singh, T. K., Fox, P. F., and Healy, A. (1997). Isolation and identification of further peptides in the diafiltration retentate of the water-soluble fraction of Cheddar cheese. *J. Dairy Res, 64,* 433-443.

[79] Saito, T., Nakamura, T., Kitazawa, H., Kawai, Y.and Itoh, T. (2000). Isolation and structural analysis of antihypertensive peptides that exist naturally in Gouda cheese. *J. Dairy Sci, 83,* 1434-1440.

[80] U.S. Department of Agriculture, Agricultural Research Service (2008). USDA National Nutrient Database for Standard Reference Release, 21.Nutrient Data Laboratory.

[81] Lin, H., Boylston, T. D., Chang, M. J., Luedecke, L. O., and Shultz, T. D. (1995). Survey of the conjugated linoleic acid contents of dairy products. *J. Dairy Sci, 78,* 2358-2368.

[82] Pierre, A., Michel, F., Le Graet, Y., and Berrier, J. (1999). Soft goat cheeses at different ripening stages: cheese structure, composition and non solvent water. *Lait, 79 (5),* 489-501.

[83] Lucas, A., Hulin, S., Michel, V., Gabriel, C., Chamba, J. F., Rock, E. and Coulon, J. B. (2006). Relations entre les conditions de production du lait et les teneurs en composés d'intérêt nutritionnel dans le fromage: étude en conditions réelles de production. *INRA Prod. Anim, 19 (1),* 15-28.

[84] Lucas, A., Rock, E., Chamba, J. F., Verdier-Metz, I., Brachet, P., and Coulon, J. B. (2006). Respective effects of milk composition and the cheese-making process on cheese compositional variability in components of nutritional interest. *Lait, 86,* 21-41.

[85] Fresno, J. M., Tornadijo, M. E. Carballo, J., Gonzalez Prieto, J., and Bernardo, A. (1996). Characterization and biochemical changes during the ripening of a Spanish craft goat's milk cheese (Armada variety). *Food Chem. 55 (3),* 225-230.

[86] Casalta, E., Noel, Y., Le Bars, D., Carre, C., Achilleos, C., and Maroselli, M. X. (2001). Caractérisation du fromage Bastelicaccia. *Lait, 81 (4),* 529-546.

[87] Martin Hernandez, C., Amigo, L., Martin-Alvarez, P., and Juarez, M. (1992). Differentiation of milks and cheeses according to species based on the mineral content. *Z. Lebensm. Unters. Forsch. 194,* 541-544.

[88] Macedo, A. and Malcata, F. X. (1997). Changes of mineral concentrations in Serra cheese during ripening and throughout the cheese making season. *J. Sci. Food Agric. 74 (3)* 409–415.

[89] Pollman, R. M. (1984). Mise en évidence des adultérations du fromage râpé en utilisant les indices de calcium, phosphore, magnésium et lactose. *J. Assoc. Off. Anal. Chem, 67 (6),* 1062-1066.

[90] Sanjuan, E., Saavedra, P., Millan, R., Castelo, M., and Fernandez Salguero, J. (1998). Effect of ripening and type of rennet on the mineral content of Los Pedroches cheese. *J. Food Qual, 21,* 3.

[91] Santoro (1992). Ripening of Canestrato Pugliese cheese Part IV Evolution of free amino acids. *Rivista della Societa Italiana di Scienza dell'Alimentazione 21 (1),* 7-14.

[92] Ciqual, Ireland, J.J., Favier, J.C., and Feinberg, M. (2002). Répertoire général des aliments. Tome 2. Table de composition des produits laitiers, 2sd édition. Ed: Inra Edition, Technique and Documentation, Paris. ISBN: 2-7380-1051-2, 2-7430-0482-7, Goat cheeses, (pp. 303-324). *Pyrenees cheese from ewe's milk,* (pp. 245-246). Roquefort (pp. 286-288).

[93] Benjamin, S. and Spener, F. (2009). Conjugated linoleic acid as functional food: an insight into their health benefits. *Nutr. Metab. 6,* 36-48.

[94] Lopez, C., Madec, M. N., and Jimenez-Flores, R. (2010). Lipid rafts in the bovine milk fat globule membrane revealed by the lateral segregation of phospholipids and heterogeneous distribution of glycoproteins. *Food Chem, 120,* 22-33.

In: Cheese: Types, Nutrition and Consumption
Editors: Richard D. Foster, pp. 289-300

ISBN 978-1-61209-828-9
©2011 Nova Science Publishers, Inc.

Chapter 15

CHEESE TYPES

Jee-Young Imm[1] and In-Hyu Bae[2]

[1]Department of Foods and Nutrition, Kookmin University, Seoul, Korea
[2]Department of Animal Science, Sunchon National University, Sunchon, Korea

ABSTRACT

Classification of more than 500 cheeses is very difficult task. Although classification of cheeses based on single criterion is not perfect or satisfactory grouping of cheese would be necessary to understand similarities and differences of a variety of cheeses. Cheese can be commonly classified by texture (water content) or rind and further classified by ripening microorganism such as bacteria, mold or combination. The most common classifications for cheese are fresh, soft, semi-soft, firm and hard. Within the same classification they have similarities in taste and textures. Fresh cheese includes world famous mozzarella, cottage, those are particularly used for Pizza and Italian dishes. Brie and Camembert belongs to pungent soft cheese. Semi-hard cheeses are recognized by texture of "not too hard" and" not too firm." Blue cheese such as Roquefort, Gorgonzola is characterized by distinctive blue greens color and strong flavor. Emmental and Gruyeres cheeses are representative firm Swiss cheese and contain medium size holes formed by propionic fermentation. World reknown Cheddar cheese also belongs to this class. Hard cheese such as Grana Padano and Pecorino Romano cheeses have the lowest water content and typical grainy texture. They have long aging time and produced for grating purpose.

1. INTRODUCTION

Cheeses refer to milk coagulum generated by milk clotting enzymes or acidulants. The basic nature of cheeses is a casein gel matrix containing inert fat molecules. The ancient cheese making is originated as a food preservation method. Cheese making methods are rather complex because they are evolved through long history. The variables in manufacturing stages, such as milk preparation (standardization, pasteurization), coagulation (acidification) and pos-coagulation also, created different cheese types and enormous cheese varieties [1].

The classification of cheeses by single criterion is very difficult task since they have diverse chemical compositions, texture and flavor profiles. Cheeses can be classified based on origin, hardness (water content) or rind and further classified by ripening microorganism, such as bacteria, mold, or combination. Cheeses are separated into natural cheeses and processed cheese. Generally, cheeses mean natural cheeses, and processed cheeses are made by heating and stirring of more than two natural cheeses in the presence of melting salt. Many countries have their own regulations for the specifications of processed cheese such as allowable moisture content and concentration of melting salt and, etc [2]. Natural cheeses are separated into fresh, soft, semi-hard, firm, and hard cheeses depending upon moisture content. This classification far from adequate because there is no objective criterion to judge softness and hardness of body and furthermore, this classification hardly tells about cheeses themselves [3]. In this chapter, cheeses are grouped by the combination of most common criterions, moisture level and type of ripening microorganisms for convenience.

2. FRESH CHEESES

Fresh cheeses have soft, juicy and creamy texture. They contain more whey compared to other cheese classes. Fresh cheeses are generally packed into containers right after making and are consumed without ripening. Fresh cheeses are very popular in Europe and so called as Fromage Blanc (means "white cheese") in France, Quark (sometimes called quarg) in Germany and Mascarpone (means "better than good") in Italy as shown in Fig.1. In terms of flavor fresh cheeses tend to have more acidic flavor than other cheeses because acid are used to make curd.

Quark is typically made from skim milk or partially skimmed cow's milk as shown in Fig 1. After pasteurization, it is cultured with lactic acid starter and rennet. The heat treatment in acidic condition resulted by prolonged starter actions leads to coprecipitation of whey protein and caseins [4]. Cottage cheese (also called as pot cheese, Dutch cheese, and schmierkase) is traditionally made by acid coagulation of skim milk either by starter culture or by direct acidification. In US, Cottage cheese is otherwise called as soft uncured cheese and it is prepared by mixing creaming mixture with cottage cheese dry curd [5]. The cottage cheese curds have flaky and granular shape, so they are called as popcorn cheese. The uniformity of curds with a meat like texture without being too firm, rubbery or tough were considered as ideal Cottage cheese [6].

Neufchatel and cream cheeses are produced from homogenized and pasteurized milk or cream. For commercial production, milk is usually fortified to have solids content greater than 20%. The milk is incubated until pH reached 4.5-4.8 [7] The way of productions are similar to Cottage cheese but the method of whey drainage and cream incorporation are different Also, distinct individual curd cannot be found in Neufchatel [8].

Mozzarella is one of the most famous fresh cheeses in the world and used as a key ingredient in pizza. Mozzarella was traditionally made from milk of water buffalo, but now almost all the Mozzarella is made also from whole or partly skimmed cow's milk [9]. The most important characteristic of Mozzarella cheese is resilient stringy texture. This texture can be acquired from lengthy stretching during cooking process. The rate of acid development and the pH range at the time of stretching were critical for melting quality of Mozzarella cheese [10]. Mozzarella has very thin soft skins and does not have holes.

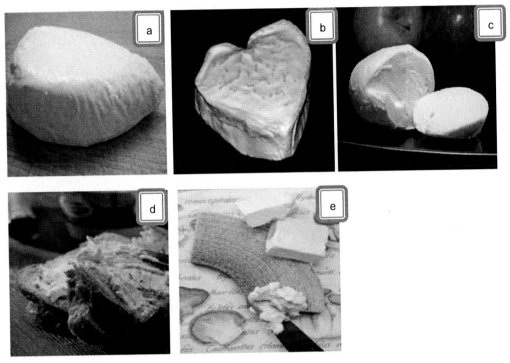

Figure 1. Fresh cheeses. [a] Quark [b] Neufchatel [c] Mozzarella (source: http://en.wikipedia.org) [d] Ricotta [e] Mascarpone (source: Encyclopedia of cheese).

Ricotta (Céracée, Recuite, Schottenziger) is a soft cheese and originally developed from the process of Mozzarella making. Ricotta is known as whey cheese since whey protein is recovered from heat precipitation [11]. Literally, ricotta means "recooked". Ricotta cheese can be made from a variety of milks including sheep, goat, cow or water buffalo's milk. The incorporation of fat with the coagulated albumin resulted in improved body and texture. Ricotta cheese is suitable for baking lasagna and ravioli because of creamy and smooth texture and mild flavor. Mascarpone is very similar to whole milk Ricotta except cream addition followed by heating about 85°C. This is a reason for buttery flavor of Mascarpone.

3. Soft Cheeses

Different from previous classe, cheese ripening leads to significant changes in flavor and texture of different cheese varieties. Soft cheeses include surface-ripened cheeses and this surface ripening takes place by moulds and bacteria. The Brie and Camembert are typical mould surface-ripened cheeses and they are ripend quickly because of rapid growth of surface mold [12]. Traditionally, Camembert cheese was produced with *Penicillim Camemberti* but currently both Brie and Camembert are being made with *Penicillim Caseicolum* [13]. Although yeasts and moulds are dominant in initial ripening stages *Brevibacterium linens* and other coryneforms produced yellow crust with surfuric flavor in mature Brie and Camembert cheese [14]. As ripening proceeds enzymes released from *surface moulds* turn *crumbly* texture of Camembert cheese into creamier texture. Brie cheese is a soft, surface-ripened French cheese and usually produced from cow's milk. Brie de Meaux is uncooked French cheese which made with raw cow's milk. Brie shares basic cheese processing with Camembert but internal ripening and characteristic flavor are different from each other.

Tilsiter, Limburger, Muenster and Taleggio are considered as bacteria smear surface-ripened cheeses. Bacteria including *Brevibacterium, Arthrobacter, Micrococcus* and *Corynebacterium* became dominant at the end of ripening period [13]. The naturally occurring *Brevibacterium linens* are uniformly spread by "smearing step" during cheese making. Therefore, the surfaces of cheese must be rubbed typically with a brine solution. Muenster is a semisoft, whole-milk German cheese. It is a brine salted cheese and distinctive orange-yellow rind.

Limburger cheese also semisoft, surface-ripened cheese originated from Belgium. Although yeasts and micrococci grow on Limberger cheese *Br. Lines* is a major contributor for the development of pungent flavor and yellow pigment [15]. The proteolytic activity of surface flora creates pH gradient from surface to interior and this pH gradient might be a reason for characteristic texture of surface-ripened cheese cheeses. The characteristic ammonia odor reflects surface proteolysis during ripening [16].

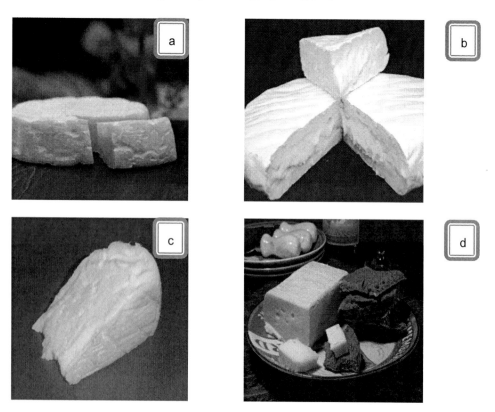

Figure 2. Soft cheeses. [a] Brie (source: Encyclopedia of cheese) [b] Camembert [c] Muenster [d] Limburger (source: http://en.wikipedia.org).

4. SEMI HARD CHEESES

Different from white surface mold cheeses such as Camembert and brie blue cheeses have a characteristic green blue veins within cheese mass. This unique appearance puts them in a separate category [14]. Roquefort, Gorgonzola, and Stilton are belongs to this group and the fungi, *penicillium roquefortii* or *penicillium glaucum* are involved in cheese making along with other yeasts and bacteria. The addition of *P. roqueforti* or *P. glaucum* spores into milk or curds produces blue pigment in cheese. Air circulation during ripening is important for mold to grow. Accoring to French regulation "Roquefort" can only be used for cheese made in the Roquefort area with ewe's milk [17]. *P. roquefortii* is resistant to lactic acid bacteria and their metabolites [18] and it is a source of proteolytic and lipolytic enzymes which responsible for flavor and texture development.

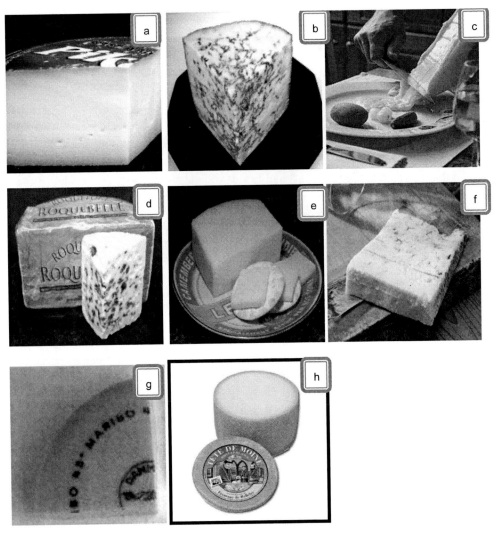

Figure 3. Semi-hard cheeses. [a] Gouda [b] Stiltion [c] Raclette [d] Roquefort [e] Danbo (source: http://en.wikipedia.org) [f] Gorgonzola (source: Encyclopedia of cheese) [g] Maribo (source: http://www.geocities.co.jp) [h] Tete de Moine (source: http://www.jukkolanjuustola.fi).

Gouda is a semi-hard Holland cheese produced with whole milk. Traditionally, Gouda cheese is ripened without packaging at 10-18°C. Ripening takes at least 40 days to obtain characteristic mild flavor and elastic structure [19]. The appearance of Gouda cheese is similar to Edam cheese but Gouda usually has greater fat content. The high fat level of Gouda cheese provides soft and less fracturable texture with increased smoothness. Based on the sensory evaluation of Gouda cheese, most American consumers prefer smooth and cohesive texture over firm and elastic texture of Gouda cheese [20].

Stilton is a mold ripened semi-hard English blue cheese and *P. roquefortii* plays in important role in ripening stage. The molds are added at the beginning of manufacture and typical blue appearance is expressed in 3 weeks [21]. Stilton has delicate and mild flavor than Roquefort and has narrow blue-green veins.

Maribo is a semi-hard Denish cheese which has mild flavor. It has yellow-brown rind and irregular holes and is usually coated with paraffin wax [22]. Gorgonzola is a blue veined Italian cheeses and is produced based on controlled denomination of origin (DOC). Larger size with a blue-green appearance of Gorgonzola is a chracteritic differentiated from other blue cheeses. Zarmpoutis, McSweeney, and Fox [23] compared the extent of proteolysis in blue-veined cheese varieties including Stilton, Gorgonzola, Danablu, Cashel, and Chetwynd. Although all cheeses showed significant proteolysis, Gorgonzola had higher levels of amino acids than the other cheeses.

Danbo is smear ripened cheese with medium-sized holes. It is produced with fat level of 20, 30, and 45%. Danbo cheese usually consumed after 2-3 month ripening but a few varieties allows 12 month maturation and can be grated [24]. Sensory and rheological analysis indicated that low fat Danbo (20% fat) had firmer and elastic texture. However, there was no difference in the extent of proteolysis. Therefore, the extent proteolysis in low fat Danbo should be controlled in order to reduce bitterness and to obtain pleasant texture [25]. Tete de Moine is a semi-hard Swiss cheese which has sharp flavor along with sweet beef hint. The name means "monk's head" and it actually looks like little drum [26].

5. FIRM CHEESES

Swiss styles of cheese are belongs to this class. Swiss type cheeses are originally produced at Emmental in Switzerland. In US, Canada, and Australia "Swiss cheese" means several cheese varieties resemble Emmental [27]. Swiss type cheese has large round holes known as "eyes." Although cheese eye formation is started during preripening stage by starters, propionic acid fermentation is a major contributor in characteristic cheese eyes formation [28]. Since eye formation is a critical step in Swiss cheese, the acceptability of Swiss cheese is closely related to size, number, and uniformity of 'eye" [29]. A soft and elastic texture also influence quality of Swiss cheese. In this context, size of curds and brine step are also important in soft and elastic texture and eye formation. Gruyere is the second most popular Swiss cheese. Apparently, Gruyere looks similar to Emmental but it is much smaller. Gruyere has sharper flavor expressed as rancid, sulphury and animal-like flavor [30]. Gruyere required longer maturation period than Emmental and has known as key ingredient in fondue [31].

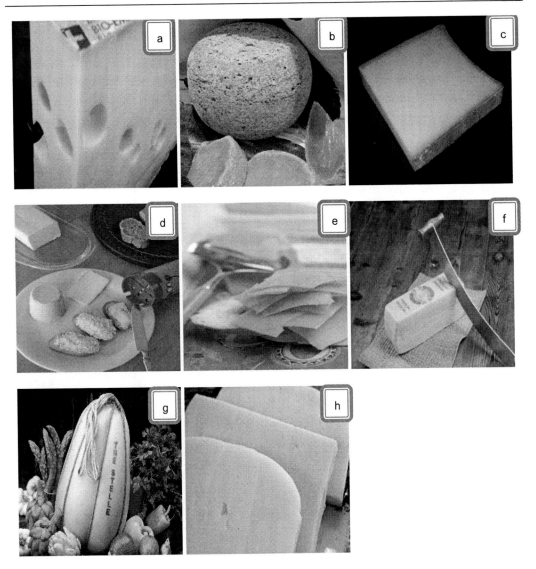

Figure 4. Firm cheeses. [a] Emmental [b] Mimolette [c] Beaufort [d] Sapsago (source: http://en.wikipedia.org) [e] Cheddar [f] Gruyeres (source: Encyclopedia of cheese) [g] Provolone (source: http://www.theworldwidegourmet.com) [h] Havarti (source: http://www.practicallyedible.com)

Cheddar cheese is world famous English hard cheese made from whole cow's milk. "Cheddaring" is a unique process found in Cheddar cheese manufacture. It involves turing, flipping and pushing the curds with regular intervals. During cheddaring whey is continuously removed from cheese and it renders to fibrous structure [32]. Cheddar cheese is also very popular in US and often called as American cheese or American Cheddar cheese. Drake et al. [33] defined sensory language for Cheddar cheese flavor and its flavor is characterized by sulfur, brothy, and nutty.

Mimolette is traditionally produced in France and has grey rind and orange interior originated from annatto, the natural pigment. The grey crust is produced by the action of cheese mite during ripening. Recently, mite in Mimolette cheese was identified as *Acarus siro*

L. and its morphological characteristics was examined using cryogenic scanning electron microscopy [34].

Cheshire is one of the oldest hard cheeses made from raw cow's milk in England. Cheshire has lower curd pH and mineral content than those of Cheddar. The low pH disrupts submicellar casein units and the size of protein aggregate of Cheshire was relatively smaller than other hard cheeses [35]. Provolone is an Italian cheese produced with cow's milk. It is classified as semi-hard or hard cheese depending upon aging period. Before the cheeses are sold washing is required because *Aspergillus* and *Penicillium* moulds grow on surfaces of cheese during aging [36]. Havarti is a Danish semi-hard cow's milk cheese with small holes. The preference of reduced fat Harvati-type cheese were evaluated by Finnish consumers. According to results, consumers expected pale appearance, sticky texture [37].

Sapsago cheese originated from Swizeland and made from skim milk. It is very hard texture and made for grating purpose. Traditionally dried clover species, *Melilotus coerulea* are added for flavor generation. It also called as Schabziger cheese [38].

6. HARD CHEESE

Hard cheeses typically have dry, crumbly texture and intense flavor as a result of long muturation. The water content in cheese is inversely proportional to aging period. Hard cheeses typically have a 30-35 % while fresh cheeses have 70-80% water content. Many hard cheeses commonly dried for grating purposes.

Grana cheese is a well known Italian cheese. More than 70% of total milk production is used for cheese manufacture and 55% of the total milk production is Protected Designation of Origin (PDO) cheeses such as Grana Padano, Asiago, Parmigiano-Reggiano, and Gorgonzola [39]. The name "Grana" derived from granular body and texture. Grana cheeses are introduced to the United in a name of "Parmesan." Grana pandano cheese generally made after partial skimming. Typically, natural whey culture and rennet are used as a starter and coagulant, respectively [40]. The thermophillic lactic acid bacteria come from whey starter culture act as a dominant microflora during cheese making and early aging stage [41]. Parmigiano-Reggiano is also made with cow's milk using natural whey culture. Parmigiano-Reggiano is famous for very rich fruity, sweet, and nutty aroma and crumbly grainy texture [42].

Pecorino is the trivial Italian word for sheep milk cheese. Depending on the source of milk, cheeses are called as Pecorino, Vacchino (cow's milk), and Caprino (goat milk), respectively.

Pecorino Romano is the most famous Pecorino cheese. The unique flavor of Pecorino Romano is mainly due to different enzyme compositions in lamb rennet paste. The rennet pastes prepared from lab had greater chymosin and lipolytic acivity than commercial rennet Trained sensory specialists considered cheese prepared with lamb rennet paste was more piquant than the one with commercial rennet [43]. Pecorino Tuscano is a cheese made of raw sheep milk. It's size is smaller than Romano and only manufactured between september and June, when sheep milk is available. Asiago cheese is another POD product of Italy. "Asiago d'Allevo variety is made from skimmed raw milk. The length of maturation varies generally from 3 to 18 month [44]. The aged Asiago cheese is widely used in salads, soups, and pastas.

Sbrinz is extra hard Swiss cheese produced with whole milk and claimed to be the oldest European cheese. It also has good grating and melting quality with savory mellow taste [45].

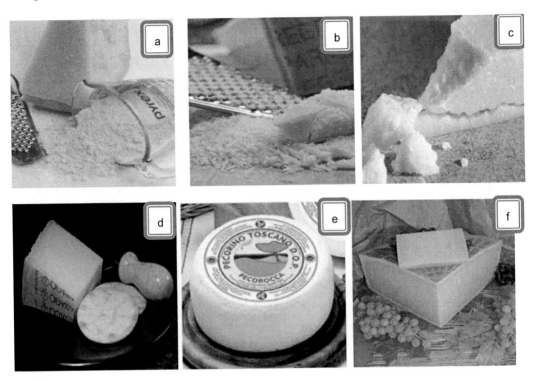

Figure 5. Hard cheeses. [a] Grana Padano [b] Parmigiano-Reggiano [c] Pecorino Romano [d] Asiago (source: http://en.wikipedia.org) [e] Pecorino Toscano (source: http://www.cibo360.it) [f] Sbrinz (source: http://www.schoepfer.fr)

CONCLUSION

Innumerable types of cheeses are produced in all over the world. Every cheese has its own style, texture and flavor. Many factors including source and composition of milk, processing conditions, maturation are crucial to determine sensory quality of cheeses and most factors are interrelated. Recently, there have been attempts to characterize unique quality traits of cheese varieties only produced in small quantity and in restricted areas. New research findings regarding biochemical pathways of microorganisms, microbial genetics, cheese chemistry and functionality will facilitate better process control and efficient production of cheese.

REFERENCES

[1] Coker, C. J., Crawford, R. A., Johnston, K. A., Singh, H., and Creamer, L. K. (2005). Towards the classification of cheese variety and maturity on the basis of statistical analysis of proteolysis data-a review. *Int. Dairy J.*, 15, 631-643.

[2] Kosikowski, F.V. and Mistry, V.V. (1997). Process cheese and related products. In: Cheese and Fermented Milk Foods: Origins and Principles (edited by F.V. Kosikowski). pp. 328–352. Westport: F.V. Kosikoswki and Associates.

[3] Kosikowski, F.V. and Mistry, V.V. (1997). Fundamentals of cheese making and ripening. In: Cheese and Fermented Milk Foods: Origins and Principles (edited by F.V. Kosikowski). pp. 109–126. Westport: F.V. Kosikoswki and Associates.

[4] Gambelli, L., Manzi, P., Panfili, G., Vivanti, V., and Pizzoferrato, L. (1999). Constituents of nutritional relevance in fermented milk products commercialised in Italy. *Food Chem.*, 66, 353-358.

[5] Code of Federal Regulations. 2004. Code of Federal Regulations, title 21. Vol. 2: Food and drugs. U.S. Government Printing Office. http://www.access.gpo.gov/cgi-bin/cfrassemble.cgi?title=200721

[6] Bodyfelt, F. W., and Potter, D. 2009. Sensory evaluation of creamed cottage cheese. In: The Sensory Evaluation of Dairy Products. (edited by S. Clark, M. Costello, M. A. Drake, and F. Bodyfelt). pp. 167-190. Van Nostrand Reinhold, New York, NY.

[7] Brighenti, M., Govindasamy-Lucey, S., Lim, K., Nelson, K., and Lucey, J. A. (2008). Characterization of the rheological, textural, and sensory properties of samples of commercial US cream cheese with different fat contents. *J. Dairy Sci.*, 91, 4501-4517.

[8] Dahlberg, A. C. (1927). A new method of manufacturing cream cheese of the Neufchatel type. *J. Dairy Sci.*, 10, 106-116.

[9] Coppola, S., Parente, E., Dumontet, S., and La Peccerella, A. (1988). The microflora of natural whey cultures utilized as starter in the manufacture of Mozzarella cheese from water-buffalo milk. *Le Lait*, 68, 295-310.

[10] Kindsstet, P. S. (2004). Mozzarella cheese: 40 years of scientific advancement. *Int. J. Dairy Technol.* 57, 85-90.

[11] Pizzillo, M., Claps, S., Cifuni, G., Fedele. V, and Rubino, R. (2005). Effect of goat breed on the sensory, chemical and nutritional characteristics of ricotta cheese. *Livestock Prod. Sci.* 94, 33-40.

[12] Schlesser, J. E., Schmidt, S. J., and Speckman, R. (1992). Characterization of chemical and physical changes in Camembert cheese during ripening. *J. Dairy Sci.*, 75, 1753-1760.

[13] Corsetti, A., Rossi, J., and Bobbetti , M. (2001). Intercations between yeasts and bacteria in the smear surface-ripened cheeses. *Int. J. Food Microbiol.*, 69, 1-10.

[14] Sable, S., and Cottenceau, G. (1999). Current knowledge of soft cheeses flavor and related compounds. *J. Agric. Food Chem.* 47, 4825-4836.

[15] Tuckey, S. L., and Sahasrabudhe, M. R. (1957). Studies in the ripening of Limberger cheese. *J. Dairy Sci.*, 40, 1329-1337.

[16] Lawrence, R. C., Creamer, L. K., and Gilles, J. (1987). Texture development during cheese ripening. *J. Dairy Sci.*, 70, 1748-1760.

[17] Sanders, G. Roquefort. (1953) In: Cheese Variety and descriptions. pp. 109–111. U.S. Dept. of Agriculture, Washington D.C.

[18] Frisvad, J. C. (1981). Physiological criteria and mycotoxin production as aids in identification of common asymmetric penicillia. *Appl. Environ. Microbiol.* 41, 568-579.

[19] Berola, N. C., Califano, A. N., Bevilacqua, A. E., and Zaritzky, N. E. Effects of ripening conditions on the texture of Gouda cheese. *Int. J. Food Sci. Technol.*, (2000). 35, 207-214.

[20] Yates, M. D., and Drake, M. A. (2007). Texture properties of Gouda Cheese. *J. Sensory Sci.,* 22, 493-506.

[21] Ercolini, D., Hill, P. J., and Dodd, C. E. R. (2003). Bacterial community structure and location in Stilton cheese. *Appl. Environ. Mirobiol.,* 69, 3540-3548.

[22] Brito, C., Astete, M. A., Pinto, M., and Molina, L. H. (2000). Maribo cheese manufactured with concentrated milk: characteristics, maturation and yield. *Int. J. Dairy Technol.,* 53, 6-12.

[23] Zarmpoutis, I. V., McSweeney, P. L. H. and Fox, P. F. (1997). Proteolysis in blue-veined cheese: An intervarietal study. *Irish J. Agric. Food Res.,* 56, 219-229.

[24] Sorensen, J., and Benfeldt, C. (2001). Comparison of ripening characteristics of Danbo cheeses from two daries. *Int. Dairy J.,* 11, 355-362.

[25] Madsen, J. S., and Ardö, Y. (2001). Exploratory study of proteolysis, rheology and sensory properties of Danbo cheese with different fat contents. *Int. Dairy J.,* 11, 423-431.

[26] Ehlers, S., Hurt, J. (2008) In: The Complete Idiot's Guide to Cheese of the World. pp. 72–79. Alpha, USA.

[27] Liggett, R. E., Drake, M. A., and Delwiche. (2008). Impact of flavor attributes on consumer liking of Swiss cheese. *J. Dairy Sci.,* 91, 466-476.

[28] Eskelinen, J. J., Alavuotunki, A. P., Hæggström, E., and Alatossava, T. (2007). Preliminary study of ultrasonic structural quality control of Swiss-type cheese. *J. Dairy Sci.,* 90, 4071-4077.

[29] Mocquot, G. (1979). Reviews of the progress of dairy science: Swiss-type cheese. *J. Dairy Res.,* 46, 133-160.

[30] Muir, D. D., Hunter, E. A., Banks, J. M., and Horne, D. S. (1995). Sensory properties of hard cheese: Identification of key attributes. *Int. Dairy J.,* 5, 157–177.

[31] Sanders, G. Gruyere. (1953) In: Cheese Variety and descriptions. pp. 55-56. U.S. Dept. of Agriculture, Washington D.C.

[32] Shakeel-ur-Rehman, Drake, M. A., and Farkye, N. Y. (2008). Difference between Cheddar manufactured by the mill-curd and stirred-curd methods using different commercial starters. *J. Dairy Sci.,* 91, 76-84.

[33] Drake, M. A., McIngvale, S. C., Gerard, P. D., Cadwallader, K. R., and Civille, G. V. (2001). Development of a descriptive language for Cheddar cheese. *J. Food Sci.* 66, 1422–1427.

[34] Melnyk, J. P., Smith, A., Scott-Dupree, C., Marcone, M. F., and Hill, A. (2010). Identification of cheese mite species inoculated on Mimolete and Mibenkase cheese through cryogenic scanning electron microscopy. *J. Dairy Sci.,* 93, 3461-3468.

[35] Lawrence, R. C., Heap, H. A., and Gilles, J. (1984). A controlled approach to cheese technology. *J. Dairy Sci.,* 67, 1632-1645.

[36] Battistotti, B., Bottazzi, V., Piccinardi, A., Volpato, G. (1983) In: Cheese: A Guid to the World of Cheese and Chessmaking. pp. 139-140. Fact on file Publications, New York, Bicester, England.

[37] Ritvanen, T., Lilleberg, L., Tupasela, T., and Suhonen U. (2010). The characteristics of the most-liked reduced fat Harvati-type cheeses. *J. Dairy Sci.,* 93, 5039-5047.

[38] Sanders, G. Gruyere. (1953) In: Cheese Variety and descriptions. p. 113. U.S. Dept. of Agriculture, Washington D.C.

[39] Cassandro, M., Comin, A., Ojala, M., Zotto, R. D., Marchi, M. D., Gallo, L., Carnier, P., and Bittante, G. (2008). Genetic parameters of milk coagulation properties and their

relationships with milk yield and quality traits in Italian Holstein cows. *J. Dairy Sci.*, 91, 371-376.

[40] Gaiaschi, A., Beretta, B., Poiesi, C., Conti, A., Giuffrida, M. G., Galli, C. L., and Restani, P. Proteolysis of β-casein as a marker of Grana Padano cheese ripening. *J. Dairy Sci.*, 84, 60-65.

[41] Giraffa, G., and Neviani, E .(1999). Different Lactobacillus helviticus strain populations dominate during Grana Padano cheesemaking. Food Microbiol. 16, 205-210.

[42] Qian, M., and Reineccius, G. Identification of aroma compounds in Parmigiano-Reggino cheese by gas chromatography/olfactory. *J. Dairy Sci.*, 85, 1362-1369.

[43] Addis, M., Piredda, G., Pes, M., Salvo, R. D., Scintu, M. F., and Pirisi, A. (2005). Effect of the use of three different lam paste rennets on lipolysis of the PDO Pecorino Romano cheese. *Int. Dairy J.*, 15, 563-569.

[44] Segato, S., Balzan, S., Elia, C. A., Lignitto, L., Granata, A., Magro, L., Cotiero, B., Andrighetto, I., and Novelli, E. (2007). Effect of period of milk production and ripening on quality traits of Asiago cheese. *Italian J. Anim. Sci.* 6, 469-471.

[45] Battistotti, B., Bottazzi, V., Piccinardi, A., Volpato, G. (1983) In: *Cheese: A Guid to the World of Cheese and Chessmaking.* pp. 147-148. Fact on file Publications, New York, Bicester, England.

In: Cheese: Types, Nutrition and Consumption
Editor: Richard D. Foster, pp. 301-307
ISBN 978-1-61209-828-9
©2011 Nova Science Publishers, Inc.

Chapter 16

WORLD PRODUCTION AND CONSUMPTION OF CHEESE

Suk-Ho Choi[1] and Se-Jong Oh[2]

[1]Department of Animal Science and Biotechnology, Sangji University, Wonju, Korea
[2]Department of Animal Science, Chonnam National University, Gwangju, Korea

ABSTRACT

World production of industrial cheeses has reached 17.0 million tons in 2009. The countries in Europe and northern America produced and consumed about 80% of cheeses in the world. Cheese production and consumption worldwide steadily increased during the period from 2000 to 2007 due both to demand for commodity cheeses, such as Mozzarella, Cheddar, and other cheeses of prospering fast food outlets and restaurants and to rising incomes in both non-EU European countries, such as Russia, Belarus and Ukraine, and developing countries, such as Brazil, Republic Korea. Cheese production and consumption of New Zealand and Australia stagnated and decreased, which can be attributed to both to stagnating milk supplies and to decreasing cheese export. The cheese production and consumption were negatively affected by the financial crisis and following economic depression in 2008. The cheese trade outpaced cheese production during the period from 2000 to 2009. EU, New Zealand and Australia are leading cheese exporters, while Russia and Japan are noticeable cheese importers. Cheese importing countries are located rather widely throughout the world.

1. INTRODUCTION

The early records of cheese making are inscribed in the kings' tombs of ancient Egypt. The names of the present cheese varieties which have been established since the age of Roman reached 400 to 2,000 depending on how to differentiate them. The International Dairy Federation described 510 different cheeses in a catalogue [1]. The types of cheeses were affected by numerous factors, e.g. mammal species from milk are obtained, microbial cultures, coagulants, curd scalding, cheese sizes, pressing and ripening procedures. Cheeses are both excellent nutritional sources for growing youths and delectable side dishes of alcoholic beverages for adults. Cheeses can be easily incorporated into various foods including fast foods, e.g. pizza, hamburger, pita, sandwiches, pastas, and main dishes. Great varieties of cheeses available at the market provide affluent dining custom and also indicate a high cultural level of the regions and countries. There are more than 300 varieties of cheeses available in U.S. marketplaces [2], while 350 more than 400 cheeses are listed in France [3].

Production and consumption of cheeses which have been dominated by the developed countries, such as Europe, Northern America and Oceania due to the dining habits, life-styles, high income levels, and affluent milk supply from dairy farms steadily increased so far. While the cheese market of the developed countries become matured, adoption of the western lifestyle, income rise and increase in international cheese trade will promote cheese consumption further in Asia, Latin America and Africa. Trends in production, consumption, and trade of cheeses in the world during the time from 2000 to 2009 and differences between countries regarding popular cheese varieties were described in this chapter.

2. CHEESE PRODUCTION

World production of natural cheeses is estimated at around 20 million tons in 2009 [4]. Cow milk cheeses produced from milk delivered to dairies (i.e. industrial cheeses) represent more than 80% of the global cheese production. The rest is made up of farm and home-made cheeses, cheeses from other milk (sheep, goat, and buffalo). Europe and Northern America represent 80% of the world natural cheese production.

World production of industrial cheeses has slowed down since 2007 and reached 17.0 million tons in 2009 as shown in Fig 1. The compound annual growth rate during the period from 2007 to 2009 was 0.5% which was much lower than that of 3.5% during the period from 2000 to 2007. EU 27 was leading producer throughout the period from 2000 to 2009 and produced 51% of world cheese in 2009. Northern America including USA and Canada was the second largest producer which churned out 29% of world cheese. The cheese production of other regions including South America, other Europe, Oceania, Asia, Central America and Africa has increased slightly during the period, which is due to 118% increase in cheese production of other Europe countries, among which Russia, Ukraine and Belarus have increased cheese production at the compound annual growth rate of 7.8%, 18.6%, and 14.1% during the period from 2000 to 2009, respectively (Table 1).

USA was the top cheese producing country in the world and has increased cheese production steadily during the period from 2000 to 2009 [4]. The cheese varieties produced high quantities in USA are Mozzarella (32.3%), Cheddar (31.7%) and Cream/Neufchatel (7.6%) in 2009 [2]. Nineteen European countries were included in 28 cheese producing countries worldwide as shown in Table 1 and the other 9 countries were USA, Brazil, Argentina, Canada, Australia, New Zealand, Turkey, Mexico and Israel. The countries which have increased cheese production more than 20% during the period from 2000 to 2009 were USA, Germany, Brazil, Poland, Russia, Ukraine, Ireland, Austria, Belarus, Israel and Lithuania. However, cheese production in Australia and New Zealand has slightly decreased during the same time, which can be attributed to both to stagnating milk supplies and to the preferences in European and other world regions for cheese products of domestic origin [5].

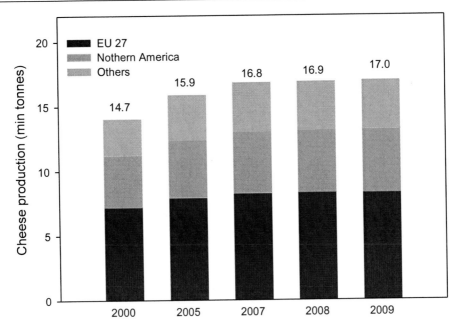

Figure 1. World production of industrial cheese [4].

Table 1. Industrial cheese production in selected countries [4] (in thousand tons)

Country	2000	2009	Country	2000	2009
USA	3,746	4,585	New Zealand	289	270
Germany	1,686	2,088	Greece	143	195
France	1,612	1,693	Switzerland	167	178
Italy	927	1,059	Turkey	129	153
Netherlands	684	714	Ireland	99	146
Brazil	445	614	Austria	119	146
Poland	404	610	Mexico	134	142
Argentina	443	509	Belarus	41	134
Russia	221	436	Spain	111	126
Canada	292	331	Israel	99	121
Australia	375	330	Czech Republic	92	109
UK	302	323	Sweden	127	108
Denmark	306	321	Finland	98	105
Ukraine	67	312	Lithuania	40	94

3. CHEESE CONSUMPTION

Twenty two countries in Europe and Northern America are among the 28 countries which are listed in order of cheese consumption in Table 2. The other important cheese consuming countries are Argentina, Japan, Mexico, Australia, Korea and New Zealand. Most leading cheese consuming countries have significantly increased cheese consumption during the period from 2001 to 2007 and contributed to overall increase in cheese production. Cheese consumption of Argentina had increased 37% during period from 2001 to 2007. Global cheese consumption decelerated its growth in 2008 and stagnated in 2009 due to economic depression.

Table 2. Cheese consumption of selected countries [11]

Country	2003	2007	Country	2003	2007
USA	4,435	4,819	Mexico	204	-
Germany	1,791	1,824	Switzerland	149	171
France	1,473	1,551	Sweden	158	166
Italy	1,268	1,232	Austria	158	156
Russia	800	-	Australia	158	156
UK	641	744	Portugal	106	107
Argentina	322	442	Finland	87	104
Canada	376	417	Norway	70	71
Poland	394	408	Ireland	42	12
Spain	377	330	Korea	58	74
Greece	310	-	Slovakia	50	53
Netherlands	279	295	South Africa	35	-
Czech Republic	151	176	Croatia	29	37
Japan	239	-	New Zealand	28	26

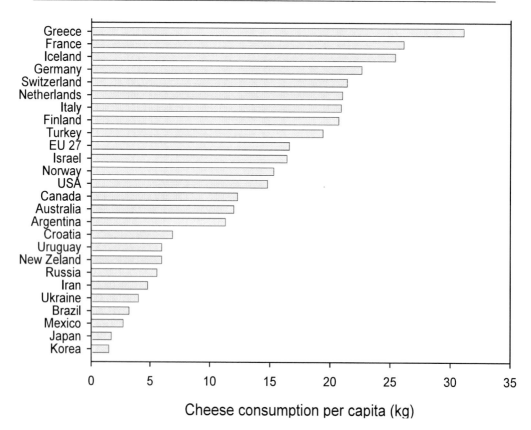

Figure 2. Per capita cheese consumption of selected countries in 2009 [4].

Cheese consumption has been affected by the demand from food service rather than the demand from private households [5, 6, 7]. During the period from 2004 to 2007, the consumption of cheese continued to grow in EU, North America and Russia. The trend to fast food was in favor of the commodity cheeses, e.g. Mozzarella and Cheddar, which were incorporated to the fast foods, such as pizza, hamburger and etc. However, the market of specialty cheeses stagnated during the period. The top favorite cheeses in America are Mozzarella, Cheddar and Cream cheeses [8]. In Britain, Cheddar accounted for more than 50% of all cheese sales. Switzerland's favorite cheese was Mozzarella in 2006 followed by Gruyere, often used in fondue [9]. Natural cheese consumption of Korea continued to increase during the period from 1987 to 2008 and reached 51,812 tons which accounted for 72% of total cheese consumption in 2009 [10], which was mainly due to sales increase of pizza delivery outlets and restaurants.

Global cheese consumption decelerated its growth and stagnated in 2008 and 2009. The annual growth rates of cheese consumption of EU27 and USA during the years of 2008 and 2009 were 0.9% and 1.5%, respectively. Most other countries experienced mixed developments due to weak economic conditions, but Mexico showed robust annual growth of 16.7% [4]. As the market of developed countries become matured, any further development in cheese consumption with these markets is likely to be marginal. Meanwhile, developing markets, such as Asia, Latin America, and Africa, with rising incomes are projected to display superior growth rates in cheese consumption [12].

The per capita cheese consumption of the countries in Europe and northern America was ranked high in order as shown in Fig 2. Greece was the top cheese consuming country whose per capita cheese consumption reached 31.1 kg in 2009 followed by France, Iceland, and German. In Greece, Feta accounts for three-quarters of this consumption [13]. Emmental used mainly as a cooking ingredient and Camembert are the most sold cheeses in France where more than 400 cheese varieties are produced and listed. The industry estimates that there are now more than 300 varieties of cheese available in the U.S. marketplace. By far the two most popular cheeses in the United States are Mozzarella (4.8kg per capita) and Cheddar (4.6kg per capita). A small growing category is Hispanic cheese, which continued a upward clime in 2009, but consumption level remains modest at 0.3 kg per capita. The other countries with high per capita cheese consumption outside of Europe and northern America are Turkey, Israel, and Iran in Asia, Argentina and Uruguay in South America, and Australia and New Zealand in Oceania.

4. CHEESE TRADE

The total trade of cheese rose 41% during the period from 2000 to 2007 and reached to 1.8 million tons in 2007. The trade sharply decreased in 2008 and then bounced back in 2009. The percentage of trade to production of cheese increased from 8.9% in 2000 to 10.9% in 2009. EU 27 is a leading cheese supplier to the world market, holding a 31% export market share in 2009 [4]. The European cheeses are exported to Russia, USA, Japan, Middle East, and Northern Africa. Leading member states in the EU cheese export are Germany, Netherlands, France, and Italy, together representing nearly 60% of total EU exports.

Table 3. World exports of cheese [4] (in thousand tones)

	2000	2005	2007	2008	2009
EU 27	526	554	594	551	573
New Zealand	246	264	305	247	290
Australia	246	208	217	162	162
Belarus	17	65	92	121	121
United States of America	50	58	99	106	106
Ukraine	12	116	62	77	77
Switzerland	57	52	54	62	62
Argentina	25	52	45	36	48
Uruguay	17	32	28	27	37
Rest of World	111	230	346	373	374
World	1308	1,630	1,843	1761	1,850

Table 4. World imports of cheese [4] (in thousand tones)

	2000	2005	2007	2008	2009
Russia	52	312	318	350	353
Japan	205	212	225	187	184
United States of America	192	211	200	136	130
EU 27	143	95	94	84	83
Mexico	54	79	86	68	73
Australia	38	54	65	68	65
Korea	31	44	49	47	49
Switzerland	31	32	37	41	44
Saudi Arabia	73	103	106	77	42
Rest of World	489	488	663	703	827
World	1,308	1,630	1,843	1761	1,850

New Zealand and Australia are the second and third largest exporter of cheeses, respectively. The prime destinations of New Zealand's cheeses are Asia, Australia, and Europe. Most Australian cheese goes to Asia, where Japan remains by far the most important market. Belarus and Ukraine have become emerging cheese exporters which increased cheese export more than 600% during the period from 2000 to 2009. Most of their cheeses are sent to Russia. USA exports around 30% of cheese to Mexico. Argentina and Uruguay have increased cheese export steadily during the time and most of their cheeses go to Brazil and neighboring countries in South America.

The major cheese importers accounting for 19% and 7% of imported cheeses are Russia and Japan, respectively, as shown in Table 4. Russia dramatically increased cheese import during the period from 2000 to 2005. However, cheese imports of Japan slightly increased before 2007 and then decreased after 2007. Cheese imports of other countries not listed in Table 4 continued to increase during the period from 2005 to 2009, indicating that developing countries in Asia and Africa have become emerging markets of cheese.

CONCLUSION

Production of industrial cheeses in the world increased steadily during the period from 2000 to 2007 due to demand for commodity cheeses by fast food services and increased cheese consumption of non-EU Europe countries. Cheese trade also increased sharply during the same time and outpaced cheese production. However, less favorable economic condition in 2008 and 2009 caused stagnation of production, consumption and trade of cheeses. Future economic recovery of the developed countries, adoption of Western eating habits, and rising incomes of the developing countries are expected to promote production and consumption of world cheeses.

REFERENCES

[1] IDF (1981) *IDF catalogue of cheese*. Doc. 141. International Dairy Federation.
[2] United States Departmet of Agriculture. (2010) *Dairy Products* 2009 Summary.
[3] Wikipedia (2010) List of Frech cheeses. *http://en.wikipedia.org/wiki/List_of French _cheeses#Other_French_cheeses*.
[4] IDF (2010) The world dairy situation 2010. *Bull. Inter Dairy Federat.* No. 446/2010.
[5] IDF (2006) The world dairy situation 2006, *Bull. Inter. Dairy Federat.* No. 409/2006.
[6] IDF (2005) The world dairy situation 2005. *Bull. Inter. Dairy Federat.* No. 399/2005.
[7] IDF (2007) The world dairy situation 2005. *Bull. Inter. Dairy Federat.* No. 414/2007.
[8] Row, R (2010) Cheese - global consumption *http://www.suite101.com/content/cheese.*
[9] Giles, W. 2007. Swiss cheeses consumption rises to record on mozzarella demand. *http://www.bloomberg.com/apps/news?pid=newsarchiverandsid=aCINly4mP9hoandre fer=germany.*
[10] Korea Dairy Industries Association (2010) Dairy products statistics. *http://www.koreadia.or.kr/statistics/sub05:html.*
[11] Global Industry Analysts, Inc. 2010. Global cheese consumption to reach 21 million metric tons by 2015. *http://www.preweb.com/releases/cheesecheddar/organicmartisan/ prweb 3489924.htm.*
[12] Wikipedia (2010) Cheese. *http://en.wikipedia.org/wiki/cheese.*
[13] International Dairy Food Association (2010) Cheese sales and trends. *http://www. idfa.or/news--views/media.*

INDEX

A

Abraham, 5, 30, 93, 99
access, 90, 224, 298
accounting, 20, 306
ACE-inhibitory peptides, xiv, 221, 225, 226, 230, 232, 233, 238, 241
acetaldehyde, 16, 22, 212, 214
acetic acid, 20, 25, 136, 252
acetone, 22, 213, 227, 230
acidic, ix, 1, 5, 213, 234, 258, 260, 281, 290
acidity, 4, 46, 90
active site, 96, 223, 224
adaptability, 13
adaptation, 15, 32, 39
additives, 19, 35, 250, 252
adsorption, 265, 268
adults, 158, 302
adverse effects, xii, 106, 113, 158
Africa, 142, 302, 305, 306
agar, 25, 28, 29
age, 23, 52, 53, 58, 68, 141, 161, 175, 176, 199, 261, 277, 281, 301
age-related diseases, 277
aging process, 90, 189
agriculture, 82, 83, 157, 171
alanine, 135, 137, 191, 214
albumin, 149, 269, 291
alcohols, xiii, 191, 196, 207, 214, 215, 216
aldehydes, xiii, 207, 208, 214, 216
alkaloids, 95, 97, 98, 102, 103, 104
amine, 152, 261, 268
amino, xiv, 19, 22, 24, 42, 54, 96, 113, 136, 137, 139, 142, 159, 190, 191, 192, 196, 197, 198, 199, 201, 209, 211, 214, 215, 222, 223, 224, 226, 230, 232, 234, 238, 247, 255, 256, 257, 258, 260, 261, 267, 268, 269, 270, 272, 273, 274, 280, 281, 283, 287, 294
ammonia, 211, 215, 292
ammonium, 112, 165
angiotensin converting enzyme, ix, xiv, 2, 221, 223, 242, 244
angiotensin converting enzyme (ACE), xiv, 221
angiotensin II, xiv, 221, 223
antagonism, 18, 177
antibiotic, 41, 97, 99, 146
anti-carcinogenic, xiv, 148, 267
anti-microbial, xiv, 110, 146, 149, 267
antioxidant, x, 44, 58, 222, 271, 272, 277
antitumor, xi, 89, 92, 94, 100
aorta, 239, 242
apoptosis, 277
Apulia Region, vii, xii, 119, 120
Argentina, 33, 302, 303, 304, 305, 306
arginine, 113, 224
aromatic compounds, 190, 196
aromatic hydrocarbons, 58, 65, 66, 68, 69
aromatics, 217, 224
Artisan, x, 43, 66
ascorbic acid, 33, 256, 280
Asia, 302, 305, 306
aspartate, 135, 136, 201, 214
assessment, 31, 37, 38, 67, 85, 141, 177, 202, 226
atherosclerosis, xi, 105, 275, 277
attachment, 277, 279
Austria, 87, 144, 302, 303, 304
authentication, ix, x, xi, 71, 72, 87
authenticity, 81, 87, 186, 202
authorities, 78, 79, 82, 83, 84, 85, 86
awareness, 3, 72, 86, 168

B

bacterial pathogens, 108, 147
bacteriocins, 17, 146
bacteriostatic, x, 44, 58, 63
bacterium, 25, 33, 90
base, 4, 41, 112, 114, 164, 165, 198, 235
beef, 64, 284, 294
beer, 79, 97, 100
Belarus, xv, 301, 302, 303, 306
Belgium, 28, 87, 142, 292
beneficial effect, 23, 148, 177, 268, 273
benefits, xiv, 2, 3, 4, 18, 32, 106, 165, 222, 258, 263, 267, 271, 286, 287
benzo(a)pyrene, 58, 63, 65, 67
beverages, 2, 22, 34, 38, 302
bile, 3, 11, 17, 36, 286
bioavailability, xiv, 44, 133, 221, 237, 271
biochemical processes, 146, 272
biochemistry, 99, 199
biological activities, 103, 269, 271
biological activity, xiv, 95, 221, 241, 268, 271, 274
biopolymer, 188, 194, 204
biopolymers, 13, 185
biosynthesis, 32, 94, 95, 96, 98, 101, 102, 103, 104, 274
blood, xiv, 24, 112, 148, 158, 160, 166, 167, 221, 223, 227, 237, 238, 239, 240, 241, 244, 251, 257, 263, 265, 268, 271, 274, 279, 280
body fat, 148, 275, 284
body mass index, 160
body weight, 148, 239, 279
bone, 158, 159, 166, 168, 279
bone resorption, 159, 168
bones, 133, 279
bradykinin, xiv, 221, 223, 271
brain, 95, 101, 239, 276
Brazil, xv, 65, 301, 302, 303, 306
breakdown, 69, 211, 213, 214, 231, 232, 268
brevis, 4, 11, 147, 176, 274
brittleness, 258, 260
buffalo, 36, 141, 142, 173, 175, 186, 290, 291, 298, 302

C

calcium, xi, 12, 13, 15, 36, 40, 105, 106, 109, 110, 114, 115, 116, 133, 148, 158, 159, 161, 162, 163, 166, 167, 168, 171, 177, 209, 211, 267, 268, 269, 271, 278, 279, 280, 281, 285, 287
cancer, 94, 148, 153, 274, 275, 277, 281, 284
carbohydrate, 213, 269
carbohydrates, xiii, 153, 184, 190, 192, 196, 197, 207, 280, 281, 284
carbon, 98, 122, 124, 130, 215, 216, 249, 265, 273, 276
carbon dioxide, 249, 265, 273
carcinoma, 148, 237, 242
cardiovascular disease, 106, 112, 148, 149, 159, 166, 167, 280
caries, 24, 30, 279
casein, x, xi, xii, 19, 25, 43, 46, 48, 54, 66, 68, 69, 105, 109, 110, 114, 117, 119, 123, 124, 133, 142, 161, 162, 163, 169, 188, 189, 192, 194, 195, 196, 198, 209, 210, 214, 215, 221, 222, 225, 237, 242, 259, 268, 269, 270, 271, 272, 278, 279, 283, 289, 296, 300
cattle, 46, 64, 67, 79, 92
cell culture, 11, 102
cell division, 94, 95
cell line, 177, 237, 242
cell lines, 177, 242
cell signaling, 277
certificate, 76, 86
certification, 72, 75
challenges, xii, 17, 31, 32, 88, 106, 111
Charlemagne, xi, 89
Cheddar type scalded cheeses, ix, 1
chemical, ix, xii, xiii, 1, 6, 16, 18, 24, 32, 40, 44, 46, 51, 53, 55, 58, 61, 64, 66, 67, 68, 69, 86, 95, 96, 98, 102, 110, 117, 118, 119, 121, 122, 123, 124, 125, 137, 140, 164, 177, 179, 182, 183, 184, 185, 186, 188, 189, 191, 192, 194, 195, 196, 198, 201, 203, 204, 226, 242, 248, 249, 265, 290, 298
children, 24, 107, 128
cholesterol, xiv, 23, 148, 153, 178, 222, 247, 248, 249, 251, 252, 254, 255, 256, 257, 258, 259, 260, 261, 262, 263, 264, 265, 266, 267, 268, 274, 275, 276, 277, 281, 284
chromatography, xiv, 104, 123, 147, 207, 215, 217, 228, 229, 233, 234, 235, 241, 245, 300
chymotrypsin, 222, 238
circulation, 148, 293
classes, 100, 290
classification, xv, 40, 146, 289, 290, 297
climate, 74, 130, 142
CO2, 122, 124, 211, 214

colon, 11, 242, 276, 277
colonization, 144, 150
color, v, xv, 29, 68, 80, 121, 263, 289
commercial, x, 2, 7, 11, 23, 33, 37, 39, 41, 43, 52, 53, 54, 65, 66, 69, 75, 97, 118, 140, 181, 218, 222, 229, 231, 244, 263, 264, 272, 283, 284, 290, 296, 298, 299
commodity, xiii, xv, 72, 157, 301, 305, 307
community, 73, 79, 88, 158, 176, 180, 299
competition, 45, 72, 75, 95
complexity, 192, 196, 201
compliance, 84, 86
complications, 111, 160
comprehension, 72, 86
compression, 59, 60
configuration, 224, 275
conservation, x, 44, 53, 58, 69, 158, 165, 189, 199, 200
constituents, 127, 153, 158, 221, 283
consumers, xiv, 2, 23, 44, 45, 47, 51, 55, 58, 61, 63, 72, 78, 82, 106, 107, 111, 113, 140, 162, 165, 171, 208, 218, 226, 247, 248, 249, 256, 259, 262, 263, 294, 296
consumption, ix, xiii, xv, 3, 5, 11, 23, 30, 97, 134, 144, 147, 148, 153, 157, 158, 159, 162, 164, 168, 189, 223, 251, 256, 259, 261, 267, 274, 275, 279, 280, 281, 285, 301, 302, 303, 304, 305, 307
containers, 18, 290
contamination, 58, 59, 62, 66, 95, 97, 128, 142, 250
control group, 24, 239
cooking, 109, 117, 163, 175, 210, 257, 258, 263, 291, 305
cooling, 110, 125, 161
coronary heart disease, 248, 284
correlation, 66, 72, 159, 192, 201, 231, 248
correlations, 30, 191, 192, 196
cost, 184, 248, 249
covering, 44, 92, 164, 176, 240
crust, 292, 295
crystals, 110, 158, 195
cultivation, 122, 130
culture, xii, xiv, 6, 11, 12, 18, 20, 25, 28, 29, 31, 33, 37, 40, 41, 53, 72, 90, 96, 101, 102, 109, 111, 115, 143, 144, 150, 179, 181, 207, 210, 232, 233, 259, 268, 271, 272, 273, 280, 290, 296
customers, 76, 173
CVD, 271, 274, 275, 280, 281

cysteine, 94, 135, 136, 215, 273
cytochrome, 97, 99, 101
cytochrome p450, 97, 99
cytokines, 177, 275
Czech Republic, 303, 304

D

dairies, 122, 174, 176, 179, 302
dairy industry, 184, 218
database, 116, 205
decay, 184, 187, 193, 201, 203
defects, 107, 109, 110, 256, 257, 260, 263
degradation, xiv, 19, 25, 40, 54, 96, 100, 169, 208, 214, 216, 221, 223, 231, 233, 234, 237, 271, 273
dehydration, 98, 107
Denmark, xi, 87, 89, 90, 303
dental caries, 24, 30, 285
Department of Agriculture, 207, 218, 286
depression, xv, 301, 304
derivatives, 94, 96, 98, 102, 140, 275
detectable, 190, 217, 269
detection, 128, 217, 234
developed countries, 113, 302, 305, 307
developing countries, xv, 301, 306, 307
deviation, 49, 50, 60, 124, 227
diabetes, 30, 240
dialysis, 215, 225
diet, x, xiv, 43, 52, 53, 67, 68, 111, 114, 122, 130, 141, 153, 157, 158, 159, 160, 163, 168, 208, 216, 240, 267, 269, 271, 274, 278, 279, 280, 281, 282, 283
dietary fat, 153, 284
diffusion, 18, 34, 140, 165, 166, 167, 188, 189, 194, 195, 204
digestibility, 128, 198, 268, 269
digestion, 123, 237, 238, 239, 241, 243, 268, 270, 282
digestive enzymes, 222, 238, 271
dipeptides, 25, 224
discrimination, 103, 217
diseases, 106, 112, 114, 147, 148, 151, 159, 167, 222
dispersion, 161, 162, 203, 204
dissociation, 110, 209, 251, 252, 255
dissolved oxygen, 17, 37, 41
distillation, 215, 216, 249
distilled water, 226, 239

distribution, xiii, 97, 109, 127, 145, 183, 186, 193, 195, 196, 209, 287
diversity, 29, 75, 151, 152, 153
DNA, 95, 97, 146, 181
dosage, 239, 240
dough, 150, 154, 155
drainage, 44, 257, 290
drugs, 160, 223, 242, 271, 298
dry matter, 48, 131, 139, 147, 164, 165, 186, 261
drying, x, 43, 58, 128, 133, 175, 226

E

egg, 154, 248, 262, 284
Egypt, 48, 105, 301
elaboration, 59, 60, 61, 92, 99
emulsifying agents, 115, 161
encapsulation, 13, 15, 36, 41
energy, 106, 148, 149, 183, 202, 249, 269, 275, 279
engineering, xi, 90, 95
England, xi, 57, 89, 296, 299, 300
entrapment, xiv, 13, 247, 273
environment, ix, 1, 3, 5, 15, 17, 45, 74, 149, 163, 177, 209, 211, 281
environmental conditions, x, 2, 5, 12, 14, 25, 102, 182
enzyme, ix, xiv, 2, 24, 34, 36, 38, 40, 52, 96, 98, 109, 199, 210, 221, 222, 223, 224, 226, 227, 229, 230, 237, 238, 239, 240, 241, 242, 243, 244, 245, 270, 282, 292, 293, 296
EPA, 263, 264
equilibrium, 202, 231, 278
equipment, 184, 209, 225
ester, 257, 265
ethanol, 22, 191, 192, 197, 214, 215, 226, 230, 252
ethnicity, 267
ethyl acetate, 227, 229
European Union (EU), x, xv, 55, 71, 73, 78, 80, 83, 86, 88, 146, 149, 301, 302, 305, 306, 307
eukaryotic, 94, 104, 153
Europe, xv, 2, 57, 72, 174, 261, 290, 301, 302, 303, 305, 306, 307
European Commission, 82, 88
European Community, 171, 174, 186
evaporation, 175, 195, 200, 216, 227
evidence, xi, 54, 78, 80, 83, 92, 105, 159, 160, 177, 178, 187, 193, 237, 254

evolution, xiii, 67, 179, 182, 183, 185, 188, 189, 194
exchange rate, 203, 204
excretion, 99, 158, 159, 167, 168, 285
experimental condition, 44, 45, 47, 48, 59, 125
exporters, xv, 301, 306
exports, 305, 306
exposure, 5, 17, 110
expulsion, 108, 210, 280
extraction, xii, 119, 139, 184, 200, 215, 216, 218, 225, 226, 229, 242, 249, 265
extracts, 70, 95, 96, 122, 125, 140, 165, 201, 225, 226, 228, 229, 233, 238, 240, 242, 283
extrusion, 13, 14, 16, 20, 21

F

FAA, 272, 273
factories, xiii, 58, 144, 145, 171
farmers, 51, 78, 82, 140, 145
farms, 122, 130, 173, 302
fast food, xv, 301, 302, 305, 307
fat reduction, 182, 256
fatty acids, xiii, xiv, 16, 20, 21, 48, 54, 67, 70, 106, 123, 127, 132, 138, 139, 143, 147, 148, 153, 178, 208, 215, 247, 249, 256, 263, 267, 268, 274, 275, 281, 283, 284
fermentation, xiii, xv, 11, 13, 19, 22, 25, 39, 41, 103, 107, 109, 114, 118, 132, 143, 145, 146, 180, 186, 190, 191, 222, 261, 289, 294
fermented dairy products, ix, 1, 42, 152, 285
Finland, 6, 303, 304
fish, 2, 248, 249, 262, 264
fish oil, 2, 248, 249, 262, 264
flight, 234, 235
flora, ix, 1, 22, 92, 292
flour, 150, 154, 155
flowers, 55, 70, 208
food additives, 19, 250, 252
food industry, 2, 3, 58, 88, 254
food preservation techniques, x, 43, 58
food products, x, 71, 86, 95, 113, 167, 178, 182, 184, 248, 251, 263, 264
food safety, 109, 110, 113, 152
force, 2, 73, 202
formation, xi, xii, xiii, 22, 25, 42, 93, 98, 102, 105, 106, 110, 111, 114, 133, 161, 163, 175, 176, 178, 181, 192, 207, 210, 215, 216, 218, 231, 233, 241, 249, 272, 273, 279, 294
formula, 124, 164, 227, 230

Index

fragility, 158, 159
fragments, 235, 238, 270, 276
France, xi, 32, 57, 66, 87, 89, 171, 205, 242, 261, 290, 295, 302, 303, 304, 305
fraud, 75, 80
freezing, 13, 166
French kings, xi, 89
fructose, 22, 40
fruits, 55, 158, 210, 217
functional food, 2, 37, 41, 42, 149, 262, 268, 271, 287
fungi, 92, 95, 96, 98, 146, 147, 152, 176, 211, 272, 293
fungus, 90, 99, 104, 147, 211

G

GABA, 273, 274, 281, 283
gastrointestinal tract, 4, 11, 36, 182
gel, 161, 188, 189, 194, 196, 279, 283, 289
genes, 98, 104, 147, 151, 275
genetic factors, x, 43, 45
genetics, 46, 160, 297
genotype, x, 43, 46, 47, 51
genus, x, 4, 19, 31, 40, 43, 93, 146, 147, 153
geographical origin, 73, 74, 76, 77, 121, 130, 141, 142
geometry, 189, 194, 204
Germany, 57, 87, 114, 115, 124, 125, 200, 290, 302, 303, 304, 305
glucose, 22, 135, 136, 138, 148, 192, 197, 249
glue, 213
glutamate, 135, 136, 137, 165, 191, 214, 274
glutamic acid, 97, 224, 269, 273
glutamine, 97, 202
glycerol, 135, 137, 138, 139, 192, 197, 215
glycine, 201, 226, 229
glycoproteins, 276, 287
goat milk, xii, 34, 47, 58, 68, 119, 121, 122, 123, 124, 126, 127, 128, 129, 130, 134, 140, 181, 235, 236, 273, 280, 283, 296
grazing, 67, 148
Greece, 52, 87, 303, 304, 305
growth, ix, xiii, 1, 2, 4, 5, 6, 12, 13, 16, 17, 18, 20, 25, 28, 29, 33, 42, 90, 92, 93, 97, 99, 102, 106, 107, 108, 109, 110, 112, 114, 117, 146, 152, 153, 171, 178, 179, 210, 259, 260, 275, 279, 281, 286, 291, 302, 304, 305
growth rate, 2, 106, 302, 305
guidelines, xi, 105, 159, 191, 196, 205

H

hardness, 47, 61, 162, 163, 257, 258, 260, 290
health, ix, xiii, xiv, 1, 2, 3, 4, 18, 23, 24, 32, 33, 44, 58, 72, 93, 107, 114, 115, 128, 140, 143, 147, 148, 151, 152, 153, 154, 158, 159, 160, 165, 166, 178, 208, 221, 222, 256, 258, 263, 267, 268, 270, 271, 274, 275, 276, 277, 279, 280, 281, 283, 285, 286, 287
health effects, 147, 152, 268, 285
health problems, 93, 178
heterogeneity, 189, 194
heterogeneous systems, 186, 188, 204
high fat, 4, 261, 274, 294
high-risk populations, 107
history, xi, xii, 75, 89, 143, 144, 150, 160, 289
homocysteine, 268, 280
host, 3, 4, 269, 284
human, ix, xiii, xiv, 1, 4, 11, 17, 23, 32, 33, 36, 44, 51, 58, 73, 74, 80, 97, 143, 147, 148, 151, 153, 157, 158, 160, 203, 217, 222, 237, 239, 240, 242, 243, 245, 248, 267, 268, 269, 270, 272, 275, 280, 283, 284, 285, 286
human body, 11, 158, 203, 272
human health, xiii, 23, 44, 58, 143, 147, 148, 151, 222, 268
human milk, 272, 284
human subjects, 239, 240
humidity, 18, 20, 34, 90, 92, 95, 192, 270
hydrocarbons, 58, 65, 66, 68, 69, 216
hydrogen, 17, 251, 281
hydrogen peroxide, 17, 281
hydrolysis, 139, 222, 227, 229, 230, 231, 237, 238, 272
hydroxyl, 95, 254, 271, 281
hypertension, xi, xiv, 30, 105, 106, 114, 115, 159, 160, 166, 221, 223, 224, 239, 240, 270, 280, 283
hypotensive, 232, 237, 270

I

ideal, ix, 1, 15, 18, 290
identification, xii, 25, 29, 38, 40, 59, 119, 152, 179, 233, 234, 243, 286, 298
identity, 3, 79, 80, 141, 234, 261
image, xiv, 106, 163, 184, 267
imitation, 112, 116, 164, 166, 167, 266
immobilization, 13, 16, 252

immortality, xiii, 157
immune response, 23, 281
immune system, 23, 107, 177, 268, 281
immunity, 23, 270
immunoglobulins, 149, 269
in vitro, xiv, 101, 148, 221, 224, 227, 228, 233, 237, 238, 239, 270, 272, 284, 286
in vivo, xiv, 95, 221, 224, 236, 237, 239, 240, 276, 284
incidence, 94, 148
India, 48, 205
individuals, xiii, 47, 72, 85, 106, 160, 171, 178, 179, 239, 240, 267, 279
induction, 30, 203
industry, xi, 2, 3, 17, 58, 88, 90, 93, 95, 113, 145, 162, 184, 218, 252, 254, 255, 256, 258, 305
ingredients, 73, 81, 86, 107, 112, 114, 117, 142, 145, 160, 161, 162, 164, 167, 177, 258, 262
inhibition, xiv, 95, 99, 101, 102, 221, 223, 224, 226, 227, 228, 230, 231, 233, 238, 243, 244, 270, 271, 272, 275, 276, 277
inhibitor, 20, 24, 34, 38, 94, 104, 164, 223, 224, 226, 227, 230, 237, 238, 241, 243, 251
inoculation, 6, 12, 26, 90
inoculum, 6, 12, 36, 174
interface, 161, 188, 194
intestine, ix, 1, 23, 148, 269, 279
ionization, 217, 234
ions, 12, 15, 133, 163, 234
Ireland, 57, 105, 287, 302, 303, 304
isolation, 25, 96, 103, 104, 215, 216, 233, 242
isoleucine, 135, 191, 273
isotope, 122, 124, 130, 142
Isotope Ratio Mass Spectroscopy (IRMS), xii, 119
Israel, 302, 303, 305
issues, 167, 182
Italy, vii, xi, xii, 52, 57, 63, 64, 67, 68, 87, 88, 89, 119, 120, 123, 124, 129, 142, 171, 173, 174, 179, 183, 186, 192, 199, 200, 231, 290, 296, 298, 303, 304, 305

J

Japan, xv, 94, 301, 303, 304, 305, 306

K

ketones, xiii, 207, 215, 216, 261
kidney, 101, 160
kidneys, 160, 239
Korea, xv, 247, 267, 289, 301, 303, 304, 305, 306, 307
koumiss, 25, 42

L

labeling, xi, 71, 72, 81
lactation, 66, 67, 69, 140, 268
lactic acid, xi, xii, xiv, xv, 12, 17, 18, 22, 25, 29, 30, 32, 33, 35, 37, 40, 41, 42, 89, 90, 97, 111, 114, 135, 136, 137, 139, 143, 146, 147, 151, 179, 180, 181, 209, 211, 221, 222, 232, 244, 261, 267, 272, 276, 282, 283, 286, 290, 293, 296
lactobacillus, 11, 180, 249
lactoferrin, 149, 269, 282
lactose, 20, 23, 37, 48, 109, 118, 123, 133, 149, 190, 191, 192, 196, 197, 207, 210, 213, 221, 255, 279, 285, 287
Latin America, 2, 302, 305
laws, 74, 81
LDL, 148, 274, 275
lead, 2, 46, 109, 110, 122, 148, 209, 249, 274, 278
leakage, 223, 259
leucine, 135, 191, 227, 273
light, xi, 79, 90, 114, 124, 176
linoleic acid, xiii, 24, 29, 30, 32, 36, 39, 46, 63, 66, 67, 143, 147, 151, 153, 178, 268, 274, 275, 284, 286, 287
lipases, 52, 53, 66, 215
lipids, xiii, xiv, 59, 147, 153, 184, 185, 187, 188, 193, 207, 208, 211, 267, 274, 275, 276, 277, 281, 284
lipolysis, 20, 22, 34, 54, 62, 64, 65, 90, 109, 118, 176, 198, 207, 209, 260, 275, 277, 279, 300
lipoproteins, 274, 276
liquid chromatography, 104, 233, 234, 235, 241, 245, 283
liquid phase, 216, 276
Listeria monocytogenes, 53, 146, 153
lithium, 25, 112
Lithuania, 302, 303
liver, 95, 96, 97, 99, 262, 263, 264, 266
livestock, 93, 173, 178
local conditions, 81, 130
localization, 184, 244
lysine, 137, 202, 224, 273

Index

M

macromolecules, 185, 186
magnetic field, 125, 183, 184, 200, 201, 202
magnetic moment, 183, 202
magnetic resonance, xiii, 142, 183
magnetic resonance spectroscopy, xiii, 183
magnetization, 183, 186, 187, 193, 201, 202, 203
majority, 17, 82, 92, 96, 137, 210
mammals, 93, 158
management, 45, 51, 64, 75, 173
manipulation, 34, 121, 181
manufacturing, ix, 1, 4, 5, 6, 11, 18, 22, 54, 72, 78, 86, 109, 110, 145, 149, 153, 164, 171, 174, 175, 176, 179, 188, 199, 231, 273, 278, 289, 298
marketing, 44, 140, 165, 171, 177
marketplace, 113, 305
Maryland, 33, 115, 285
MAS, xii, 119, 122, 124, 125, 138, 139, 141
mass, 68, 77, 96, 114, 124, 158, 159, 160, 162, 163, 217, 233, 234, 241, 293
mass spectrometry, 217, 233, 235, 241
materials, xv, 18, 37, 41, 59, 60, 62, 65, 74, 76, 77, 80, 158, 165, 184, 203, 252, 257, 267
matrix, xiii, 5, 11, 13, 15, 19, 34, 178, 183, 188, 194, 211, 215, 225, 234, 239, 260, 289
matter, v, 48, 59, 61, 66, 83, 107, 131, 139, 147, 164, 165, 176, 186, 261
measurement, 125, 166, 185, 186, 203, 204, 229, 230, 263, 278
measurements, 30, 123, 141, 184, 185, 186, 189, 196, 199, 200, 202, 203, 204
meat, 74, 79, 144, 151, 158, 290
media, 25, 27, 29, 33, 40, 94, 229, 230, 307
medical, 2, 151, 152, 212
melting, 110, 117, 160, 162, 163, 176, 249, 290, 291, 297
meta-analysis, 153, 284
metabolism, 90, 99, 148, 159, 207, 210, 214, 277, 280
metabolites, ix, xi, xiii, 1, 13, 15, 17, 89, 92, 93, 95, 99, 100, 102, 103, 121, 139, 183, 190, 192, 196, 197, 199, 281, 293
metabolized, 213, 214, 259, 279
metals, xii, 119, 128, 132
methanol, 192, 197, 216
methodology, 6, 181, 251, 264
Mexico, 302, 303, 304, 305, 306
mice, 23, 95, 97
microbiota, 92, 153
microorganism, xv, 34, 52, 53, 249, 269, 272, 289, 290
microorganisms, xii, xiii, xiv, 4, 19, 24, 31, 38, 97, 104, 107, 108, 109, 112, 143, 146, 147, 148, 171, 207, 208, 211, 214, 215, 222, 249, 268, 269, 277, 281, 290, 297
microstructure, 115, 117, 162, 182, 186, 266, 284
migration, 184, 195, 211, 260, 278
milk fat globule membrane (MFGM), xiv, 267
milk quality, x, 43, 44, 45, 173
misuse, 75, 79
mixing, 92, 107, 110, 125, 161, 201, 252, 254, 257, 258, 262, 263, 264, 290
model system, 217, 242
models, 11, 23, 31, 42, 148, 178, 187, 277
modifications, 5, 11, 192, 196, 198, 216
moisture, xii, 55, 59, 90, 107, 109, 113, 119, 124, 131, 161, 164, 174, 175, 176, 178, 180, 184, 186, 210, 214, 239, 259, 261, 285, 290
moisture content, 55, 109, 113, 131, 164, 174, 175, 184, 290
mold, xi, xv, 89, 90, 99, 102, 109, 146, 210, 211, 259, 260, 278, 289, 290, 291, 293, 294
molds, xiv, 90, 92, 207, 260, 294
molecular mass, 68, 96, 234
molecular structure, 94, 184, 203
molecular weight, xiii, 183, 226, 228, 234, 238, 271
molecules, 94, 96, 184, 185, 186, 188, 189, 194, 195, 196, 203, 204, 233, 237, 289
monosodium glutamate, 165
morphology, 184, 186, 188, 194
mortality, 160, 284
motivation, xiii, 157
moulding, 44, 186
mucosa, 52, 133
multiples, 191, 197
muscle strength, 149
mutagenesis, 94, 95
mycotoxins, xi, 89, 93, 95, 97, 99, 100, 101, 102, 103, 286

N

NaCl, 107, 108, 111, 112, 113, 116, 124, 125, 131, 152, 162, 163, 164, 169, 178, 182, 210, 230
National Research Council, 171, 262

nausea, 94, 112
near infrared spectroscopy, 278, 285
negative effects, 256, 277
Netherlands, 34, 116, 117, 123, 152, 303, 304, 305
neutral, 257, 261
New Zealand, xv, 118, 301, 302, 303, 304, 305, 306
niacin, 256, 268, 280, 286
nitrogen, 18, 54, 96, 122, 124, 130, 216, 225, 242
NMR, viii, xii, xiii, 119, 120, 121, 122, 125, 135, 136, 137, 138, 139, 141, 183, 184, 185, 186, 187, 188, 190, 191, 192, 193, 194, 196, 197, 198, 199, 200, 201, 202, 203, 204, 205, 206
non-starter lactic acid bacteria (NSLAB), xv, 18, 29, 267
North America, 2, 3, 261, 305
nuclear magnetic resonance, xiii, 142, 183
Nuclear Magnetic Resonance, xii, 119, 121, 141, 183
nuclei, 183, 184, 202, 203
nucleus, 184, 202
nutraceutical, 268, 284
nutrient, ix, xi, 105, 166, 178, 255, 268, 269, 280
nutrients, xiv, 13, 15, 18, 106, 221, 247, 249, 255, 256, 261, 262, 263, 265, 267, 269, 279
nutrition, ix, xiii, 2, 51, 143, 147, 148, 151, 157, 168, 208, 269, 280, 283, 285
nutritional status, 286

O

obesity, 274, 275
Oceania, 302, 305
oil, 74, 110, 145, 150, 155, 161, 163, 178, 212, 248, 249, 251, 257, 262, 263, 264, 265, 266
oleic acid, 48, 132, 148, 274, 275
oligosaccharide, 16, 249
optimization, 256, 262
organ, 94, 160, 166
organic food, x, 71, 86
organic solvents, 249, 252, 255
organism, 92, 158
organoleptic properties, x, 43, 113, 162, 283
osteoporosis, 148, 149, 158, 159, 167, 168, 268, 279
oxidation, 5, 22, 96, 139, 148, 215, 257, 263, 275
oxygen, 4, 5, 11, 18, 33, 37, 38, 41, 90, 95, 122, 130

P

palm oil, 251, 265
parallel, 84, 85, 98, 158, 186, 202
parity, 66, 67, 69
Parliament, 81, 144
pasta, xiii, 15, 17, 64, 65, 143, 174, 175, 176, 178, 186
pasteurization, 53, 127, 148, 208, 209, 216, 271, 280, 289, 290
pasture, 45, 52, 70, 120, 128, 148, 153, 173, 208
pathogens, 17, 107, 108, 146, 147, 177, 178, 208, 276, 284
pathways, xi, xiii, 23, 37, 90, 94, 191, 196, 207, 214, 223, 297
PCA, 61, 62
PCR, 153, 179, 286
pepsin, 52, 54, 222, 238, 269
peptide, 25, 26, 98, 210, 222, 223, 224, 231, 232, 233, 234, 238, 239, 240, 241, 244, 269, 271, 272
peptides, ix, xiv, 1, 2, 19, 24, 26, 34, 38, 39, 40, 177, 214, 221, 222, 223, 224, 225, 226, 228, 229, 230, 231, 232, 233, 234, 235, 236, 237, 238, 239, 240, 241, 242, 243, 244, 245, 247, 267, 268, 269, 270, 271, 272, 273, 274, 279, 280, 281, 282, 283, 286
permeability, 18, 242
pH, ix, xii, 1, 3, 4, 5, 6, 11, 13, 17, 22, 27, 30, 46, 48, 49, 59, 66, 90, 95, 108, 109, 110, 114, 119, 123, 124, 125, 126, 127, 131, 152, 161, 162, 163, 175, 177, 196, 200, 209, 211, 227, 230, 259, 278, 279, 285, 290, 291, 292, 296
phenolic compounds, 139, 192
phenylalanine, 192, 224
phosphate, xii, 22, 40, 105, 110, 113, 133, 158, 161, 165, 191, 209, 211, 227, 269, 278, 279, 281, 285
phosphates, 110, 163, 168
phospholipids, 276, 277, 287
phosphorous, 254, 278, 279
phosphorus, xi, 105, 106, 133, 158, 159, 285
physical properties, 16, 18
physical structure, 141, 188, 194, 201
physicochemical characteristics, 46, 59, 68, 180
Physiological, 167, 237, 242, 298
placebo, 24, 159, 240, 241
plants, 57, 122, 130, 142, 153, 158, 208, 222
Poland, 57, 302, 303, 304
polar, 161, 233, 277

polycyclic aromatic hydrocarbon, 58, 65, 66, 68
polymorphism, 46, 68
polypeptide, xiv, 221
polyphosphates, 110, 117
population, xiii, 3, 6, 23, 147, 157, 159, 160, 166, 167, 177, 181, 239, 281
population group, 147, 160
Portugal, 52, 304
positive correlation, 159, 248
potassium, xii, 106, 111, 112, 114, 115, 116, 117, 123, 159, 162, 163, 165, 168, 227, 278, 285
potato, xiii, 143, 150, 212
precipitation, 230, 252, 279, 291
preparation, 52, 53, 73, 74, 82, 86, 116, 134, 149, 150, 154, 227, 260, 267, 268, 269, 271, 279, 289
preservation, x, 43, 58, 107, 140, 145, 289
preservative, xii, 105, 107
prevention, 23, 24, 94, 148, 151, 153, 159, 168, 268, 275, 277, 284
probe, 125, 184, 200, 201, 278, 279, 285
probiotic, ix, xiii, xv, 1, 2, 3, 4, 5, 6, 7, 8, 11, 12, 13, 14, 16, 17, 18, 20, 22, 23, 24, 25, 26, 27, 28, 29, 30, 31, 32, 33, 34, 35, 36, 37, 38, 39, 40, 41, 42, 171, 177, 181, 182, 229, 243, 267, 268, 271, 281, 283, 286
producers, x, xiii, 43, 72, 75, 76, 77, 78, 80, 82, 91, 145, 171
proline, 137, 202, 224, 238, 271
Protected Designation of Origin (PDO), x, 43, 45, 51, 71, 72, 91, 103, 296
Protected Geographical Indication (PGI), xii, 45, 51, 143, 144, 149
Protected Geographical Origin (PGO), x, 71
protection, 4, 12, 14, 16, 33, 73, 75, 76, 77, 81, 82, 83, 84, 85, 88, 145, 146, 151, 153, 179
protein hydrolysates, 234, 240
protein structure, 161, 162, 188, 194, 196, 222, 259
protein synthesis, 30, 95, 102, 277
proteinase, 210, 211
proteins, xiii, xiv, 59, 94, 95, 107, 108, 109, 110, 147, 149, 159, 161, 163, 175, 177, 184, 185, 186, 188, 192, 193, 198, 203, 207, 209, 210, 221, 222, 223, 224, 228, 232, 233, 234, 237, 238, 241, 242, 243, 247, 267, 268, 269, 276, 277, 280, 281, 282, 285
proteolysis, xiv, 16, 18, 20, 22, 30, 31, 34, 36, 37, 38, 39, 40, 54, 56, 64, 65, 66, 69, 109, 118, 180, 181, 182, 195, 198, 199, 207, 208, 209, 210, 211, 214, 221, 222, 225, 230, 231, 232, 242, 243, 244, 260, 270, 271, 272, 273, 277, 292, 294, 297, 299
proteolytic enzyme, 40, 52, 109, 222, 238, 244, 272, 280, 282
protons, 139, 185, 186, 188, 189, 192, 194, 195, 200, 201, 202, 203, 204
public health, 107, 160
pure water, 124, 185
purification, xiv, 100, 221, 233, 236
purines, 94, 99

Q

quality control, 142, 184, 201, 299
quantification, xiv, 29, 221, 233, 235

R

race, 64, 80, 267
radiation, 202, 203
radio, 201, 202
rancid, 55, 209, 212, 213, 215, 257, 277, 294
raw materials, 74, 76, 77, 80
reactions, xiii, 61, 192, 207, 211, 214, 215, 238, 245, 249, 252
recovery, 29, 242, 251, 252, 307
recycling, 248, 251, 252, 253, 254, 255, 262, 263, 264, 265
regulations, xi, 71, 72, 73, 88, 161, 290
relaxation, 141, 184, 185, 186, 187, 188, 189, 193, 194, 196, 199, 200, 201, 202, 203, 204
relevance, 104, 298
reliability, 25, 225
renin, 223, 240
repetitions, 199, 200
reputation, 74, 75, 76, 78, 79, 144
requirements, xiii, 4, 51, 53, 76, 77, 78, 82, 83, 85, 86, 99, 157, 171, 176, 177, 178, 179, 267
researchers, 20, 24, 162, 177, 225, 226, 271, 272, 273, 274
residues, 24, 224, 238
resistance, 4, 11, 17, 88, 146, 147, 160, 177, 237, 272, 286
resolution, xiii, 125, 141, 183, 184, 185, 196, 199, 200, 201, 202, 235
resources, 69, 73, 75, 88, 233
response, 23, 93, 181, 208, 218, 251, 264
restaurants, xv, 301, 305

rheology, 117, 162, 182, 299
riboflavin, 106, 256, 280, 286
risk, 2, 30, 44, 66, 97, 104, 107, 112, 116, 147, 148, 158, 159, 160, 222, 248, 271, 275, 281, 283, 285
risk factors, 30, 116
risks, xi, 105, 140, 152, 168
RNA, 95, 97
Royal Society, 116, 285
rules, 73, 76, 78, 81, 82, 88
rural development, 51, 75, 151
Russia, xv, 144, 301, 302, 303, 304, 305, 306

S

safety, xiii, 4, 44, 53, 108, 109, 110, 113, 115, 143, 152, 232
saliva, 24, 281
salt concentration, 11, 162, 166, 257
salt substitutes, 112, 116
salts, xi, xii, 11, 17, 105, 106, 107, 109, 110, 112, 114, 115, 116, 118, 159, 160, 161, 163, 164, 165, 166, 167, 177, 178, 281
saponin, 249, 265
saturated fat, xi, xiv, 105, 132, 148, 248, 267, 268, 274
saturated fatty acids, 132, 148, 274
scanning electron microscopy, 296, 299
science, 205, 242, 258, 299
secretion, 269, 271, 281
sensitivity, 183, 216
sequencing, 104, 147, 234
serum, 148, 149, 153, 188, 189, 190, 230, 241, 248, 269, 276, 279, 284
serum albumin, 149, 269
services, v, 80, 83, 88, 307
sesquiterpenoid, 96, 103
shape, 80, 92, 144, 149, 204, 276, 290
sheep, ix, xi, xii, 47, 51, 53, 56, 58, 63, 64, 65, 67, 69, 89, 90, 104, 142, 143, 144, 145, 147, 149, 150, 153, 173, 210, 260, 271, 272, 274, 275, 283, 291, 296, 302
shelf life, 4, 6, 107, 109, 161, 162, 226
showing, 25, 78, 80, 95, 110, 120, 136, 137, 230
side chain, 24, 214
side effects, 223, 240
signals, 135, 136, 137, 139, 184, 190, 191, 192, 196, 197
Single Gloucester, x, 71, 87
skin, 144, 158

Slovakia, xii, 143, 144, 149, 150, 152, 154, 304
smoking, x, 43, 44, 45, 58, 59, 60, 61, 62, 65, 66, 67, 144, 274
sodium, ix, xi, xii, 12, 15, 17, 105, 106, 107, 108, 109, 110, 111, 112, 113, 114, 115, 116, 117, 125, 134, 157, 158, 159, 160, 161, 162, 163, 164, 165, 166, 167, 168, 178, 182, 186, 191, 197, 200, 223, 227, 252, 254, 278, 280, 285
solid phase, 22, 65, 139, 216
solubility, xiv, 109, 163, 227, 247, 248
solution, 5, 11, 15, 20, 36, 82, 83, 123, 124, 144, 145, 178, 184, 186, 188, 234, 239, 292
solvents, 225, 234, 249, 252, 255
somatic cell, 66, 123, 208
South Africa, 142, 304
South America, 32, 302, 305, 306
Spain, xi, 43, 51, 52, 53, 57, 58, 87, 89, 90, 92, 173, 221, 303, 304
species, x, xi, 3, 6, 18, 20, 25, 29, 32, 41, 43, 45, 46, 51, 52, 55, 56, 80, 89, 93, 97, 102, 103, 111, 122, 127, 130, 158, 160, 173, 176, 181, 202, 209, 211, 232, 273, 274, 275, 281, 287, 296, 299, 301
specifications, 73, 78, 84, 85, 86, 88, 290
spectroscopy, xiii, 101, 121, 141, 183, 184, 201, 279
spin, 192, 201, 202
stability, xii, 5, 13, 24, 32, 102, 105, 106, 113, 144, 152, 192, 227, 237, 286
stabilization, 94, 162
stabilizers, 254
Staffordshire Cheese, x, 71
standard deviation, 49, 50, 60, 188, 227
standardization, 53, 289
starch, 15, 35, 107, 163, 254
state, xiii, 14, 16, 21, 78, 183, 184, 185, 186, 188, 192, 194, 201
states, 72, 141, 174, 183, 184, 193, 202, 305
steel, 145, 154
stomach, 52, 55, 210
storage, xiii, 3, 4, 6, 12, 13, 18, 24, 40, 44, 53, 92, 95, 107, 109, 113, 140, 161, 176, 184, 185, 186, 190, 196, 199, 200, 207, 211, 214, 251, 258, 260, 261, 262, 263, 266, 268, 271, 278
streptococci, 41, 92
stress, 13, 17, 30, 158, 273
stretching, 164, 186, 291
stroke, 116, 160
structure, x, xiii, 43, 46, 94, 95, 96, 98, 99, 102, 104, 113, 141, 161, 164, 166, 168, 174, 175,

176, 178, 182, 183, 184, 185, 188, 189, 192, 194, 195, 196, 201, 203, 222, 224, 243, 248, 250, 259, 277, 282, 285, 286, 294, 295, 299
structure formation, 175, 176
style, 274, 283, 297, 302
substitutes, 112, 116, 148, 211, 263, 266
substitution, xii, 106, 112, 114, 116, 163
substrate, 6, 19, 95, 96, 97, 192, 223, 227, 229, 230, 238
substrates, 24, 102, 214, 223, 224, 227, 244
sulfur, 159, 209, 211, 216, 268, 269, 295
supplier, 122, 305
suppression, 125, 201, 277
survival, 4, 5, 11, 15, 17, 30, 33, 34, 35, 36, 38, 39, 40, 41, 176, 177, 179, 181, 281
suspensions, 90, 163
sustainability, xi, 71, 72
sustainable development, xiii, 171
Sweden, 303, 304
Switzerland, 30, 35, 37, 117, 231, 294, 303, 304, 305, 306
synthesis, 29, 30, 95, 97, 100, 101, 102, 103, 158, 232, 271, 274

T

target, 160, 166, 223, 249, 270
techniques, ix, x, xiv, 2, 5, 13, 14, 29, 36, 41, 43, 58, 59, 72, 121, 146, 184, 185, 199, 203, 207, 208, 217, 221, 225, 226, 233, 269
technologies, 113, 231, 249, 275
technology, x, xii, 2, 11, 13, 20, 34, 35, 44, 58, 64, 118, 143, 144, 174, 175, 176, 231, 248, 249, 258, 264, 273, 299
temperature, xiv, 11, 12, 17, 18, 20, 25, 34, 38, 58, 59, 61, 90, 95, 109, 123, 145, 152, 164, 174, 175, 185, 192, 200, 201, 207, 210, 211, 214, 216, 225, 226, 230, 232, 239, 249, 250, 251, 252, 254, 257, 258, 262, 263, 264, 270
tension, 239, 257
terpenes, 208, 216
territory, 72, 75, 80, 85, 127, 140, 144, 175
textural character, 59, 60, 176, 180
texture, x, xiv, xv, 4, 6, 11, 15, 30, 31, 35, 44, 54, 56, 57, 58, 59, 61, 64, 65, 68, 107, 109, 110, 111, 112, 162, 163, 164, 165, 166, 167, 168, 176, 177, 178, 182, 184, 192, 194, 195, 209, 222, 247, 248, 249, 256, 257, 258, 259, 260, 261, 264, 266, 270, 274, 276, 289, 290, 291, 292, 293, 294, 296, 297, 298

therapy, 160, 283
threonine, 191, 273
tissue, 23, 158, 177, 242, 244
total cholesterol, 148, 257
tourism, xiii, 143, 150
toxicity, 41, 93, 95, 97, 100, 254
toxin, xi, 89, 95, 96, 99, 100, 101, 102, 103, 104, 249
trade, xv, 75, 91, 218, 260, 301, 302, 305, 307
trademarks, 75, 79
traits, 66, 177, 297, 300
transformation, 75, 80, 96, 102, 140, 192, 203
transformations, xiv, 221, 239
transport, 158, 238, 271, 277, 280
treatment, 15, 17, 30, 94, 127, 130, 164, 174, 175, 180, 184, 199, 215, 223, 232, 249, 250, 265, 271, 273, 290
trial, 35, 37, 159, 251, 252, 257, 258, 263, 264, 275, 286
triglycerides, 127, 132, 139, 148, 153, 274
trypsin, 222, 238, 272
tryptophan, 98, 104, 136, 214, 224, 273
Turkey, 1, 15, 302, 303, 305
turnover, 92, 158, 159
type 2 diabetes, 30, 240, 283
tyrosine, 135, 136, 192, 214, 224
Tyrosine, 273

U

UK, 34, 116, 117, 266, 267, 282, 303, 304
Ukraine, xv, 301, 302, 303, 306
uniform, 79, 121, 150, 258
United, 87, 90, 151, 164, 296, 305, 306, 307
United Kingdom, 87, 151
United States, 90, 164, 305, 306, 307
urea, xii, 119, 123
urine, 158, 159, 168
Uruguay, 305, 306
USA, 2, 32, 34, 35, 37, 41, 115, 118, 123, 124, 167, 168, 200, 223, 256, 261, 262, 267, 299, 302, 303, 304, 305, 306
USDA, 272, 286
UV, 94, 95

V

vacuum, 5, 6, 18, 124, 216, 249, 260
valine, 135, 137, 191

variables, 252, 289
variations, 20, 46, 54, 153, 172, 198, 199, 225, 227, 258, 285
varieties, ix, xi, 1, 5, 6, 17, 19, 22, 45, 70, 79, 86, 89, 90, 101, 102, 106, 107, 108, 160, 207, 208, 209, 210, 213, 218, 222, 225, 227, 228, 231, 232, 243, 258, 267, 270, 272, 283, 290, 291, 294, 297, 301, 302, 305
vector, 182, 202, 203
vegetable oil, 110, 275
vessels, 123, 144, 223
viscosity, 161, 162, 163, 249, 251, 254, 263
vitamin A, 106, 280
vitamin B1, 106, 268, 280, 285
vitamin B12, 106, 268, 280, 285
vitamin D, 159, 177
vitamins, xi, xiii, xiv, 2, 105, 143, 147, 177, 221, 247, 255, 264, 267, 268, 277, 280, 281

W

Washington, 218, 219, 220, 298, 299
water diffusion, 189, 194
water evaporation, 175, 200
well-being, 2, 23
West Country farmhouse Cheddar cheese, xi, 71
Western countries, xi, 105
WHO, 3, 33
Wisconsin, 68, 117, 118, 168
wood, 57, 59, 60, 61, 62, 144, 145
workers, 95, 97, 98
worldwide, xv, 75, 146, 160, 250, 301, 302
WTO, 83, 85

Y

yeast, 24, 155, 211, 214, 269
Yeasts, 92, 211
yield, 45, 46, 47, 48, 51, 67, 69, 181, 182, 227, 254, 255, 299, 300

Z

zinc, xiv, 221, 223, 278